CAMPBELL'S

CORE ORTHOPAEDIC PROCEDURES

CAMPBELL'S

CORE ORTHOPAEDIC PROCEDURES

S. Terry Canale, MD

Harold B. Boyd Professor and Chairman, Department of Orthopaedic Surgery
University of Tennessee–Campbell Clinic
Memphis, Tennessee

James H. Beaty, MD

Professor, Department of Orthopaedic Surgery
University of Tennessee–Campbell Clinic
Memphis, Tennessee

Frederick M. Azar, MD

Professor, Department of Orthopaedic Surgery
University of Tennessee–Campbell Clinic
Chief of Staff, Campbell Clinic
Memphis, Tennessee

ELSEVIER

ELSEVIER

1600 John F. Kennedy Blvd.
Ste 1800
Philadelphia, PA 19103-2899

CAMPBELL'S CORE ORTHOPAEDIC PROCEDURES   ISBN: 978-0-323-35763-0

Notices

International Standard Book Number: 978-0-323-35763-0

Executive Content Strategist: Dolores Meloni
Content Development Manager: Taylor Ball
Publishing Services Manager: Patricia Tannian
Senior Project Manager: John Casey
Design Manager: Renee Duenow
Illustrations Manager: Karen Giacomucci

Printed in China

Last digit is the print number: 9 8 7 6 5 4 3 2 1

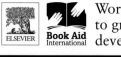

CONTRIBUTORS TO *CAMPBELL'S OPERATIVE ORTHOPAEDICS*, 12TH EDITION

WILLIAM E. ALBERS, MD
Assistant Professor
University of Tennessee–Campbell Clinic
Department of Orthopaedic Surgery and Biomedical
    Engineering
Memphis, Tennessee

FREDERICK M. AZAR, MD
Professor
Director, Sports Medicine Fellowship
University of Tennessee–Campbell Clinic
Department of Orthopaedic Surgery and Biomedical
    Engineering
Chief-of-Staff, Campbell Clinic
Memphis, Tennessee

JAMES H. BEATY, MD
Professor
University of Tennessee–Campbell Clinic
Department of Orthopaedic Surgery and Biomedical
    Engineering
Memphis, Tennessee

JAMES H. CALANDRUCCIO, MD
Associate Professor
Director, Hand Fellowship
University of Tennessee–Campbell Clinic
Department of Orthopaedic Surgery and Biomedical
    Engineering
Memphis, Tennessee

FRANCIS X. CAMILLO, MD
Associate Professor
University of Tennessee–Campbell Clinic
Department of Orthopaedic Surgery and Biomedical
    Engineering
Memphis, Tennessee

S. TERRY CANALE, MD
Harold H. Boyd Professor and Chair
University of Tennessee–Campbell Clinic
Department of Orthopaedic Surgery and Biomedical
    Engineering
Memphis, Tennessee

DAVID L. CANNON, MD
Associate Professor
University of Tennessee–Campbell Clinic
Department of Orthopaedic Surgery and Biomedical
    Engineering
Memphis, Tennessee

KEVIN B. CLEVELAND, MD
Instructor
University of Tennessee–Campbell Clinic
Department of Orthopaedic Surgery and Biomedical
    Engineering
Memphis, Tennessee

ANDREW H. CRENSHAW, JR., MD
Professor
University of Tennessee–Campbell Clinic
Department of Orthopaedic Surgery and Biomedical
    Engineering
Memphis, Tennessee

JOHN R. CROCKARELL, JR., MD
Associate Professor
University of Tennessee–Campbell Clinic
Department of Orthopaedic Surgery and Biomedical
    Engineering
Memphis, Tennessee

GREGORY D. DABOV, MD
Assistant Professor
University of Tennessee–Campbell Clinic
Department of Orthopaedic Surgery and Biomedical
    Engineering
Memphis, Tennessee

RAYMOND J. GARDOCKI, MD
Assistant Professor
University of Tennessee–Campbell Clinic
Department of Orthopaedic Surgery and Biomedical
    Engineering
Memphis, Tennessee

JAMES L. GUYTON, MD
Associate Professor
University of Tennessee–Campbell Clinic
Department of Orthopaedic Surgery and Biomedical
    Engineering
Memphis, Tennessee

JAMES W. HARKESS, MD
Associate Professor
University of Tennessee–Campbell Clinic
Department of Orthopaedic Surgery and Biomedical
    Engineering
Memphis, Tennessee

ROBERT K. HECK, JR., MD
Associate Professor
University of Tennessee–Campbell Clinic
Department of Orthopaedic Surgery and Biomedical
    Engineering
Memphis, Tennessee

SUSAN N. ISHIKAWA, MD
Assistant Professor
Co-Director, Foot and Ankle Fellowship
University of Tennessee–Campbell Clinic
Department of Orthopaedic Surgery and Biomedical
    Engineering
Memphis, Tennessee

MARK T. JOBE, MD
Associate Professor
University of Tennessee–Campbell Clinic
Department of Orthopaedic Surgery and Biomedical
    Engineering
Memphis, Tennessee

DEREK M. KELLY, MD
Associate Professor
Assistant Director, Residency Program
University of Tennessee–Campbell Clinic
Department of Orthopaedic Surgery and Biomedical
    Engineering
Memphis, Tennessee

DAVID G. LAVELLE, MD
Associate Professor
University of Tennessee–Campbell Clinic
Department of Orthopaedic Surgery and Biomedical
    Engineering
Memphis, Tennessee

SANTOS F. MARTINEZ, MD
Instructor
University of Tennessee–Campbell Clinic
Department of Orthopaedic Surgery and Biomedical
    Engineering
Memphis, Tennessee

ANTHONY A. MASCIOLI, MD
Assistant Professor
University of Tennessee–Campbell Clinic
Department of Orthopaedic Surgery and Biomedical
    Engineering
Memphis, Tennessee

MARC J. MIHALKO, MD
Assistant Professor
University of Tennessee–Campbell Clinic
Department of Orthopaedic Surgery and Biomedical
    Engineering
Memphis, Tennessee

WILLIAM W. MIHALKO, MD
Professor, H.R. Hyde Chair of Excellence in Rehabilitation
    Engineering
Director, Biomedical Engineering
University of Tennessee–Campbell Clinic
Department of Orthopaedic Surgery and Biomedical
    Engineering
Memphis, Tennessee

ROBERT H. MILLER III, MD
Associate Professor
University of Tennessee–Campbell Clinic
Department of Orthopaedic Surgery and Biomedical
    Engineering
Memphis, Tennessee

G. ANDREW MURPHY, MD
Associate Professor
Co-Director, Foot and Ankle Fellowship
University of Tennessee–Campbell Clinic
Department of Orthopaedic Surgery and Biomedical
    Engineering
Memphis, Tennessee

ASHLEY L. PARK, MD
Clinical Assistant Professor
University of Tennessee–Campbell Clinic
Department of Orthopaedic Surgery and Biomedical
    Engineering
Memphis, Tennessee

EDWARD A. PEREZ, MD
Associate Professor
Director, Trauma Fellowship
University of Tennessee–Campbell Clinic
Department of Orthopaedic Surgery and Biomedical
    Engineering
Memphis, Tennessee

BARRY B. PHILLIPS, MD
Associate Professor
University of Tennessee–Campbell Clinic
Department of Orthopaedic Surgery and Biomedical
    Engineering
Memphis, Tennessee

DAVID R. RICHARDSON, MD
Assistant Professor
University of Tennessee–Campbell Clinic
Department of Orthopaedic Surgery and Biomedical
    Engineering
Memphis, Tennessee

E. GREER RICHARDSON, MD
Professor Emeritus
University of Tennessee–Campbell Clinic
Department of Orthopaedic Surgery and Biomedical
    Engineering
Memphis, Tennessee

MATTHEW I. RUDLOFF, MD
Assistant Professor
University of Tennessee–Campbell Clinic
Department of Orthopaedic Surgery and Biomedical
    Engineering
Memphis, Tennessee

JEFFREY R. SAWYER, MD
Associate Professor
Director, Pediatric Orthopaedic Fellowship
University of Tennessee–Campbell Clinic
Department of Orthopaedic Surgery and Biomedical
    Engineering
Memphis, Tennessee

THOMAS W. THROCKMORTON, MD
Associate Professor
Director, Residency Program
University of Tennessee–Campbell Clinic
Department of Orthopaedic Surgery and Biomedical
    Engineering
Memphis, Tennessee

PATRICK C. TOY, MD
Assistant Professor
University of Tennessee–Campbell Clinic
Department of Orthopaedic Surgery and Biomedical
    Engineering
Memphis, Tennessee

WILLIAM C. WARNER, JR., MD
Professor
University of Tennessee–Campbell Clinic
Department of Orthopaedic Surgery and Biomedical
    Engineering
Memphis, Tennessee

JOHN C. WEINLEIN, MD
Assistant Professor
University of Tennessee–Campbell Clinic
Department of Orthopaedic Surgery and Biomedical
    Engineering
Memphis, Tennessee

A. PAIGE WHITTLE, MD
Associate Professor
University of Tennessee–Campbell Clinic
Department of Orthopaedic Surgery and Biomedical
    Engineering
Memphis, Tennessee

KEITH D. WILLIAMS, MD
Associate Professor
Director, Spine Fellowship
University of Tennessee–Campbell Clinic
Department of Orthopaedic Surgery and Biomedical
    Engineering
Memphis, Tennessee

DEXTER H. WITTE, MD
Clinical Assistant Professor of Radiology
University of Tennessee–Campbell Clinic
Department of Orthopaedic Surgery and Biomedical
    Engineering
Memphis, Tennessee

GEORGE W. WOOD II, MD
Professor
University of Tennessee–Campbell Clinic
Department of Orthopaedic Surgery and Biomedical
    Engineering
Memphis, Tennessee

PREFACE

The purpose of this text, as the title suggests, is to describe the "core" procedures from *Campbell's Operative Orthopaedics*. These include some of the most frequently used procedures at our clinic, as well by orthopaedic surgeons worldwide. We picked what we considered to be the top 100 procedures without regard to specialization or complexity. These procedures are described in no certain order, but generally follow the outline in *Campbell's Operative Orthopaedics*, edition 12.

The text is intended for orthopaedic residents and fellows and orthopaedic generalists and specialists. It is meant to be a source that is easily accessible in print, online, or via downloadable applications so that the user can find information about a specific procedure at the moment of need. For that reason, only detailed information about the surgical technique itself is included, and indications, contraindications, outcomes, complications, and alternate treatments are not given here.

We have had many requests over the years for a practical, transportable, easily accessible volume of the most popular procedures used at the Campbell Clinic — so, here it is. We hope you like it and find it helpful.

ACKNOWLEDGMENTS 〉

Our thanks to Kay Daugherty and Linda Jones, medical editors at the Campbell Foundation, and to Taylor Ball, Content Development Manager; John Casey, Senior Project Manager; and Dolores Meloni, Executive Content Strategist at Elsevier.

CONTENTS

PART X TRAUMA

PART XI   HAND AND WRIST

PART XII   FOOT AND ANKLE

A. LOCAL ANESTHESIA

B. HALLUX VALGUS

VIDEO CONTENTS

BONE GRAFT HARVEST: TIBIA, FIBULA, ILIAC CREST

Andrew H. Crenshaw, Jr. • G. Andrew Murphy

REMOVAL OF A TIBIAL GRAFT 〉

- To avoid excessive loss of blood, use a tourniquet (preferably pneumatic) when the tibial graft is removed. After removal of the graft, the tourniquet can be released without disturbing the sterile drapes.
- Make a slightly curved longitudinal incision over the anteromedial surface of the tibia, placing it so as to prevent a painful scar over the crest.
- Without reflecting the skin, incise the periosteum to the bone.
- With a periosteal elevator, reflect the periosteum medially and laterally exposing the entire surface of the tibia between the crest and the medial border. For better exposure at each end of the longitudinal incision, incise the periosteum transversely. The incision through the periosteum is I shaped.

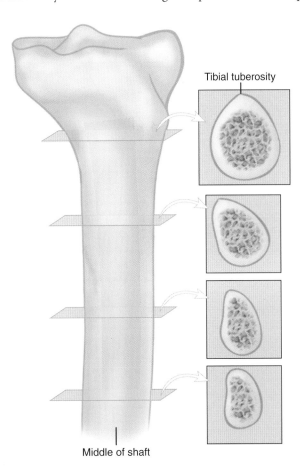

Tibial tuberosity

Middle of shaft

Figure 1-1

- Because of the shape of the tibia, the graft is usually wider at the proximal end than at the distal end. This equalizes the strength of the graft because the cortex is thinner proximally than distally. Before cutting the graft, drill a hole at each corner of the anticipated area (Figure 1-1).
- With a single-blade saw, remove the graft by cutting through the cortex at an oblique angle, preserving the anterior and medial borders of the tibia. Do not cut beyond the holes, especially when cutting across at

the ends because overcutting here weakens the donor bone and may serve as the initiation point of a future fracture. This is particularly true at the distal end of the graft.

- As the graft is pried from its bed have an assistant grasp it firmly to prevent it from dropping to the floor.
- Before closing the wound, remove additional cancellous bone from the proximal end of the tibia with a curet. Take care to avoid the articular surface of the tibia or in the case of a child, the physis.
- The periosteum over the tibia is relatively thick in children and can usually be sutured as a separate layer. In adults it is often thin, and closure may be unsatisfactory. Suturing the periosteum and the deep portion of the subcutaneous tissues as a single layer is recommended.
- If the graft has been properly cut, little shaping is necessary. Our practice is to remove the endosteal side of the graft because (1) the thin endosteal portion provides a graft to be placed across from the cortical graft; and (2) the endosteal surface, being rough and irregular, should be removed to ensure good contact of the graft with the host bone.

REMOVAL OF FIBULAR GRAFTS 〉

Three points should be considered during the removal of a fibular graft: (1) the peroneal nerve must not be damaged; (2) the distal fourth of the bone must be left to maintain a stable ankle; and (3) the peroneal muscles should not be cut (Figure 1-2).

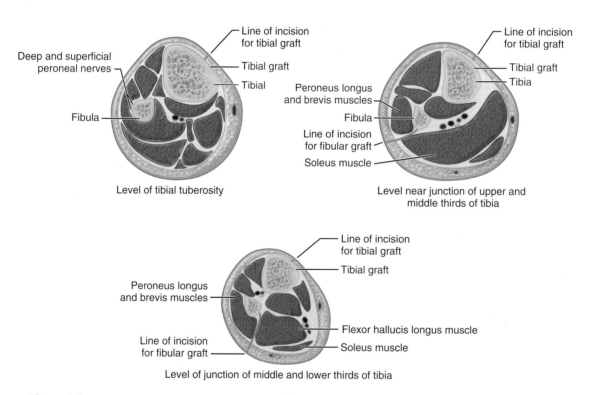

Figure 1-2

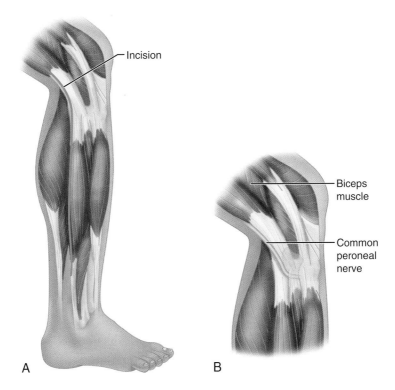

Figure 1-3   A   B

- For most grafting procedures, resect the middle third or middle half of the fibula using a Henry approach (Figure 1-3).
- Dissect along the anterior surface of the septum between the peroneus longus and soleus muscles. Identify the common peroneal nerve at the fibular head.

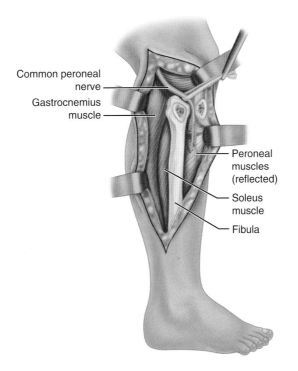

Figure 1-4

- Reflect the peroneal muscles anteriorly after subperiosteal dissection (Figure 1-4).
- Begin the stripping distally and progress proximally so that the oblique origin of the muscle fibers from the bone tends to press the periosteal elevator toward the fibula.

- Drill small holes through the fibula at the proximal and distal ends of the graft.
- Connect the holes by multiple small bites with the bone-biting forceps to osteotomize the bone otherwise the bone may be crushed. A Gigli saw, an oscillating power saw, or a thin air-powered cutting drill can be used. An osteotome may split or fracture the graft. The nutrient artery enters the bone near the middle of the posterior surface and may occasionally require ligation.
- If the transplant is to substitute for the distal end of the radius or fibula, resect the proximal third of the fibula through the proximal end of the Henry approach and take care to avoid damage to the peroneal nerve.
- Expose the nerve first at the posteromedial aspect of the distal end of the biceps femoris tendon and trace it distally to where it winds around the neck of the fibula. In this location the nerve is covered by the origin of the peroneus longus muscle. With the back of the knife blade toward the nerve, divide the thin slip of peroneus longus muscle bridging it. Displace the nerve from its normal bed into an anterior position.
- As the dissection continues, protect the anterior tibial vessels that pass between the neck of the fibula and the tibia by subperiosteal dissection.
- After the resection is complete, suture the biceps tendon and the fibular collateral ligament to the adjacent soft tissues.

REMOVAL OF AN ILIAC BONE GRAFT ⟩

Harvesting autograft bone from the ilium is not without complications. Hernias have been reported to develop in patients from whom massive full-thickness iliac grafts were taken. Muscle-pedicle grafts for arthrodesis of the hip have also resulted in a hernia when both cortices were removed. With this graft, the abductor muscles and the layer of periosteum laterally are removed with the graft. Careful repair of the supporting structures remaining after removal of an iliac graft is important and represents probably the best method of preventing hernias. Full-thickness windows made below the iliac crest are less likely to lead to hernia formation. In addition to hernia formation, nerve injury, arterial injury, or cosmetic deformity can be a problem after harvesting of iliac bone. The lateral femoral cutaneous and ilioinguinal nerves are at risk during the harvesting of bone from the anterior ilium. The superior cluneal nerves are at risk if the dissection is carried farther than 8 cm lateral to the posterior superior iliac spine (Figure 1-5).

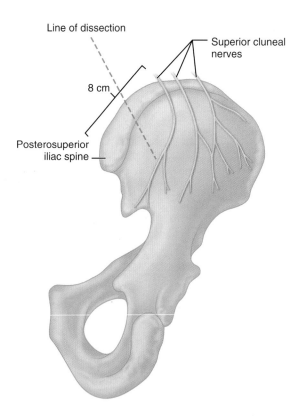

Figure 1-5

The superior gluteal vessels can be damaged by retraction against the roof of the sciatic notch. Removal of large full-thickness grafts from the anterior ilium can alter the contour of the anterior crest, producing significant cosmetic deformity. Arteriovenous fistula, pseudoaneurysm, ureteral injury, anterior superior iliac spine avulsion, and pelvic instability have been reported as major complications of iliac crest graft procurement.

- Make an incision along the subcutaneous border of the iliac crest at the point of contact of the periosteum with the origins of the gluteal and trunk muscles. Carry the incision down to the bone.
- When the crest of the ilium is not required as part of the graft, split off the lateral side or both sides of the crest in continuity with the periosteum and the attached muscles. To avoid hemorrhage, dissect subperiosteally.
- If a cancellous graft with one cortex is desired, elevate only the muscles from either the inner or the outer table of the ilium. The inner cortical table with underlying cancellous bone may be preferable owing to body habitus.

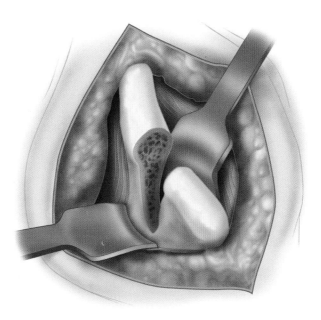

Figure 1-6

- For full-thickness grafts, also strip the iliacus muscle from the inner table of the ilium (Figure 1-6).
- When chip or sliver grafts are required remove them with an osteotome or gouge from the outer surface of the wing of the ilium taking only one cortex.
- After removal of the crest, considerable cancellous bone may be obtained by inserting a curet into the cancellous space between the two intact cortices.
- When removing a cortical graft from the outer table, first outline the area with an osteotome or power saw. Then peel the graft up with slight prying motions using a broad osteotome. Wedge grafts or full-thickness grafts may be removed more easily with a power saw and this technique also is less traumatic than when an osteotome and mallet are used. For this purpose, an oscillating saw or an air-powered cutting drill is satisfactory. Avoid excessive heat by irrigating with saline at room temperature.

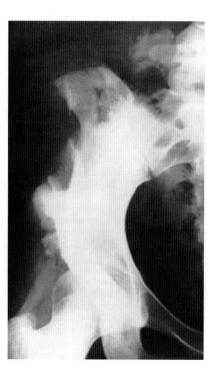

Figure 1-7

- Avoid removing too much of the crest anteriorly, which would leave an unsightly deformity posteriorly. shows a defect in the ilium after a large graft was removed (Figure 1-7). The anterior border of the ilium that included the anterior superior iliac spine was preserved but because the defect was so large, deformity was visible even under clothing. The unsightly contour was improved by removing more bone from the crest posteriorly.

- After removal of the grafts, accurately appose and suture the periosteum and muscular origins with strong interrupted sutures.

- Bleeding from the ilium is sometimes profuse; avoid using Gelfoam and bone wax and rely instead on wound packing and local pressure. Gelfoam and bone wax are foreign materials. Bone wax is said to retard bone healing and Gelfoam in large amounts has been associated with sterile serous drainage from wounds. Microcrystalline collagen has been reported to be more efficient in reducing blood loss from cancellous bone than either thrombin powder or thrombin-soaked gelatin foam. Gentle wound suction for 24 to 48 hours combined with meticulous obliteration of dead space is satisfactory for the management of these wounds.

- When harvesting bone from the posterior ilium, an incision parallel to the superior cluneal nerves and perpendicular to the posterior iliac crest has been recommended.

TOTAL HIP ARTHROPLASTY: STANDARD POSTEROLATERAL APPROACH

TECHNIQUE 2

James W. Harkess • John R. Crockarell, Jr.

The posterolateral approach is a modification of the posterior approaches described by Gibson and by Moore. The approach can be extended proximally by osteotomy of the greater trochanter with anterior dislocation of the hip (see section on trochanteric osteotomy). The approach can be extended distally to allow a posterolateral approach to the entire femoral shaft. We use the posterolateral approach for primary and revision total hip arthroplasty.

EXPOSURE AND REMOVAL OF THE FEMORAL HEAD ⟩

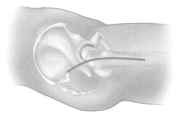

Figure 2-1

- With the patient firmly anchored in the straight lateral position, make a slightly curved incision centered over the greater trochanter. Begin the skin incision proximally at a point level with the anterior superior iliac spine along a line parallel to the posterior edge of the greater trochanter. Extend the incision distally to the center of the greater trochanter and along the course of the femoral shaft to a point 10 cm distal to the greater trochanter. Adequate extension of the upper portion of the incision is required for reaming of the femoral canal from a superior direction, and the distal extent of the exposure is required for preparation and insertion of the acetabular component from an anteroinferior direction (Figure 2-1).
- Divide the subcutaneous tissues along the skin incision in a single plane down to the fascia lata and the thin fascia covering the gluteus maximus superiorly.
- Dissect the subcutaneous tissues from the fascial plane for approximately 1 cm anteriorly and posteriorly to make identification of this plane easier at the time of closure.
- Divide the fascia in line with the skin wound over the center of the greater trochanter.
- Bluntly split the gluteus maximus proximally in the direction of its fibers, and coagulate any vessels within the substance of the muscle.
- Extend the fascial incision distally far enough to expose the tendinous insertion of the gluteus maximus on the posterior femur.
- Bluntly dissect the anterior and posterior edges of the fascia from any underlying fibers of the gluteus medius that insert into the undersurface of this fascia. Suture moist towels or laparotomy sponges to the fascial edges anteriorly and posteriorly to exclude the skin, prevent desiccation of the subcutaneous tissues, and collect cement and bone debris generated during the operation.
- Insert a Charnley or similar large self-retaining retractor beneath the fascia lata at the level of the trochanter. Take care not to entrap the sciatic nerve beneath the retractor posteriorly.
- Divide the trochanteric bursa and bluntly sweep it posteriorly to expose the short external rotators and the posterior edge of the gluteus medius. The posterior border of the gluteus medius is almost in line with the femoral shaft and the anterior border fans anteriorly.
- Maintain the hip in extension as the posterior dissection is performed. Flex the knee and internally rotate the extended hip to place the short external rotators under tension.
- Palpate the sciatic nerve as it passes superficial to the obturator internus and the gemelli. Complete exposure of the nerve is unnecessary unless the anatomy of the hip joint is distorted.

- Palpate the tendinous insertions of the piriformis and obturator internus and place tag sutures in the tendons for later identification at the time of closure.
- Divide the short external rotators, including at least the proximal half of the quadratus femoris, as close to their insertion on the femur as possible. Maintaining the length of the short rotators facilitates their later repair. Coagulate vessels located along the piriformis tendon and terminal branches of the medial circumflex artery located within the substance of the quadratus femoris. Reflect the short external rotators posteriorly while protecting the sciatic nerve.
- Bluntly dissect the interval between the gluteus minimus and the superior capsule. Insert blunt cobra or Hohmann retractors superiorly and inferiorly to obtain exposure of the entire superior, posterior, and inferior portions of the capsule.

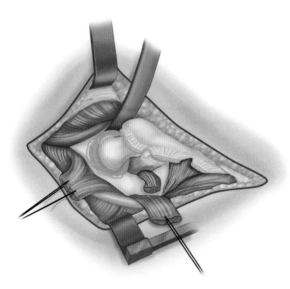

Figure 2-2

- Divide the entire exposed portion of the capsule immediately adjacent to its femoral attachment. Retract the capsule and preserve it for later repair (Figure 2-2).
- To determine leg length, insert a Steinmann pin into the ilium superior to the acetabulum and make a mark at a fixed point on the greater trochanter. Measure and record the distance between these two points to determine correct limb length after trial components have been inserted. Make all subsequent measurements with the limb in the identical position. Minor changes in abduction of the hip can produce apparent changes in leg-length measurements.

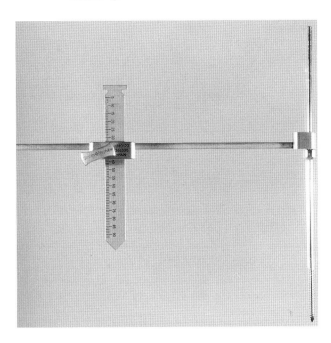

Figure 2-3

- We currently use a device that enables the measurement of leg length and offset. A sharp pin is placed in the pelvis above the acetabulum or iliac crest and measurements are made at a fixed point on the greater trochanter. An adjustable outrigger is calibrated for measurement of leg length and femoral offset (Figure 2-3).
- Dislocate the hip posteriorly by flexing, adducting, and gently internally rotating the hip.
- Place a bone hook beneath the femoral neck at the level of the lesser trochanter to lift the head gently out of the acetabulum. The ligamentum teres is usually avulsed from the femoral head during dislocation. In younger patients however, it may require division before the femoral head can be delivered into the wound.
- If the hip cannot be easily dislocated, do not forcibly internally rotate the femur because this can cause a fracture of the shaft. Instead, ensure that the superior and inferior portions of the capsule have been released as far as possible anteriorly. Remove any osteophytes along the posterior rim of the acetabulum that may be incarcerating the femoral head. If the hip still cannot be dislocated without undue force (most often encountered with protrusio deformity), divide the femoral neck with an oscillating saw at the appropriate level and subsequently remove the femoral head segment with a corkscrew, or divide it into several pieces.
- After dislocation of the hip, deliver the proximal femur into the wound with a broad, flat retractor.
- Excise residual soft tissue along the intertrochanteric line and expose the upper edge of the lesser trochanter.

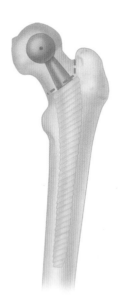

Figure 2-4

- Mark the level and angle of the proposed femoral neck osteotomy with electrocautery or with a shallow cut with an osteotome (Figure 2-4). Many systems have a specific instrument for this purpose. If not, plan the osteotomy using a trial prosthesis. Use the stem size and neck length trials determined by preoperative templating.
- Align the trial stem with the center of the femoral shaft and match the center of the trial femoral head with that of the patient. The level of the neck cut should be the same distance from the top of the lesser trochanter as determined by preoperative templating.
- Perform the osteotomy with an oscillating or reciprocating power saw. If this cut passes below the junction of the lateral aspect of the neck and greater trochanter, a separate longitudinal lateral cut is required. Avoid notching the greater trochanter at the junction of these two cuts because this may predispose the trochanter to fracture.
- Remove the femoral head from the wound by dividing any remaining soft tissue attachments. Keep the head on the sterile field because it may be needed as a source of bone graft.

Exposure and Preparation of the Acetabulum

- Isolate the anterior capsule by passing a curved clamp within the sheath of the psoas tendon.
- Retract the femur anteriorly with a bone hook to place the capsule under tension.

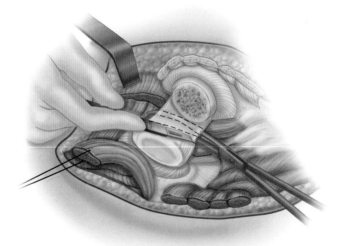

Figure 2-5

- Carefully divide the anterior capsule along the course of psoas tendon sheath between the jaws of the clamp (Figure 2-5).

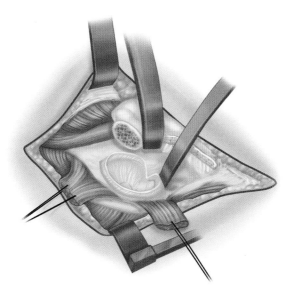

Figure 2-6

- Place a curved cobra or Hohmann retractor in the interval between the anterior lip of the acetabulum and the psoas tendon. The femur should be well retracted anteriorly to allow unimpeded access to the acetabulum. Erroneous placement of this retractor over the psoas muscle can cause injury to the femoral nerve or adjacent vessels. Place an additional retractor beneath the transverse acetabular ligament to provide inferior exposure (Figure 2-6).

- Retract the posterior soft tissues with a right-angle retractor placed on top of a laparotomy sponge to avoid compression or excessive traction on the sciatic nerve. As an alternative, place Steinmann pins or spike retractors into the posterior column. Avoid impaling the sciatic nerve or placing the pins within the acetabulum where they would interfere with acetabular preparation.

- Retract the femur anteriorly and medially and rotate it slightly to determine which position provides the best acetabular exposure. If after complete capsulotomy the femur cannot be fully retracted anteriorly, divide the tendinous insertion of the gluteus maximus, leaving a 1-cm cuff of tendon on the femur for subsequent reattachment.

- Complete the excision of the labrum. Draw the soft tissues into the acetabulum and divide them immediately adjacent to the acetabular rim. Keep the knife blade within the confines of the acetabulum at all times to avoid injury to important structures anteriorly and posteriorly.

- Expose the bony margins of the rim of the acetabulum around its entire circumference to facilitate proper placement of the acetabular component.

- Use an osteotome to remove any osteophytes that protrude beyond the bony limits of the true acetabulum.

- Begin the bony preparation of the acetabulum. The procedure for cartilage removal and reaming of the acetabulum is similar for cementless and cemented acetabular components.

- Excise the ligamentum teres, and curet any remaining soft tissue from the region of the pulvinar. Brisk bleeding from branches of the obturator artery may be encountered during this maneuver and will require cauterization.

- Palpate the floor of the acetabulum within the cotyloid notch. Occasionally, hypertrophic osteophytes completely cover the notch and prevent assessment of the location of the medial wall. Remove the osteophytes with osteotomes and rongeurs to locate the medial wall. Otherwise, the acetabular component can be placed in an excessively lateralized position.

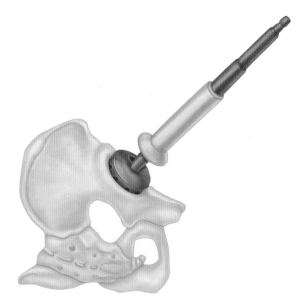

Figure 2-7

- Prepare the acetabulum with motorized reamers. Begin with a reamer smaller than the anticipated final size and direct it medially down to, but not through, the medial wall. Make frequent checks of the depth of reaming to ensure that the medial wall is not violated. This allows a few millimeters of deepening of the acetabulum with improved lateral coverage of the component (Figure 2-7).

- Occasionally, the transverse acetabular ligament is hypertrophic and must be excised to allow larger reamers to enter the acetabulum. Carefully dissect the ligament from its bony attachments anteriorly and posteriorly. Keep the knife blade superficial because branches of the obturator vessels pass beneath it and bleeding in this area can be difficult to control.

- Direct all subsequent reamers in the same plane as the opening face of the acetabulum.

- Retract the femur well anteriorly so that reamers can be inserted from an anteroinferior direction without impingement. If the femur is inadequately retracted anteriorly it may force the reamers posteriorly and excessive reaming of the posterior column occurs. Use progressively larger reamers in 1- or 2-mm increments.

- Irrigate the acetabulum frequently to assess the adequacy of reaming and to adjust the direction of the reaming to ensure that circumferential reaming occurs. Reaming is complete when all cartilage has been removed, the reamers have cut bone out to the periphery of the acetabulum, and a hemispherical shape has been produced.

- Expose a bleeding subchondral bone bed but maintain as much of the subchondral bone plate as possible.

- Curet any remaining soft tissue from the floor of the acetabulum and excise any overhanging soft tissues around the periphery of the acetabulum. Search for subchondral cysts within the acetabulum and remove their contents with small curved curets.

- Fill the cavities with morselized cancellous bone obtained from the patient's femoral head or acetabular reamings and impact the graft with a small punch.

- Before insertion of the acetabular component, ensure that the patient remains in the true lateral position. If the pelvis has been rotated anteriorly by forceful anterior retraction of the femur, the acetabular component can easily be placed in a retroverted position which may predispose to postoperative dislocation. Most systems have trial acetabular components that can be inserted before final implant selection to determine the adequacy of fit, the presence of circumferential bone contact, and the adequacy of the bony coverage of the component. Using trial components also allows the surgeon to make a mental note of the positioning of the component before final implantation.

- Proceed with implantation of cementless or cemented acetabular and femoral components.

CREDITS

Figures 2-1, 2-2, 2-6 redrawn from Capello WN: Uncemented hip replacement, Tech Orthop 1:11, 1986; also courtesy of Indiana University School of Medicine.

DIRECT ANTERIOR APPROACH FOR TOTAL HIP ARTHROPLASTY

Patrick Toy

This technique does not include the use of a special traction table (i.e., Hanna table).

- Position the patient supine on the operating room table so that the bend of the table is at the level of the symphysis pubis. This will allow extension of the hip joint and elevation of the proximal femur during preparation of the femur. Place an arm board distally on the contralateral side of the operative leg, parallel to the table so that the nonoperative hip can be abducted to allow adduction of the operative hip.

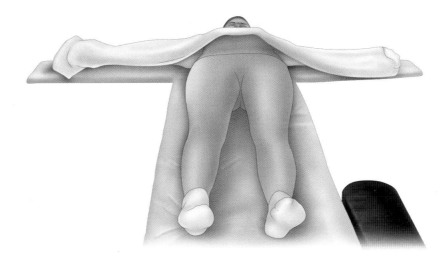

Figure 3-1

- Make an oblique incision beginning 2 to 3 cm lateral and 2 to 3 cm inferior to the anterior-superior iliac spine in line with the tensor fascia latae (TFL) muscle (Figure 3-1).
- Carry dissection distally and laterally over the TFL down through the subcutaneous tissue to the level of the fascia of the TFL. The fascia at this location is relatively translucent and the pink/red muscle may be easily observed. If one is either too far medial or lateral, the fascia is not as translucent and is white in color.

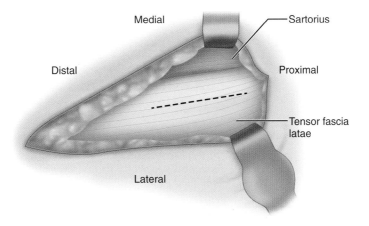

Figure 3-2

- Sharply split the fascia longitudinally in line with the muscle fibers, and carry dissection medially to develop the interval between the sartorius and TFL muscles. Because this dissection is within the tensor sheath, the sartorius muscle may not be visible (Figure 3-2).

- Carry dissection deeper in this interval between the gluteus medius and rectus femoris and place soft-tissue retractors to retract the rectus femoris medially and the gluteus medius laterally.

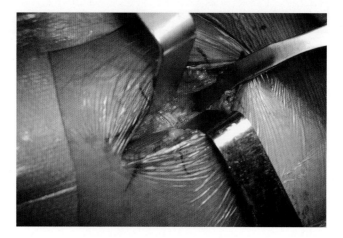

Figure 3-3

- Several large vessels lie between these two muscles (divisions of the ascending branch of the lateral femoral circumflex artery); carefully ligate or cauterize these. It is important to ligate or cauterize these in situ before dividing them because they can retract into the soft tissues and cause excessive bleeding (Figure 3-3).
- Dissect the rectus femoris muscle (on the deep side of it), just anterior to the hip capsule and carry dissection medially. Place a self-retaining retractor to retract the TFL laterally and the rectus femoris medially.
- Place a cobra retractor extracapsularly along the inferior femoral neck and another retractor in the "saddle" region (junction of the greater trochanter and the superior femoral neck).
- Use a rongeur to remove some of the anterior fat over the hip capsule to expose the capsule.

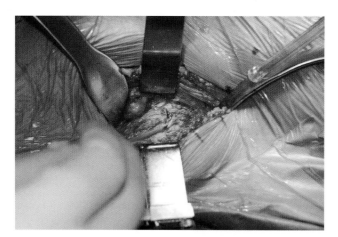

Figure 3-4

- Perform a capsulectomy or capsulotomy to allow access to the femoral neck (Figure 3-4).
- Place retractors within the capsule, and carry the capsulectomy or capsulotomy down so that the lesser trochanter is palpable with a finger; carry dissection superiorly so that the soft tissues within the saddle region are dissected free.
- Move the superior and inferior femoral neck retractors so that they are intracapsular, and make the osteotomy cut in the femoral neck.

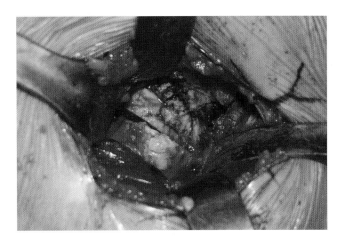

Figure 3-5

- Make two parallel cuts in the femoral neck to allow removal of a 1-cm sliver of bone ("napkin-ring" oste-otomy) for easy removal of the femoral head. Alternatively, a single osteotomy can be used, but this may make removal of the femoral head more difficult because there is not as much room as with the napkin-ring technique (Figure 3-5).

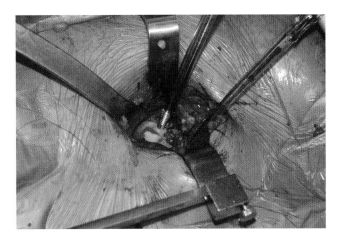

Figure 3-6

- Use a corkscrew to remove the femoral head, place retractors at the anterior aspect of the acetabulum, and sharply excise the labrum (Figure 3-6).
- Excise the pulvinar within the cotyloid fossa to expose the medial acetabular wall, and begin reaming. Continue reaming with medialization using image-intensifier guidance or by reaming down to the medial wall. If there is any concern about the depth of reaming, use image intensification to confirm the depth of the reamer, as well as its size. Under-reaming by one cup size allows a good press fit.

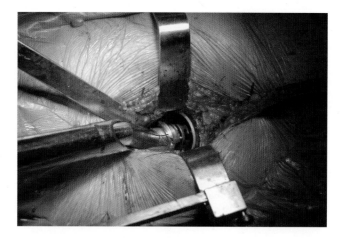

Figure 3-7

- Once medialization is complete, ream in the appropriate abduction and anteversion. Take care not to excessively antevert and abduct the cup (Figure 3-7).
- Press fit the cup into position and remove any excess osteophytes. Snap the polyethylene liner into position and use a head impactor to ensure that it is fully seated.
- Once the cup is firmly positioned, turn attention to the proximal femur. Elevation of the femur is necessary for broaching and is the most difficult step in the anterior approach.
- Move the operative hip into adduction and external rotation (abduct the nonoperative hip).

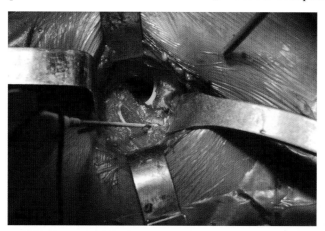

Figure 3-8

- Palpate the greater trochanter and use electrocautery to incise the capsule overlying it. Release the conjoined tendon and the obturator internus. If necessary, also release the piriformis. It is important not to release the obturator externus tendon, which is more inferior than the shortened external rotators (Figure 3-8).

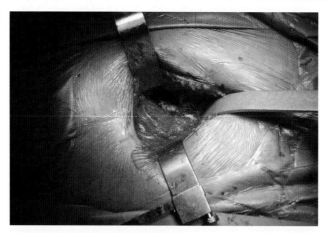

Figure 3-9

- Place a smooth retractor deep at the greater trochanter to help maintain its position in the wound. A bone hook can be used to elevate the femur into position and the retractor can be used to maintain that position. To minimize the risk of fracture, do not lever farther down on the retractor (Figure 3-9).

- Insert a canal finder instrument at the medial edge and advance it distally to open the femoral canal. Then use a box chisel to remove cancellous bone proximally.
- A broach-type stem rather than a ream-and-broach technique often is used in anterior approach THA. Insert the smallest broach, and sequentially broach the canal until the appropriate size is reached; confirm this by testing stability with internal and external rotation, as well as with image intensification.
- Place the trial components and determine the correct neck length and offset. Hip stability and limb length both can be evaluated at this time.

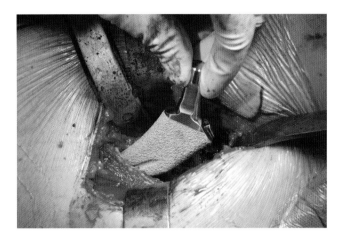

Figure 3-10

- Once the appropriate stem size is chosen, dislocate the hip, remove the broach, irrigate the proximal femur, and press-fit the femoral implant into position (Figure 3-10).
- Choose the neck length and material for the femoral head, ceramic or metal. Impact the head onto the trunion after it is clean and dry, and reduce the hip.
- If capsulotomy has been performed, repair it with no. 0 absorbable suture. Irrigate the wound and obtain hemostasis.
- Close the fascia with standard no. 0 absorbable suture, and close the subcutaneous tissue and skin in routine fashion. Apply a sterile dressing.

POSTOPERATIVE CARE ❯

Patients are often discharged the same day as their surgery, but may have an overnight stay. Administration of intravenous narcotics is uncommon, but transition to oral pain medication is often possible about 2 to 3 hours after surgery. Mobilization with physical therapy is begun 3 to 4 hours after surgery if the patient is medically stable and has no nausea or hypotension problems. When the patient can walk approximately 150 feet and ascend and descend a flight of stairs, first with and then without an assistive device, he or she is cleared for discharge. After discharge, pain is managed using a multi-modal pain control regimen. Deep vein thrombosis prophylaxis is begun postoperative day number one. Patients are encouraged to bear weight and to discontinue assistive devices as soon as they are able (physical therapist's discretion). Hip precautions are not necessary, and patients are encouraged to resume recreational activities such as golf and biking as soon as possible. Driving generally is permitted after the 1-week follow-up visit if narcotics have been discontinued. Out-patient physical therapy is continued until the patient has met his or her preoperative goals.

Three basic types of trochanteric osteotomies are currently used in hip arthroplasty: (1) the standard or conventional type, (2) the so-called trochanteric slide, and (3) the extended trochanteric osteotomy (Figure 4-1). Various modifications have been described for each type. The different types are suitable for specific purposes and should be tailored to the procedure being contemplated. Finally, the fixation method must be adapted to the type of osteotomy.

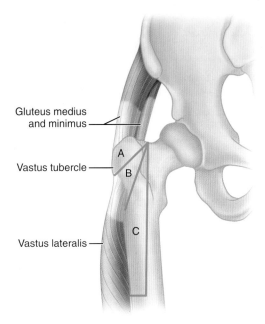

Gluteus medius and minimus

Vastus tubercle

Vastus lateralis

A
B
C

Figure 4-1

Standard Trochanteric Osteotomy

- After exposure of the hip, detach the vastus lateralis subperiosteally from the lateral aspect of the femur distal to the vastus tubercle.

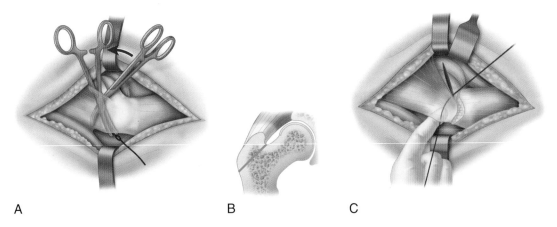

A   B   C

Figure 4-2

- With a power saw or osteotome (Figure 4-2, **A**), begin the osteotomy just distal to the vastus tubercle and direct it proximally (**B**). If a Gigli saw is used, before making the osteotomy use a finger to ensure that the saw is sufficiently anterior and that the sciatic nerve is not trapped between the saw and the bone (**C**).

- Once the trochanter has been cut, retract it proximally and release the short external rotators from the trochanteric fragment. Alternatively, if a posterior approach to the hip is used, detach the external rotators before the osteotomy is performed.

Trochanteric Slide

- Make the skin incision parallel to the posterior border of the greater trochanter.
- Incise the fascia in-line with the skin incision.
- Isolate the gluteus medius and minimus muscles anteriorly and posteriorly.
- Elevate the vastus lateralis subperiosteally from the femoral shaft and retract it anteriorly. Preserve its origin at the vastus tubercle.

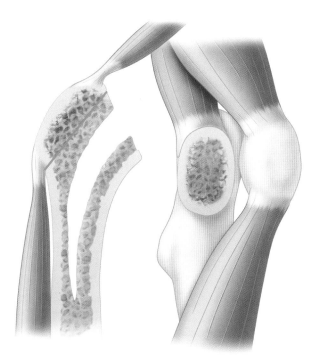

Figure 4-3

- Begin the osteotomy just medial to the tendinous insertions of the gluteus medius and minimus into the greater trochanter. The osteotomy exits distal to the vastus ridge so that the origin of the lateralis is preserved in continuity with the bony wafer (Figure 4-3).
- Divide the external rotators close to their insertion, preserving them for reattachment. Alternatively, if a posterior approach to the hip is used, detach the external rotators before the osteotomy is performed.
- Retract the osteotomized trochanter with its muscular sleeve anteriorly and hold it with a self-retaining retractor.

Extended Trochanteric Osteotomy

- Through a standard posterior approach, release the external rotators off the greater trochanter and partially release the gluteus maximus insertion.
- Elevate the vastus lateralis subperiosteally off the femur and retract it anteriorly, maintaining its origin on the vastus ridge.

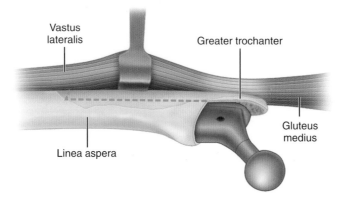

Figure 4-4

- Beginning at the base of the greater trochanter in the sagittal plane and extending distally, outline the osteotomy with multiple drill holes made with a narrow, high-speed pencil burr or oscillating saw, staying just anterior to the linea aspera (Figure 4-4).
- Continue the osteotomy distally to the point determined by preoperative templating, then carry the osteotomy anterolaterally for a distance of one-third of the femoral circumference.

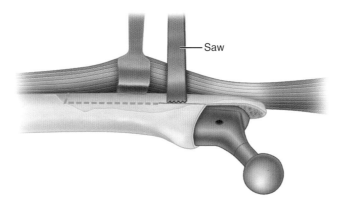

Figure 4-5

- Connect the drill holes with a high-speed pencil burr or oscillating saw, penetrating the proximal cortex and cement mantle, if present (Figure 4-5).
- Perforate the anterolateral cortex of the femur with multiple drill holes starting through the posterior limb of the osteotomy and exiting anterolaterally.

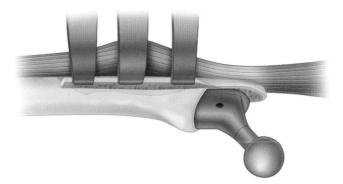

Figure 4-6

- Place wide osteotomes from posterior to anterior and lever open the previously perforated anterolateral cortex, hinging on the soft tissue (Figure 4-6).

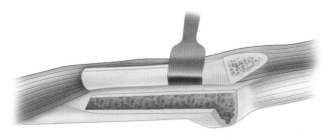

Figure 4-7

- Retract the trochanter and lateral femoral osteotomy segment, with the attached gluteus medius and minimus and the vastus lateralis, anteriorly as a single unit to provide access to the femoral canal (Figure 4-7).

Fixation of the Osteotomy

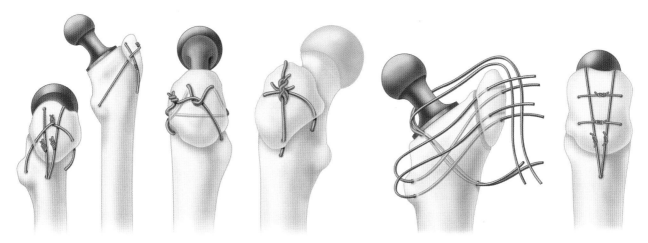

Figure 4-8

- Various wire fixation techniques using two, three, or four wires have been described (Figure 4-8).
- No. 16, 18, or 20 wire can be used, and because spool wire is more malleable, it is easier to tighten and tie or twist. A wire tightener or two sternal wire holders are used to tighten the wire. Stainless steel, cobalt-chrome alloy, or titanium alloy wire can be used, depending on the metal of the femoral component. Also, multiple filament wire or cable is available; the ends are pulled through a short metal sleeve, which is crimped after the wire has been tightened.

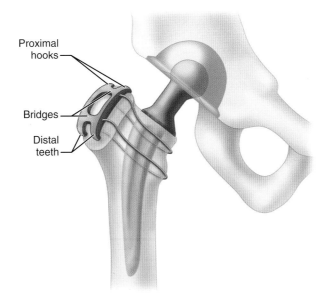

Figure 4-9

- Special care should be taken not to kink or nick the wire. In most cases, we prefer an extramedullary fixation device (Figure 4-9).

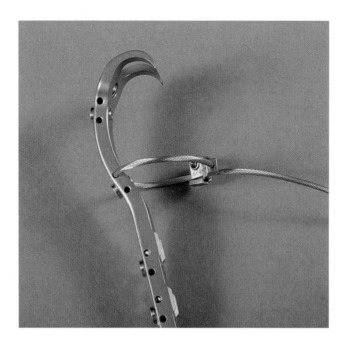

Figure 4-10

- A variety of devices featuring proximal hooks with a plate extension also are available (Figure 4-10).

POSTOPERATIVE CARE 〉

Full weightbearing on the hip should be delayed for 4 to 6 weeks if fixation is not rigid. When fixation is less stable (i.e., when the osteotomized fragment is small, osteoporotic, or retracted proximally, or if the bony bed for reattachment of the trochanteric fragment is deficient), the hip may be maintained in abduction in a spica cast or orthosis for 6 weeks.

CREDITS

Figure 4-3 redrawn from Glassman AH, Engh CA, Bobyn JD: A technique of extensile exposure for total hip arthroplasty, J Arthroplasty 2:11, 1987.

Figure 4-8 redrawn from Markolf KL, Hirschowitz DL, Amstutz HC: Mechanical stability of the greater trochanter following osteotomy and reattachment by wiring, Clin Orthop Relat Res 141:111, 1979; and from Harris WH: Revision surgery for failed, nonseptic total hip arthroplasty: the femoral side, Clin Orthop Relat Res 1709:8, 1982.

Figure 4-9 redrawn from Dall DM, Miles AW: Reattachment of the greater trochanter: the use of the trochanter cable-grip system, J Bone Joint Surg 65B:55, 1983.

Figure 4-10 courtesy of Smith & Nephew, Memphis, TN.

HIP RESURFACING

David G. Lavelle

Hip resurfacing is an attractive option for younger patients with severe hip disease. Advantages of the procedure include easier revision, decreased risk of hip dislocation, more normal walking pattern, greater hip range of motion, and earlier return to activity. Disadvantages include risk of femoral neck fracture and metal ions; resurfacing also is a more difficult procedure than total hip arthroplasty. The best candidates for hip resurfacing appear to be younger men (< 55 to 60 years) with good quality bone.

- Position the patient in the lateral position with the affected hip up. Stabilize the pelvis with a pelvic clamp or pegboard, with the pelvis oriented straight up and down. If the pelvis is leaning forward, the acetabular component may be placed in retroversion; and if it is leaning backward, the acetabular component may be placed in excessive anteversion.

Approach and Exposure

- To resurface the hip, extensive exposure is necessary to allow the acetabulum to be visible and later on in the procedure to keep the femoral head visible over its entire surface. Therefore, steps must be taken to achieve exposure not commonly used in total hip replacement surgery. Obviously, the femoral head is removed during a total hip replacement, which greatly aids in exposure.

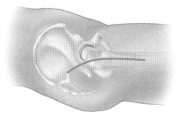

Figure 5-1

- Make a curved skin incision over the greater trochanter, angling the proximal portion posteriorly, pointing toward the posterior superior iliac spine. Carry the incision over the center of the greater trochanter and then distally over the shaft of the femur to end over the attachment of the gluteus maximus on the linea aspera (Figure 5-1).
- Divide the subcutaneous tissue in a single plane over the fascia of the gluteus maximus proximally and the fascia of the iliotibial band distally. Make a longitudinal incision over the middle to posterior third of the fascia over the greater trochanter and extend it distally over the femoral shaft. Extend the proximal end of the incision through the thin fascia over the gluteus maximus in the same direction as the skin incision. Bluntly split the fibers of the gluteus maximus muscle, taking care to find and cauterize any bleeding.
- Release the tendinous attachment of the gluteus maximus from the linea aspera to maximally internally rotate the femur to provide satisfactory exposure of the proximal femur and femoral head. If the gluteus maximus is not released, the sciatic nerve may be at risk of compression at the time of preparation of the femoral head. Place a hemostat under the gluteus maximus tendon as the tendon is divided to avoid injuring branches of the medial femoral circumflex artery and the first perforating artery. Leave a centimeter of tendon attached to the linea aspera and femoral shaft for later repair.
- Widely spread the fascial plane just divided using a Charnley or self-retaining retractor. The posterior greater trochanter and gluteus medius should be easily seen. Remove the trochanteric bursa.
- Retract the gluteus medius muscle and tendon anteriorly. A hooked instrument, such as a Hibbs retractor, is useful. Under the gluteus medius is the piriformis, which is exposed. Tag the piriformis tendon with suture, and then release it from the femur. Under and anterior to the piriformis tendon are the muscle fibers of the gluteus minimus. With an elevator, raise the gluteus medius off the capsule of the hip completely. The entire capsule of the hip should be exposed superiorly. Use of a narrow cobra retractor is helpful to see this area when it is placed under the gluteus minimus and medius.

- Expose the plane distally between the capsule and the short external rotator muscles. Release the short external rotator muscles off the femur including the quadratus femoris distally. Coagulate the vessels in this area.
- The capsule of the hip is now completely exposed posteriorly, superiorly, and inferiorly. The lesser trochanter is also visible. With the hip in internal rotation, make an incision in the capsule circumferentially, leaving at least a centimeter of capsule still attached to the femoral neck. This centimeter of capsule is later used to repair the capsule back as well as to provide protection to the intraosseous vessels needed to maintain vascularity of the femoral neck.

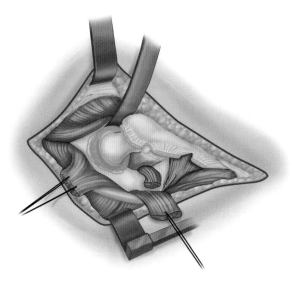

Figure 5-2

- Make two radial incisions in the posterior capsule to create a posterior capsular flap. This is helpful for retraction and later repair (Figure 5-2).
- Dislocate the femoral head and perform a complete anterior capsulotomy with sharp scissors. The inferior portion of the capsule is seen by extending and internally rotating the femur. The psoas tendon is exposed at the lesser trochanter, and the capsule is isolated just in front of the psoas tendon.

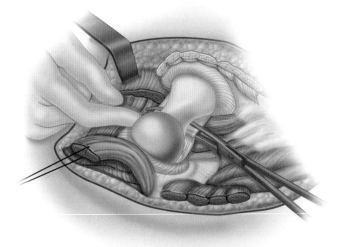

Figure 5-3

- While maintaining the scissors just posterior to the psoas tendon, incise the capsule from inferior to superior. Maintain the femur in internal rotation and apply anterior traction with a bone hook on the lesser trochanter (Figure 5-3).
- Perform the proximal end of the capsulotomy by flexing the femur 90 degrees and maintaining a narrow cobra retractor under the gluteus muscles. Incise the capsule with sharp scissors while internally rotating the femur to beyond 100 degrees. If a complete capsulotomy is not performed, exposure of the femur is compromised.

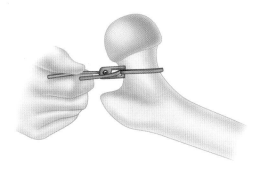

Figure 5-4

- Measure the femoral neck from superior to inferior, its longest dimension. The Birmingham Hip comes with heads in 2-mm increments. The measurement tool should loosely fit over the femoral neck to avoid undersizing the femoral component, which could cause notching of the femoral neck. Femoral neck notches may weaken the neck and predispose it to early postoperative fracture. If there is any doubt, choose the next largest size of the femoral head component (Figure 5-4).
- Once the size of the femoral component is known, the acetabular component size is also known because the acetabular component is matched with components either 6 or 8 mm larger than the femoral component. So, in the case of the femoral head measuring 52 mm, for instance, the acetabular component will need to be either 58 or 60 mm. That means the acetabulum will need to be reamed to 57 or 59 mm, respectively.
- The key to exposure of the acetabulum is to dislocate the femoral head out of the way anteriorly and superiorly. Create an anterosuperior pouch large enough for the femoral head under the gluteus muscles and above the ilium. This is done by sharply dissecting the soft tissues off the bone of the ilium, including the capsule and tendons of the rectus femoris from the superior acetabular lip and the anterior inferior iliac spine.

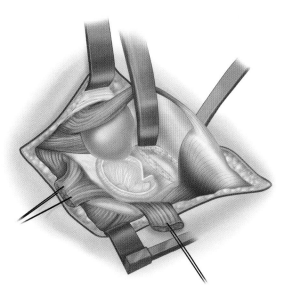

Figure 5-5

- Once the pouch has been created, dislocate the femoral head into the pouch under the gluteus muscles and retract it with a sharp, narrow Hohmann retractor driven into the ilium superior to the acetabulum and resting on the femoral neck. Additional pins may be driven into the ilium and ischium to help with the acetabular exposure. A retractor is also placed inferiorly to expose the transverse acetabular ligament. Sharply excise the labrum (Figure 5-5).
- Ream the acetabulum medially through the cotyloid notch of the acetabulum to the medial wall. Take care not to ream through the medial wall. Once medialized, the reamers are used to increase the bony acetabulum to the desired size. The acetabulum usually is underreamed by 1 mm from the desired component size.

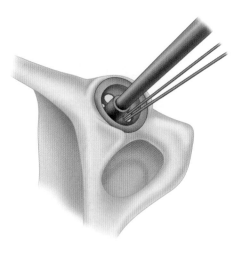

Figure 5-6

- Use an acetabular trial to assess the potential component's stability. The trial components in the Birmingham Hip Resurfacing System are 1 mm smaller than their stated size to provide for tighter fitting of the actual component (Figure 5-6).

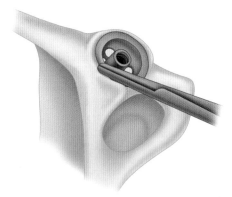

Figure 5-7

- Impact the trial into the acetabulum with a mallet, and excise osteophytes for unobstructed cup insertion. If that size trial is tight, the acetabular implant of the same size is selected. If the trial is loose, the acetabulum may be reamed 1 or 2 mm more to the next-size acetabular component that matches the appropriate size femoral head. There are two acetabular sizes per femoral head size available. The trial should be used for the larger cup size; if it is tight, that cup should be selected. Mark the edge of the trial with electrocautery inside the acetabulum to predict the depth of the implant when inserted (Figure 5-7).

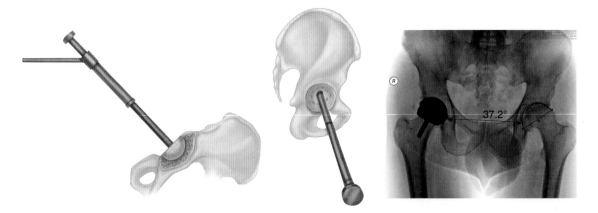

Figure 5-8

- It is critical for the long-term success of the hip that the acetabular component's orientation is done correctly. Implant the acetabular component in 10 to 20 degrees of anteversion and 35 to 45 degrees of abduction. If greater than 50 degrees of abduction is accepted or there is more than 25 degrees of anteversion, the metal femoral head component may be subjected to edge wear associated with accelerated metal debris and ion production (Figure 5-8).

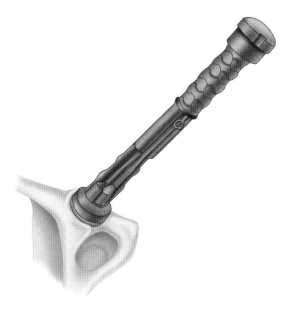

Figure 5-9

- To properly insert the acetabular cup, push the insertion tool down against the inferior portion of the wound. The mark made on the inside of the acetabular wall while the trial was in place is used to judge if the acetabular component is fully seated (there are no holes in the cup). Remove periacetabular osteophytes to the edge of the cup (Figure 5-9).

Dysplasia Cup

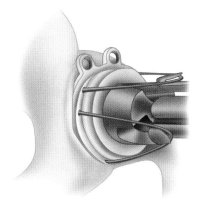

Figure 5-10

- The dysplasia cup is used when there is significant acetabular dysplasia or lateral or superior erosion of the rim of the acetabulum. The Birmingham Hip Resurfacing System includes a dysplasia cup, which is only 3 mm larger than the femoral component and has two screw holes external to the rim of the cup for superior and posterior screw fixation (Figure 5-10).

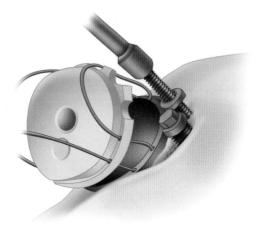

Figure 5-11

- Cup preparation and position are the same. Drill the holes for the screws using a drill guide through the threaded holes on the edge of the cup. The screws must thread into the holes in the cup and then into the iliac bone above or posterior to the acetabulum (Figure 5-11).
- Attention is now turned to the femur. Place a clean sponge in the acetabulum to protect it. The template created on radiographs before surgery shows a line drawn over the lateral shaft of the proximal femur that when continued up the femoral neck corresponds to the correct valgus orientation of the femoral component at its post that will be inserted down the middle of the femoral neck. This line, where it intersects the lateral femoral shaft, usually aligns medially with a point on the lesser trochanter. The measurement from the tip of the greater trochanter to where the line intersects the lateral femoral shaft corresponds with the measurement taken during surgery.

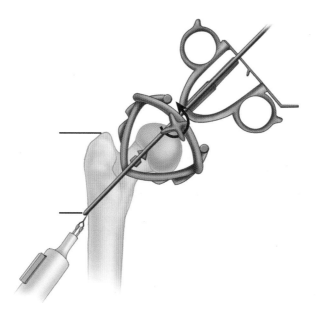

Figure 5-12

- At the time of surgery, use a spinal needle to find the tip of the lesser trochanter and then measure distally to a point on the lateral femoral cortex and mark it with a cautery. This point will then be a reference to help orient the femoral component into proper valgus alignment (Figure 5-12).

Resurfacing of Femoral Head

- To resurface the femoral head, internally rotate the femur much farther than needed to perform a total hip replacement. With the soft tissue release, which has already been discussed, this may be safely done, even though the position may seem extreme and more force than usual is required. However, fear of femoral fracture should not be great because resurfacings of the hip should be only done in patients with hard bone.

- Flex the femur to 80 to 90 degrees and then internally rotate it between 120 and 150 degrees to expose the femoral head and neck circumferentially. The anterior portion of the head is most difficult to expose. A retractor between the acetabular cup and the proximal femur lifting the femur out of the wound may be helpful.

- With the femoral head and neck exposed, remove periarticular osteophytes, taking care not to violate the bone of the femoral neck. A Kerrison rongeur may be helpful anteriorly. Take care not to strip soft tissue from the femoral neck that contains vessels supplying the femoral head.

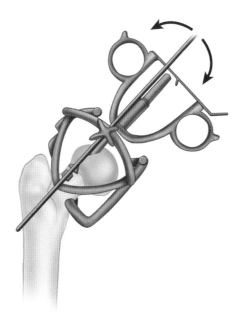

Figure 5-13

- Place a guide pin down the center of the femoral head. There are two jigs designed to help with pin placement. The jig we have most experience with is a clamp design that has two legs that clamp around the femoral neck superiorly and inferiorly. Place a long guide rod posteriorly over the femoral neck to orient the jig in a valgus position. The lateral tip of that guide rod should line up with the point marked on the lateral femoral cortex and its soft tissue mark made after measuring down from the greater trochanter. This ensures the placement of the pin down the center of the femoral neck in proper valgus alignment (Figure 5-13).

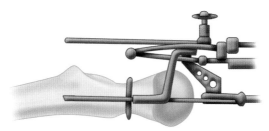

Figure 5-14

- View the guide pin from the medial side of the neck to be certain that it is not placed in retroversion. The guide pin position should be completely evaluated by its orientation to the femoral neck and not the femoral head. The pin is usually placed superior to the fovea, but, with wear, the head may become deformed (Figure 5-14).

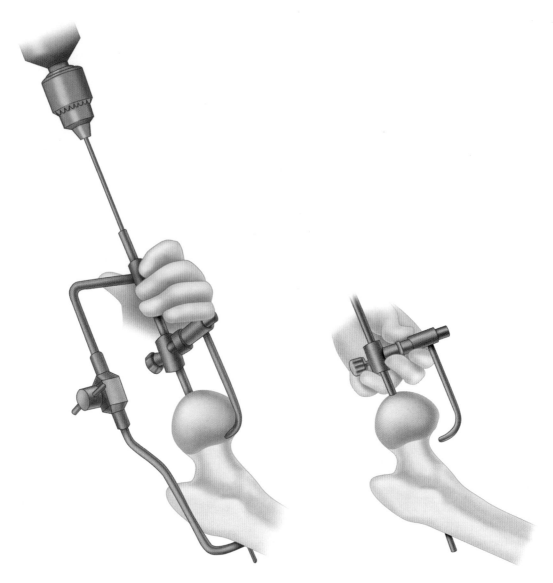

Figure 5-15

- Once the guide pin is inserted down the middle of the femoral neck in anteroposterior and lateral planes, use a cannulated reamer to ream over the pin. Remove the pin and place a large reaming guide rod into the hole in the head and neck. Take circumferential measurements with a feeler-gauge to be certain the selected head size will not notch the femoral neck, especially laterally and superiorly (Figure 5-15).

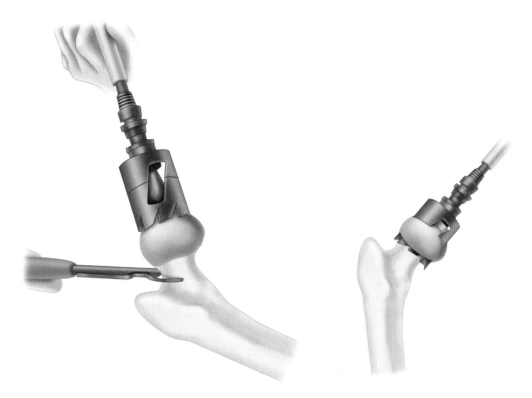

Figure 5-16

- Once this has been confirmed, ream the femoral head circumferentially with the correct size reamer. Protect the femoral neck from by with the measurement tool (Figure 5-16).

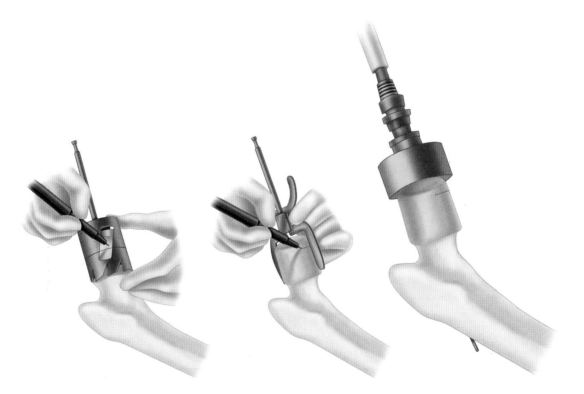

Figure 5-17

- Measure to see how far above the head-neck junction line the head needs to be resected, and ream the head to that line (Figure 5-17).

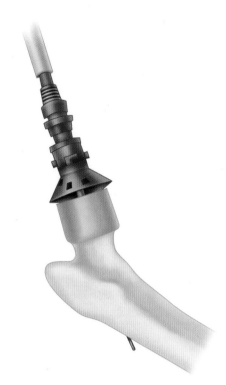

Figure 5-18

- A chamfer reamer of the correct size is used to finalize the shape of the femoral head to match the geometry of the interior of the femoral head component. Remove the reaming rod (Figure 5-18).

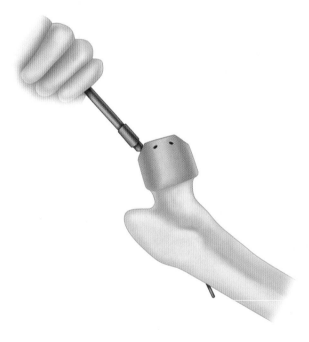

Figure 5-19

- Drill small to medium cement fixation holes into the femoral head around the chamfer and the tip of the head (Figure 5-19).

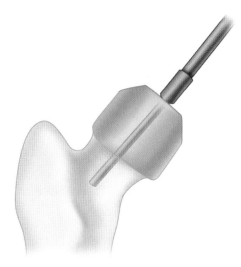

Figure 5-20

- Ream the hole in the femoral head and neck to a larger size with the appropriate head and neck reamer (Figure 5-20).

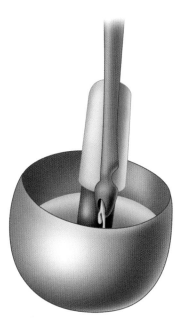

Figure 5-21

- Drill a hole into the lesser trochanter and place a metal vent in this hole to vent the proximal femur during cementing of the femoral component. This vent is attached to suction. A very viscous cement is mixed in a vacuum for a short time and then injected into the femoral component (Figure 5-21).

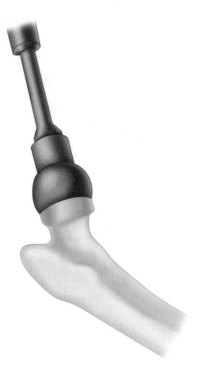

Figure 5-22

- While the cement is in a liquid state, cement the component down to the femoral head. Take care not to break the femoral neck while impacting the component down onto the head. Remove excess cement and the vent tube. Carefully reduce the hip to avoid scratching the metal head against the edge of the acetabular component (Figure 5-22).
- Close the capsule with a running absorbable suture. Repair the gluteus maximus and the piriformis. Drains are usually used, and the fascia is routinely closed.

POSTOPERATIVE CARE

Early mobilization is encouraged. Most patients are encouraged to walk the afternoon or evening of surgery. No abduction pillow is used because the femoral head is so large the risk of dislocation is small. Physical therapists are informed that the patient has a resurfaced hip and does not need hip precautions.

SURGICAL DISLOCATION OF THE HIP

James L. Guyton

TECHNIQUE 6

Surgical dislocation of the hip was described by Ganz et al. over a decade ago for the treatment of femoro-acetabular impingement (FAI) (see also Technique 8). The surgery is designed to allow full access to the acetabulum and the femoral head–neck junction while preserving the blood supply to the femoral head. The approach protects the deep branch of the medial circumflex artery as it supplies the posterolateral retinacular vessels to the femoral head. The major advantage of the approach is its extensile nature with full access to the acetabular rim, the labrum, and the femoral head–neck junction without the limitations of arthroscopy and limited anterior approaches. Surgical dislocation of the hip also has been used for open treatment of slipped capital femoral epiphysis and Pipkin fractures of the femoral head. The shortcoming of the approach also relates to its extensile nature, which requires trochanteric osteotomy with a more prolonged recovery compared with more limited exposures.

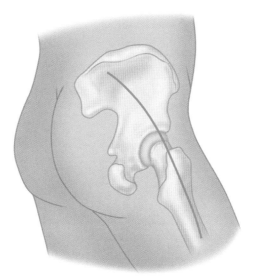

Figure 6-1

- With the patient in the lateral decubitus position, make a Kocher-Langenbeck incision and split the fascia lata accordingly (Figure 6-1). Alternatively, make a Gibson approach and retract the gluteus maximus posteriorly.
- Internally rotate the leg and identify the posterior border of the gluteus medius. Do not mobilize the gluteus medius or attempt to expose the piriformis tendon.
- Make an incision from the posterosuperior edge of the greater trochanter extending distally to the posterior border of the ridge of the vastus lateralis.

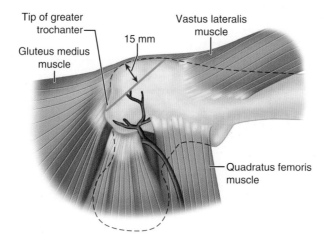

Tip of greater
trochanter

Vastus lateralis
muscle

15 mm

Gluteus medius
muscle

Quadratus femoris
muscle

Figure 6-2

- Use an oscillating saw to make a trochanteric osteotomy with a maximal thickness of 1.5 cm along this line. At its proximal limit, the osteotomy should exit just anterior to the most posterior insertion of the gluteus medius. This preserves and protects the profundus branch of the medial femoral circumflex artery (Figure 6-2).
- Release the greater trochanteric fragment along its posterior border to about the middle of the tendon of the gluteus maximus and mobilize it anteriorly with its attached vastus lateralis.
- Release the most posterior fibers of the gluteus medius from the remaining trochanteric base. The osteotomy is correct when only part of the fibers of the tendon of the piriformis have to be released from the trochanteric fragment for further mobilization.
- With the patient's leg flexed and slightly rotated externally, elevate the vastus lateralis and intermedius from the lateral and anterior aspects of the proximal femur.
- Carefully retract the posterior border of the gluteus medius anterosuperiorly to expose the piriformis tendon.
- Separate the inferior border of the gluteus minimus from the relaxed piriformis and the underlying capsule. Take care to avoid injury to the sciatic nerve, which passes inferior to the piriformis muscle into the pelvis.

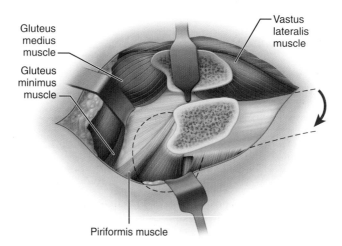

Gluteus
medius
muscle

Gluteus
minimus
muscle

Vastus
lateralis
muscle

Piriformis muscle

Figure 6-3

- Retract the entire flap, including the gluteus minimus, anteriorly and superiorly to expose the superior capsule. Further flexion and external rotation of the hip makes this step easier (Figure 6-3).

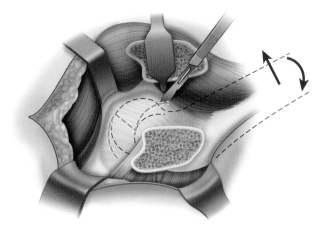

Figure 6-4

- Incise the capsule anterolaterally along the long axis of the femoral neck; this avoids injury to the deep branch of the medial femoral circumflex artery (Figure 6-4).
- Make an anteroinferior capsular incision, taking care to keep the capsulotomy anterior to the lesser trochanter to avoid damage to the main branch of the medial femoral circumflex artery. This lies just superior and posterior to the lesser trochanter.
- Elevate the anteroinferior flap to expose the labrum.
- Extend the first capsular incision toward the acetabular rim and then turn it sharply posteriorly parallel to the labrum, reaching the retracted piriformis tendon. Take care not to damage the labrum.

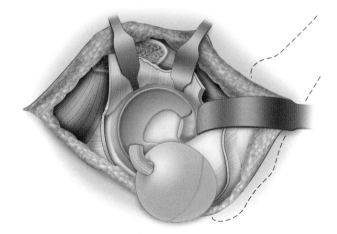

Figure 6-5

- Dislocate the hip by flexing and externally rotating the leg. Bring the leg over the front of the operating table and place it in a sterile bag. Most of the acetabulum can now be inspected (Figure 6-5).
- Manipulation of the leg allows 360 degrees access to the acetabulum and nearly 360 degrees access to the femoral head.

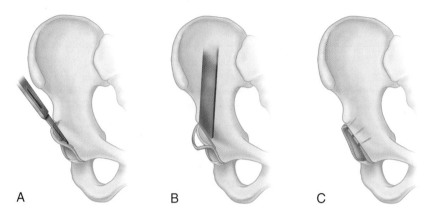

Figure 6-6

- After exposure of the acetabulum, reflect the labrum from the portion of the acetabular rim that displays overcoverage (Figure 6-6, **A**) and trim excessive bone with an osteotome or burr (**B**). If possible, reattach the labrum at the margin of the articular surface with suture anchors, re-creating the seal effect of the labrum (**C**).
- For osteochondroplasty, outline the femoral head–neck junction with a surgical marker and then cut the articular cartilage at the proximal edge of the resection with a scalpel to avoid inadvertent extension into the normal femoral head.

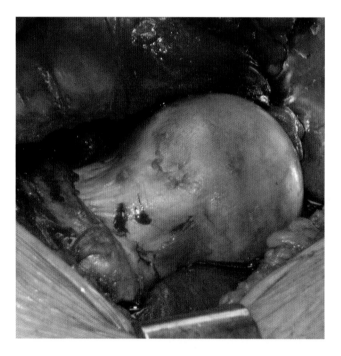

Figure 6-7

- Carefully perform the resection with small osteotomes, using a burr to complete the recontouring of the head–neck junction. Cadaver studies have shown that up to 30% of the diameter of the femoral neck can be removed from the anterolateral quadrant of the head–neck junction without substantially altering the strength of the femoral neck to axial load. A typical resection, however, is much less than 30% and is tailored to the specific anatomy encountered (Figure 6-7).

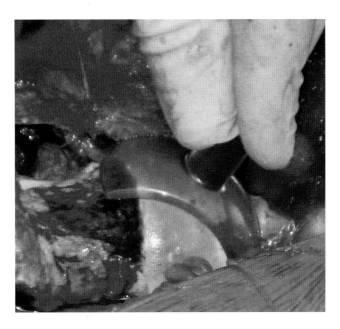

Figure 6-8

- Check the contour of the femoral head with a plastic template or spherometer to gauge the proximal extent of the osteochondroplasty where the femoral head becomes aspherical (Figure 6-8).
- Coat the exposed cancellous bone with bone wax. Reduce the hip and reproduce the position of impingement, evaluating range of motion directly and with fluoroscopy.
- Repair the capsule anatomically with nonabsorbable sutures.
- Reattach the greater trochanter with two 4.5-mm cortical screws aimed medially and distally in the region of the lesser trochanter.

POSTOPERATIVE CARE

Postoperatively, the patient is mobilized with touch-down weight bearing for 6 weeks with avoidance of active abduction and extreme flexion or rotation of the hip. After 3 weeks, pool exercises are begun, and at 6 weeks weight bearing is allowed with progressive abductor strengthening. Low-molecular-weight heparin is used for deep venous thrombosis prophylaxis for 2 weeks, followed by daily aspirin for another 4 weeks.

James L. Guyton

This approach described by Clohisy et al., Laude et al., and others has been used for patients with cam impingement. After hip arthroscopy for intraarticular or central compartment labral débridement or repair, the anterior aspect of the hip is approached through a limited Smith-Petersen approach or Hueter approach (through the sheath of the tensor fascia lata). The osteochondroplasty of the femoral head-neck junction is performed under direct vision. With traction, the anterior rim of the acetabulum can be resected with reflection of the labrum and reattachment with suture anchors, although the extent of rim exposure and resection is limited. The advantage of this approach is primarily avoiding the morbidity of surgical dislocation with a larger exposure including trochanteric osteotomy. This approach allows direct vision of the cam deformity on the femoral head–neck junction, which can be difficult to visualize and resect arthroscopically. The limitation of this approach is that only the anterior aspect of the femoral head and neck and acetabular rim can be accessed. The lateral femoral cutaneous nerve may be injured in this approach as well. Placing the incision several centimeters lateral to the anterosuperior iliac spine and approaching the anterior hip through the fascial sheath of the tensor fascia lata may lessen the risk of injury to the nerve.

- With the patient supine, perform a standard arthroscopic examination of the hip for inspection of the articular cartilage of the femoral head, acetabulum, and acetabular labrum. Débride any unstable flaps of acetabular labrum and associated articular cartilage flaps.

- After arthroscopic débridement is completed, irrigate the joint, remove the arthroscopic instruments, and release the traction.

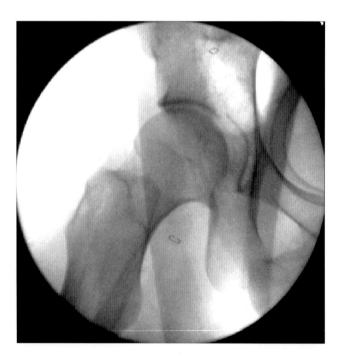

Figure 7-1

- Obtain a cross-table lateral or frog-leg lateral fluoroscopy view to ensure excellent visualization of the proximal femur, specifically the femoral head–neck junction (Figure 7-1).

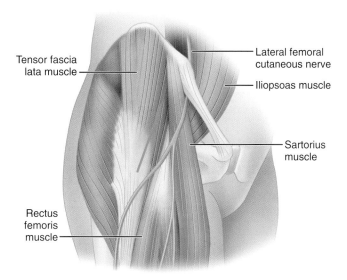

Tensor fascia lata muscle

Lateral femoral cutaneous nerve

Iliopsoas muscle

Sartorius muscle

Rectus femoris muscle

Figure 7-2

- Make a 6- to 10-cm incision, starting just inferior to the anterosuperior iliac spine and incorporating the anterior arthroscopy portal incision (Figure 7-2).
- Carry the dissection through the subcutaneous tissue laterally directly onto the fascia of the tensor fascia lata muscle.
- Incise the fascia and retract the muscle belly laterally and the fascia medially. Protect the femoral cutaneous nerve by placing the fascial incision lateral to the tensor-sartorius interval.
- Develop the interval between the tensor and sartorius, identify the rectus origin, and release the direct and reflected heads.

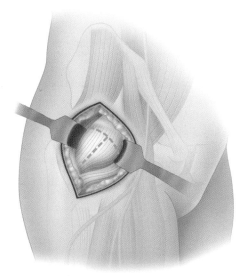

Figure 7-3

- Reflect the rectus distally, and dissect the adipose tissue and iliocapsularis muscle fibers off the anterior hip capsule (Figure 7-3).

- Make an I-shaped capsulotomy to provide adequate exposure of the anterolateral femoral head–neck junction.
- Using the normal head–neck offset anteromedially as a reference point for resection of the abnormal osteochondral lesion along the anterolateral head–neck junction, use a 0.5-inch curved osteotome to perform an osteoplasty at the head–neck junction.
- Direct the osteotome distally and posteriorly to make a beveled resection to prevent delamination of the retained femoral head articular head cartilage.

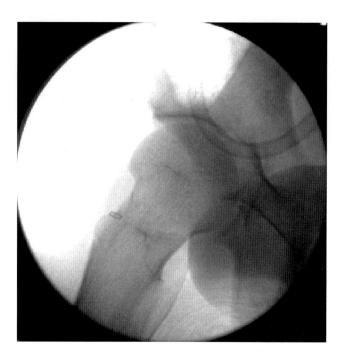

Figure 7-4

- After the anterolateral head-neck offset has been established, confirm accuracy of the resection with fluoroscopy using frog-leg lateral or cross-table lateral views in neutral and varying degrees of internal rotation (Figure 7-4).
- Examine the hip for impingement in flexion and for combined flexion and internal rotation, while palpating the anterior hip to test for residual impingement.
- If the anterior acetabular rim is overgrown secondary to labral calcification or osteophyte formation, carefully débride until adequate clearance is obtained.
- Hip motion should improve at least 5 degrees to 15 degrees in flexion and 5 degrees to 20 degrees in internal rotation.

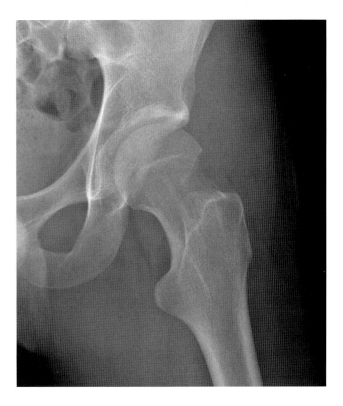

Figure 7-5

- The goal of osteoplasty is to remove all prominent anterolateral osteochondral tissue that contributes to an aspherical shape of the femoral head. If sphericity has not been achieved, perform additional resection of the femoral head–neck junction (Figure 7-5).
- Control bleeding with bone wax, irrigate the joint, and close the longitudinal and superior transverse arms of the arthrotomy with nonabsorbable suture. Close the remainder of the wound in standard fashion.

POSTOPERATIVE CARE

Patients are kept overnight in the hospital for observation. Physical therapy is instituted for toe-touch weight bearing with crutches to minimize the risk of femoral neck stress fracture. A pillow is used under the thigh to protect the rectus repair, and active flexion is avoided for 6 weeks. Abductor strengthening is begun immediately and is continued with a home exercise program. Crutches are discontinued at 6 weeks, and activities are resumed gradually as tolerated. Impact activities, such as running, are not encouraged for at least 6 months. Aspirin, 325 mg, is taken as a thromboembolic prophylaxis, and indomethacin, 75 mg sustained release, is used for heterotopic ossification prophylaxis; therapy with both is continued for 6 weeks.

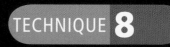
Barry B. Phillips • Marc J. Mihalko

Femoroacetabular impingement (FAI) occurs when anatomic variation of the hip causes impingement between the femoral-head junction and the acetabular rim during functional range of motion. Cam impingement occurs when a prominent head-neck junction contacts the acetabular rim during hip flexion (Figure 8-1). Pincer impingement occurs when the acetabulum has localized or global overcoverage leading to contact of the rim with the femoral head-heck junction during normal hip motion (Figure 8-2).

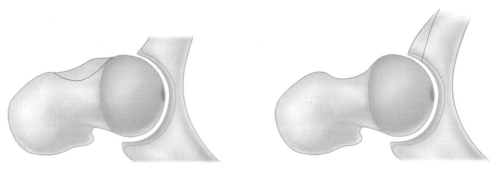

Figure 8-1   *Figure 8-2*

ARTHROSCOPIC TREATMENT OF PINCER IMPINGEMENT 〉

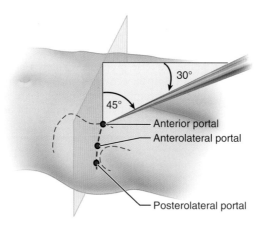

Figure 8-3

- Establish standard arthroscopic portals and examine the hip to confirm pincer impingement (Figure 8-3).

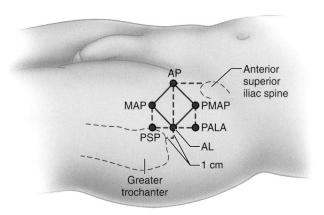

Figure 8-4

- A midanterior portal (MAP) can be used to aid in anchor placement (Figure 8-4; AL, anterolateral; AP, anterior; MAP, mid-anterior portal; PMAP, proximal mid-anterior portal; PALA, proximal accessory lateral; PSP, posterosuperior.).

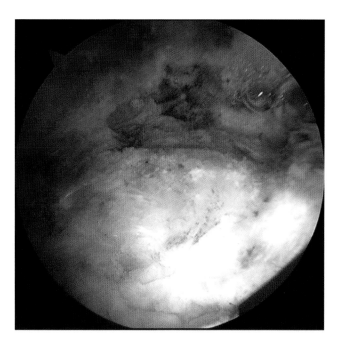

Figure 8-5

- If the pincer lesion can be seen, leave the labral-chondral junction intact and use a burr to resect the bony prominence (Figure 8-5).
- If exposure of the acetabular rim is needed to access the pincer lesion, place a banana blade through the anterior portal and take down the labrum at the labral-chondral junction in the area of the lesion.
- Place a burr in the midanterior portal and position it on the anterior wall at the level of the acetabular overcoverage. Confirm with fluoroscopy that the burr is just distal to the crossover sign, resect the rim to the appropriate level, and confirm resection of the crossover with fluoroscopy. The camera can be switched to the anterior portal and the burr to the anterolateral portal to complete the more superior rim resection.

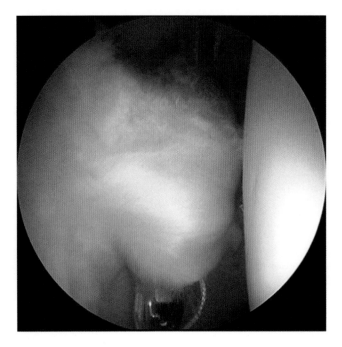

Figure 8-6

- Refix the labrum to the rim with suture anchors. Place the first anchor superiorly through the anterolateral portal, using fluoroscopy and direct observation to ensure that the joint is not penetrated. Pass one suture limb into the joint between the labrum and rim (Figure 8-6).

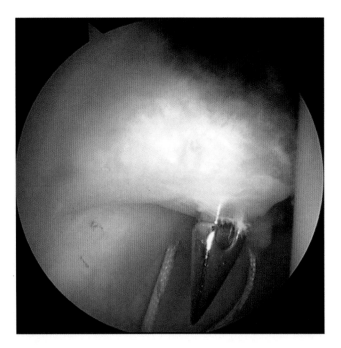

Figure 8-7

- Pass a bird beak or other penetrating grasper through the labrum, retrieve the suture, and tie it. Alternatively, loop the suture around the labrum instead of piercing the tissue (Figure 8-7).
- With the camera in the anterolateral portal, place the remaining anchors through the midanterior portal in a similar fashion.
- Remove traction from the leg, and move the hip through a range of motion to ensure there is no residual impingement.

ARTHROSCOPIC TREATMENT OF CAM IMPINGEMENT 〉

- After standard arthroscopic portal placement and examination, complete any needed central compartment procedures.
- Remove the leg from traction, and flex the hip approximately 45 degrees.
- With the camera in the midanterior portal, introduce an arthroscopic blade through a distal accessory anterolateral portal and make a T-shaped capsulotomy to allow inspection of the cam lesion. Flexion and external rotation will help expose inferior medial lesions, and extension and internal rotation will help expose superolateral lesions. Take care to avoid the retinacular vessels when treating lesions on the supero-lateral neck.

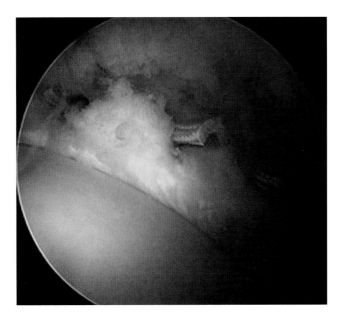

Figure 8-8

- Introduce a burr and resect the cam lesion to re-create a spherical femoral head. Use fluoroscopy to assist and confirm resection (Figure 8-8).
- Perform dynamic assessment of the hip. The hip is flexed and internally and externally rotated to ensure there is no residual impingement.
- Repair the limb of the capsulotomy that extends down the femoral neck in side-to-side fashion.

POSTOPERATIVE CARE 〉

Patients are limited to touch-down weight bearing for 2 weeks. Extremes of motion are avoided for several weeks. Physical therapy and range of motion are begun in the first 24 to 48 hours. A stationary bike can be used immediately. Impact activities are not recommended for 2 to 3 months. Return to sports may take 4 to 6 months.

CREDIT

Figure 8-4 from Robertson WJ, Kelly BT: The safe zone for hip arthroscopy: a cadaveric assessment of central, peripheral, and lateral compartment portal placement, Arthroscopy 24:1019, 2008.

CORE DECOMPRESSION FOR OSTEONECROSIS OF THE FEMORAL HEAD — PERCUTANEOUS TECHNIQUE

James L. Guyton

Core decompression is based on the belief that the procedure relieves intraosseous pressure caused by venous congestion, allowing improved vascularity and possible slowing the progression of the disease. While initial promising results of core decompression have not been matched by more recent investigations, it has been noted that the results of core decompression are better than the results of nonoperative treatment. Current literature supports the use of core decompression for the treatment of Ficat stages I and IIA small central lesions in young, nonobese patients who are not taking steroids; its results are much less predictable in Ficat stages IIB and III.

A percutaneous technique has been described for core decompression using multiple small drillings with a 3.2-mm Steinmann pin. The technique is reported to have a lower rate of femoral head collapse than traditional core decompression, with low morbidity and few or no surgical complications.

- With the patient supine on a hip fracture table, mark the position of the femoral head and prepare and drape the hip in standard fashion.

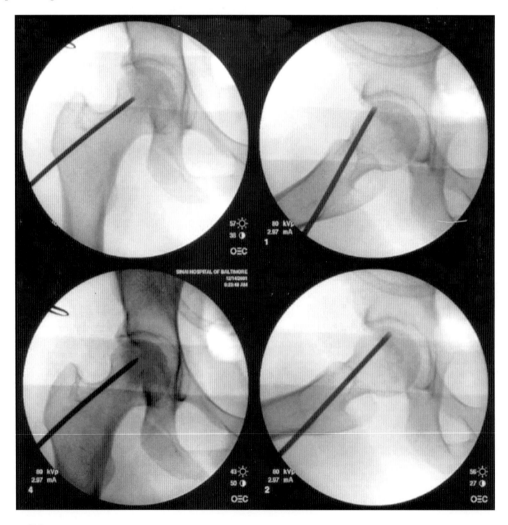

Figure 9-1

- Insert a 3.2-mm Steinmann pin laterally and percutaneously under fluoroscopic guidance (Figure 9-1).
- Advance the pin until it reaches the lateral cortex in the metaphyseal region opposite the superior portion of the lesser trochanter.

- Penetrate the femur and advance the pin through the femoral neck into the femoral head and the site of the lesion (as determined by preoperative radiographs or MR images). Use anteroposterior and lateral fluoroscopic views while advancing the pin to ensure the correct track in the medullary canal of the femoral neck.
- Using the one skin entry point, make two passes with the pin through the small lesions and three through the large lesions. Try to avoid penetration of the femoral head cartilage when advancing the pin.
- Remove the pin, and close the wound with a simple bandage or a single nylon suture.

POSTOPERATIVE CARE 〉

Physical therapy, including gait reconditioning with a cane or crutches, is encouraged. Protected weight bearing (approximately 50%) is maintained for 5 to 6 weeks and then advanced to full weight bearing as tolerated. High-impact loading such as jogging or jumping is not permitted for 12 months. If there is no radiographic evidence of collapse and the patient is asymptomatic at 12 months after surgery return to usual activities, including higher-impact loading activities such as running, is allowed.

TOTAL KNEE ARTHROPLASTY — STANDARD MIDLINE APPROACH AND BONE PREPARATION

TECHNIQUE **10**

William M. Mihalko

SURGICAL APPROACH ⟩

See also Video 10-1.

The most commonly used skin incision for primary TKA is an anterior midline incision. Variations may be considered, but in general most incisions will compromise the infrapatellar branch of the saphenous nerve and result in an area of numbness on the outer aspect of knee. This should be discussed with the patient before surgery. There are many variations on the approach to the knee deep to the subcutaneous level of dissection.

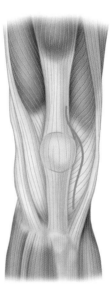

Figure 10-1

- Make a medial parapatellar retinacular incision with the knee in flexion to allow the subcutaneous tissue to fall medially and laterally, which improves exposure (Figure 10-1).
- If a preexisting anterior scar on the knee is in a usable position, incorporate it into the skin incision. If multiple previous incisions are present, choose the most lateral usable incision because the blood supply to the skin of the anterior knee tends to come predominantly from the medial side. Previous direct medial and lateral incisions and transverse incisions can generally be ignored.
- Make the skin incision long enough to avoid excessive skin tension during retraction, which can lead to areas of skin necrosis.
- Keep the medial skin flap as thick as possible by keeping the dissection just superficial to the extensor mechanism.
- Extend the retinacular incision proximally the length of the quadriceps tendon, leaving a 3- to 4-mm cuff of tendon on the vastus medialis for later closure.
- Continue the incision around the medial side of the patella, extending 3 to 4 cm onto the anteromedial surface of the tibia along the medial border of the patellar tendon.

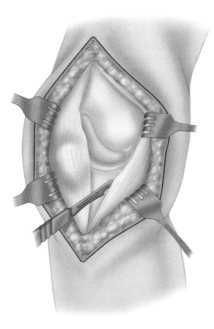

Figure 10-2

- Expose the medial side of the knee by subperiosteally elevating the anteromedial capsule and deep medial collateral ligament off the tibia to the posteromedial corner of the knee (Figure 10-2).

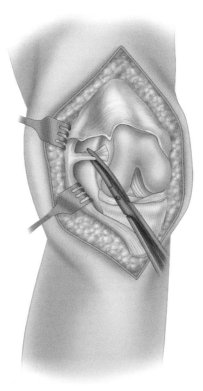

Figure 10-3

- Extend the knee, and evert the patella to allow a routine release of the lateral patellofemoral plicae. In obese patients, if eversion of the patella is difficult, develop the lateral subcutaneous flap further so that the patella can be everted underneath this tissue. Alternatively, the patella can be subluxated laterally if this provides adequate exposure (Figure 10-3).

- Flex the knee and remove the anterior cruciate ligament and the anterior horns of the medial and lateral menisci, along with any osteophytes that may lead to component malposition or soft tissue imbalance. The posterior horns of the menisci can be excised after the femoral and tibial cuts have been made. If a PCL-substituting prosthesis is to be used, the PCL can be resected at this time or can be removed later in the procedure along with the box cut made in the distal femur for the PCL-substituting femoral component.

- With PCL substitution and PCL retention, subluxate and externally rotate the tibia. External rotation relaxes the extensor mechanism, decreases the chance of patellar tendon avulsion, and improves exposure.

- Expose the lateral tibial plateau by a partial excision of the infrapatellar fat pad and retraction of the everted extensor mechanism with a levering-type retractor placed adjacent to the lateral tibial plateau.

- During all maneuvers that place tension on the extensor mechanism, especially knee flexion and patellar retraction, pay careful attention to the patellar tendon attachment to the tibial tubercle. Avulsion of the patellar tendon is difficult to repair and can be a devastating complication.

BONE PREPARATION FOR PRIMARY TKA ⟩

Bone surface preparation is based on the following principles: appropriate sizing of the individual components; alignment of the components to restore the mechanical axis; re-creation of equally balanced soft tissues and gaps in flexion and extension; and optimal patellar tracking.

- Make the distal femoral cut at a valgus angle (usually 5 to 7 degrees) perpendicular to the predetermined mechanical axis of the femur. The amount of bone removed is generally the same as that to be replaced by the femoral component. If a significant preoperative flexion contracture is present, additional resection can be done to aid the correction of the contracture. If a posterior cruciate-substituting prosthesis is used, an additional 2 mm of distal femoral resection can be done to equal the increase in the flexion gap that occurs when the PCL is sacrificed.

- The anterior and posterior femoral cuts determine the rotation of the femoral component and the shape of the flexion gap. Excessive external rotation widens the flexion gap medially and may result in flexion instability. Internal rotation of the femoral component can cause lateral patellar tilt or patellofemoral instability.

- Femoral component rotation can be determined by one of several methods. The transepicondylar axis, anteroposterior axis, posterior femoral condyles, and cut surface of the proximal tibia can all serve as reference points.

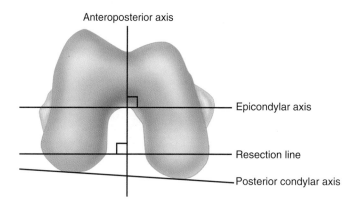

Figure 10-4

- If the transepicondylar axis is used, make the posterior femoral cut parallel to a line drawn between the medial and lateral femoral epicondyles. Determine the anteroposterior axis by drawing a line between the bottom of the sulcus of the femur and the top of the intercondylar notch and make the posterior femoral cut perpendicular to this axis (Figure 10-4).

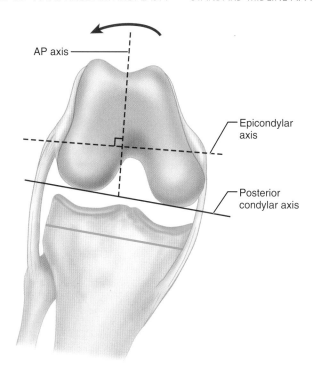

Figure 10-5

- When the posterior condyles are referenced make the cut in 3° of external rotation off a line between them. A valgus knee with a hypoplastic lateral femoral condyle may lead to an internally rotated femoral component if the posterior condyles alone are referenced (Figure 10-5).

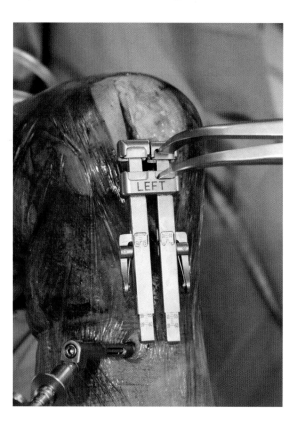

Figure 10-6

- Using the cut surface of the proximal tibia or the "gap" technique, make the posterior femoral cut parallel to the proximal tibial cut after the soft tissues have been balanced in extension. This technique is often used for mobile-bearing TKA because precise gap balancing in flexion is necessary to ensure that "spinout" of the polyethylene bearing does not occur (Figure 10-6).

- Caution should be exercised when using the gap technique because reliance on ligaments of non-anatomical length can lead to femoral component malrotation. It is important for the surgeon to be familiar with each of these reference points because reliance on a single reference could result in femoral component malrotation.

- Regardless of the method used for rotational alignment, the thickness of bone removed from the posterior aspect of the femoral condyles should equal the thickness of the posterior condyles of the femoral component. This is determined directly by measuring the thickness of the posterior condylar resection with "posterior referencing" instrumentation. "Anterior referencing" instruments measure the anteroposterior dimension of the femoral condyles from an anterior cut based off the anterior femoral cortex, to the articular surface of the posterior femoral condyles. The femoral component chosen must be equal to or slightly less than the measured anteroposterior dimension to avoid tightness in flexion.

- Posterior referencing instruments are theoretically more accurate in recreating the original dimensions of the distal femur, however anterior referencing instruments have less risk of notching the anterior femoral cortex and place the anterior flange of the femoral component more reliably against the anterior surface of the distal femur.

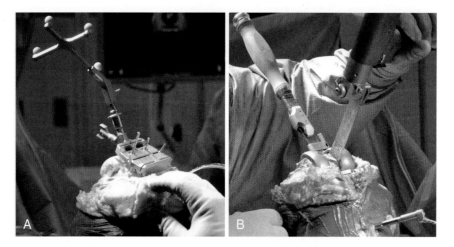

Figure 10-7

- Complete the distal femoral preparation for a PCL-retaining prosthesis by making anterior and posterior chamfer cuts for the implant (Figure 10-7, A). If a PCL-substituting design is chosen, remove the intercondylar box to accommodate the housing for the post and cam mechanism (B).

- Cut the tibia perpendicular to its mechanical axis with the cutting block oriented by an intramedullary or extramedullary cutting guide. The amount of posterior slope depends on the individual implant system being used. Many systems incorporate 3 degrees of posterior slope into the polyethylene insert, which allows the slope to be more accurately aligned using the implant rather than the cutting block. The amount of tibial resection depends on which side of the joint (more or less arthritic) is used for reference. When measured off the unaffected side of the joint, the resection should be close to the size of the implant being used, typically 8 to 10 mm. If the more arthritic side of the joint is used for reference, the amount of resection usually is 2 mm or less. Protect the patellar tendon and collateral ligaments during this portion of the procedure.

- Alternatively, the proximal tibia can be cut before completion of the distal femoral cuts.

Gap Technique

- If the distal femoral resection has not been completed, balance the flexion and extension gaps at this time by placing spacer blocks or a tensioner within the gaps with the knee in flexion and extension. Varus-valgus balance can be fine-tuned with further medial or lateral releases (see Techniques 11 to 14 for ligament balancing).

- Before any soft tissue release, remove any medial or lateral osteophytes about the tibia and femur. Remove posterior condylar osteophytes because they can block flexion and tent posterior soft tissue structures in extension, causing a flexion contracture.

- The flexion and extension gaps must be roughly equal. If the extension gap is too small or tight extension is limited. Similarly, if the flexion gap is too tight flexion is limited. Laxity of either gap can lead to instability.

- If the extension gap is smaller than the flexion gap remove more bone from the distal femoral cut surface or release the posterior capsule from the distal femur after first making sure that all posterior condylar osteophytes have been removed before raising the joint line.

- If the flexion gap is smaller than the extension gap, remove more bone from the posterior femoral condyles by making appropriate cuts for the next smaller available femoral component. Make sure this is done with anterior referencing so that the posterior condyles are shortened and the anterior cortex is not notched.

- If the flexion and extension gaps are equal but there is not enough space for the desired prosthesis, remove more bone from the proximal tibia because bone removed from the tibia affects the flexion and extension gaps equally.

- When the flexion and extension gaps are equal but lax, a larger spacer block and a thicker tibial polyethylene insert are required to obtain stability.

ARTHROPLASTY ⟩

- Make the initial exposure using your preferred surgical approach (medial parapatellar, intermedius, midvastus, subvastus) to include release of the deep medial collateral ligament off the tibia at the joint line to the posteromedial corner of the knee.

- Make the bone cuts using the preferred technique (intramedullary or extramedullary guide, computer navigation, custom cutting blocks).

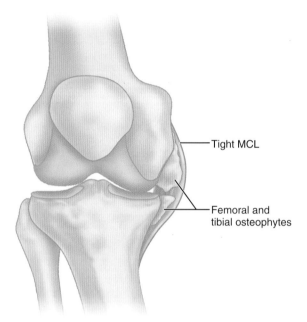

Tight MCL

Femoral and tibial osteophytes

Figure 11-1

- Remove all osteophytes on the femur and the tibia because they can tent the medial soft tissue sleeve and effectively shorten the medial collateral ligament. Be certain to check the posterior condylar region of the femur and the posteromedial aspect of the tibia since these osteophytes can contribute significantly to keeping the extension gap tight (Figure 11-1).

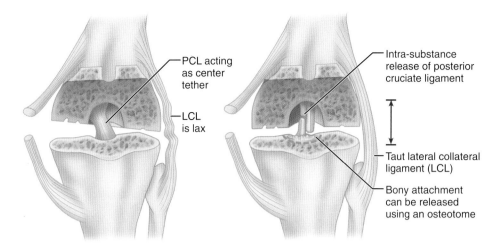

Figure 11-2

- Make sure the posterior cruciate ligament (PCL) is resected before balancing. Because the PCL is a secondary medial stabilizer, take care not to release the entire soft tissue sleeve off the tibia because it may result in medial instability (Figure 11-2). In general, less soft tissue release is needed to balance a varus knee once the PCL is resected. With a cruciate-retaining technique, the PCL is left intact.

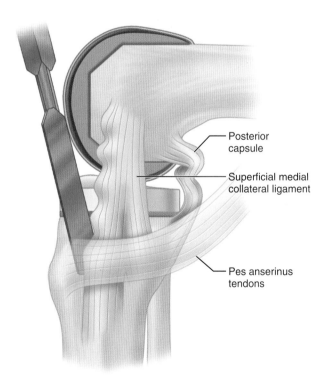

Figure 11-3

- Assess the flexion and extension gaps by your preferred means (laminar spreaders, spacer blocks, trial components and varus/valgus stress). If the medial gaps are tight in both flexion and extension, release the superficial medial collateral ligament subperiosteally off the proximal tibia but do not completely release it off the tibia distally. Recheck the gaps in flexion and extension. In a cruciate-retaining TKA with the PCL intact, the release may need to be carried out up to 6 cm distal to the joint line to effectively balance the gap (Figure 11-3).

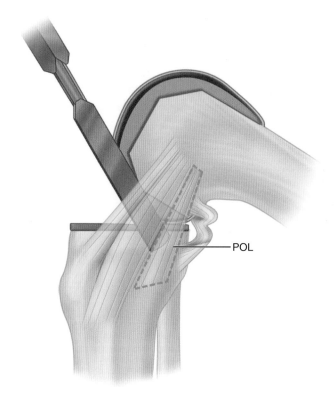

Figure 11-4

- If the extension gap is tight only medially in extension, the posterior oblique ligament (POL) portion can be subperiosteally released now or later in the soft tissue balancing procedure (Figure 11-4).

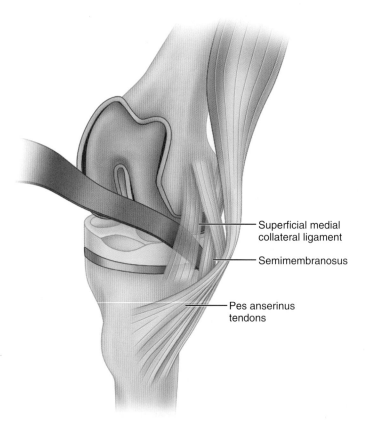

Figure 11-5

- If the extension gaps remains tight medially, the semimembranosus and posteromedial capsule can be released off of the proximal tibia (Figure 11-5).

- If the flexion gap is tight, the anterior aspect of the superficial medial collateral ligament and the pes anserinus insertion can be released.

- If the entire soft tissue sleeve is released and the medial gap is still tight (as is usually the case with severe varus deformity), consider advancing the lateral collateral ligament.

- In a PCL-retaining TKA, if the entire soft tissue sleeve is released and the medial gap is still tight, consider balancing the lateral collateral ligament (see Technique 14, Ligament Balancing: PCL-Balancing). If a posterior drawer maneuver indicates that the PCL is not functioning, consider conversion to an anterior-lipped, deep-dish insert if available with the implant system being used or consider conversion to a posterior stabilized implant.

- If after complete release of the medial soft tissue sleeve, the PCL still does not balance the tight medial cap, consider advancing the lateral collateral ligament (this usually is needed for severe varus deformity).

VALGUS DEFORMITY CORRECTION 〉

- During exposure of a knee with a valgus deformity take care not to compromise the medial soft tissue sleeve, which may already be attenuated.
- Make the bone cuts using your preferred technique (intramedullary or extramedullary guide, computer navigation, custom cutting blocks).
- Remove osteophytes to the level of the native articular margins to avoid tenting of the soft tissues.
- During exposure, release the lateral capsule from the tibia.
- The order of soft tissue release on the lateral side of the knee varies depending on the extent of fixed contracture and associated deformity.
- The structure released first depends on whether both the extension and flexion gaps are tight on the lateral side. If both are tight, release the lateral collateral ligament off the lateral epicondyle taking care to leave the insertion of the popliteus tendon intact.

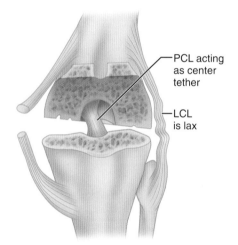

PCL acting as center tether

LCL is lax

Figure 12-1

- The posterior cruciate ligament (PCL) is a more medial structure and may be involved in coronal plane deformity in a varus knee; it less likely acts as a central tether in valgus deformity because of its more medial location. If it is involved in more severe valgus deformities, it may need to be released (Figure 12-1).
- If at any point during the balancing of the valgus knee only the extension gap is tight, release the iliotibial band by a Z-lengthening or pie-crusting of the band 2 cm above the joint line (see Technique 13). Make certain all fibers are released, and evaluate the biceps aponeurosis to make sure it is not involved in the contracture.
- Release of the posterolateral corner has been shown to effectively increase the extension space more than the flexion space and should be considered before release of the lateral collateral ligament if only a small amount of correction is needed.
- Release of the popliteus tendon will increase the flexion gap laterally more than the extension gap.

- If the knee is still not balanced in full extension after release of all of these structures, release the posterior capsule off the lateral femoral condyle, then release the lateral head of gastrocnemius if further correction is needed.
- Because it is a medial structure, the PCL often lengthens in a knee with a valgus deformity. If complete release did not balance the gaps, inspect the PCL to determine whether it is involved in the deformity.

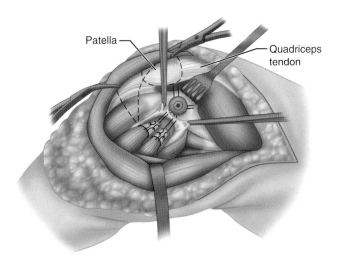

Figure 12-2

- If complete release of all of the above structures does not balance the flexion and extension gaps on the lateral side, consider advancement of the medial collateral ligament (Figure 12-2).
- If the lateral flexion gap opens more than the extension gap, make certain that the "jump height" of a posterior stabilized peg is not exceeded, if this is a possibility, consider using a constrained condylar type of implant.

A technique used for soft tissue balancing in knees with valgus deformity is pie-crusting of the lateral soft tissue sleeve. This technique allows the surgeon to direct the lengthening of soft tissue supporting structures according to which areas are taut under tension of the joint space in the operating room.

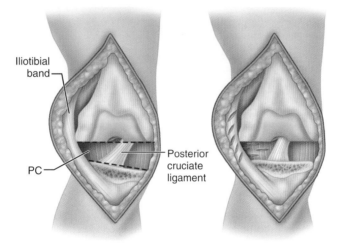

Iliotibial band

PC

Posterior cruciate ligament

Figure 13-1

- Multiple stabs are made with a scalpel blade parallel to the joint line to effectively elongate the areas of the soft tissue sleeve that are under undue tension. Multiple studies have reported good outcomes in both valgus and varus deformities with this technique (Figure 13-1).
- The advantage of pie-crusting, especially on the lateral soft tissue sleeve, is that it leaves a supporting tether that does not allow a larger gap opening on the lateral side of knee in flexion. Cadaver studies have shown that larger releases are not possible with this technique until the lateral collateral ligament is resected. Care is needed when pie-crusting is done in the posterolateral corner because the peroneal nerve is within 1.5 cm. Because the nerve is farther away when the knee is flexed, flexing the knee can help protect the nerve during pie-crusting of the posterolateral corner.
- After the distal femur is prepared using the anteroposterior and epicondylar axes as a rotational guide, cut the proximal tibia perpendicular to the mechanical axis and remove osteophytes.
- Place the knee in 90 degrees of flexion, and place tensioners medially and laterally between the posterior femoral condyles and proximal tibial cut surfaces. Careful placement of the tensioners is crucial to avoid crushing osteoporotic bone.
- Remove any retractors that are causing tension on the affected side, and replace them with rake retractors.
- Palpate the soft tissues on the affected side, and release them by pie-crusting until a rectangular flexion gap is achieved.
- Place trial components and move the knee into full extension.
- If the knee is tight medially or laterally in extension, remove the trial components and reinsert the tensioning devices with the knee in extension.
- Repeat pie-crusting with the knee in extension until a rectangular extension gap is achieved.
- Replace the trial components, and confirm coronal plane stability in flexion and extension.
- Correct any residual discrepancies in the flexion and extension gaps with pie-crusting or, if necessary, standard gap balancing techniques.

With retention of the posterior cruciate ligament (PCL), femoral rollback is accomplished by tension developed within the PCL during knee flexion. A PCL that is too tight in flexion can lead to poor postoperative knee flexion or excessive femoral rollback, which is thought to be a factor in accelerated polyethylene wear. Conversely, if the PCL does not develop adequate tension in flexion, femoral rollback does not occur. Accurate balancing of the PCL is necessary for optimal functioning and longevity of a PCL-retaining prosthesis.

- Excessive PCL tension is corrected by partial release or recession of the PCL, which is accomplished in a stepwise fashion with frequent retesting of the PCL tension.

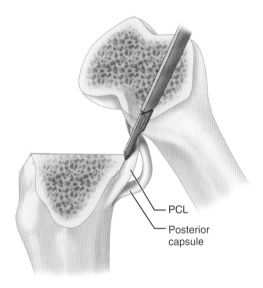

PCL

Posterior capsule

Figure 14-1

- Release the PCL from the superior surface of the bone island on the tibia (Figure 14-1).
- Release it subperiosteally in 1- to 2-mm intervals along the posterior surface of the tibia. The PCL bone island can be partially or completely removed. The PCL has a broad insertion over approximately 2 cm on the posterior surface of the proximal tibia.
- If partial release is unsuccessful in balancing the PCL, make certain that the appropriate amount of posterior slope for the implant being used was obtained in the proximal tibial cut.
- More commonly, a smaller femoral component, with anterior referencing for sizing, can be used to enlarge the flexion gap relative to the extension gap.
- Alternatively, with difficulty balancing the PCL or with PCL incompetence because of complete release, sacrifice it completely and convert to a PCL-substituting design or use a high-wall or deep-dish tibial polyethylene component, if the implant system provides that option, to prevent anterior translation of the femoral condyles with knee flexion.

COMPONENT IMPLANTATION IN TOTAL KNEE ARTHROPLASTY

William M. Mihalko

- After bone deficiencies have been treated, ligamentous balancing is satisfactory (see Technique 10), and the extensor mechanism is tracking properly, remove the trial components. Do not hyperextend the knee because the joint is unstable with the trial components removed and the posterior neurovascular structures can be injured.
- If an intramedullary guide has been used on the tibia, occlude the tibial intramedullary canal with a plug of previously resected bone distal to the level of the tibial stem. Occlude the femoral canal in a similar fashion.
- If sclerotic bone surfaces are present use a small drill to make multiple perforations into the underlying cancellous bone to allow cement intrusion.
- Clean the cut bone surfaces with a pulsatile lavage irrigator using saline that contains an added antibiotic solution such as cefazolin or genitourinary irrigant.
- Dry the surfaces with clean sponges.
- The tibial tray is usually implanted first. Apply doughy PMMA cement to the cut surface of the tibia keeping blood and fat from mixing with the cement and out of the cement-prosthesis interface. Cement applied to the implant should also ensure filling of the implant undersurface.
- Apply the cement when it no longer adheres to a gloved hand, or at a slightly earlier stage if using a cement syringe.
- Impaction of the tibial prosthesis generally results in intrusion of early dough-phase cement to a depth of 2 to 5 mm in cancellous bone. This is sufficient for long-term fixation as shown by Insall and others.
- Remove excess cement from the periphery of the component.
- Cement the femoral and patellar components in a similar fashion. Usually, all components can be cemented simultaneously, although this requires an efficient and experienced surgical team.
- Cementing of the tibia and femur also can be done by preparing two batches of cement 6 to 9 minutes apart.
- If the bone stock is osteoporotic, cement the tibial and femoral components separately and hold them carefully in place until the cement has fully hardened.
- The patella can be cemented with the femur or the tibia although the cement should be used in an early dough phase to allow adequate cement intrusion.
- Access to the posterior femoral recesses is limited after the femoral and tibial components have been implanted. To minimize the amount of cement that may have to be removed from the posterior femoral recesses, apply a small amount of cement to the posterior femoral bone surface and to the posterior condyles of the femoral implant.
- After the femoral component has been seated, carefully extend the knee with a trial tibial spacer in place to ensure complete seating of the femoral prosthesis.
- Ensure that the tibial spacer is of adequate thickness to provide varus and valgus stability in full extension. If a thinner tibial trial is substituted, hyperextension of the knee and posterior liftoff of the tibial component could result.
- Carefully search for any bone or cement debris before implantation of the final tibial polyethylene articular surface.

UNICONDYLAR KNEE ARTHROPLASTY

William M. Mihalko

If the strict indications outlined in 1989 by Kozinn and Scott were followed in practice, few patients would be candidates for unicondylar knee arthroplasty (UKA). In most reports, long-term prosthesis survival in UKA has to date been less than that in total knee arthroplasty (TKA). A few current UKA prostheses have however performed better than their predecessors with survivorship at 10 years ranging from 82% to 98%. Important selection criteria include an intact anterior cruciate ligament, unicompartmental arthritis, passively correctable deformity, and a reasonable body weight. Multiple techniques for UKA now exist from fixed bearing (inset or onlay designs), mobile bearing, and computer or robotically assisted methods (MAKOplasty, Mako Surgical Corp., Ft. Lauderdale, FL) (Fig. 16-1).

Unicompartmental · Patellofemoral · Bicompartmental

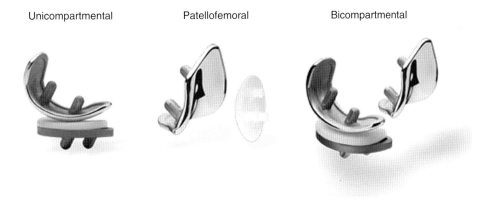

Figure 16-1

Just as in primary TKA, the differences between fixed and mobile-bearing techniques involve strict adherence to equalization of the flexion and extension gaps to avoid bearing "spit-out." The MAKOplasty technique uses preoperative CT studies to register anatomical landmarks in the operating room. The computer-assisted system then aids preparation of the bone on the femoral and tibial sides for proper implant positioning to match the preoperative plan.

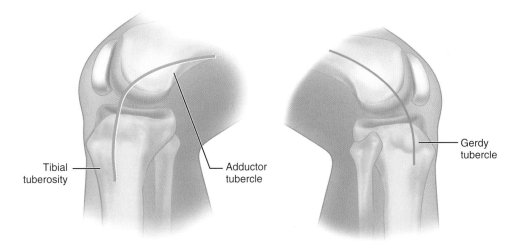

Tibial tuberosity — Adductor tubercle — Gerdy tubercle

Figure 16-2

- Make a longitudinal skin incision along the medial or lateral aspect of the patellar tendon depending on the compartment being replaced (Fig. 16-2). A medial approach can be used for a lateral unicondylar replacement but the exposure in this case must be more extensive to allow adequate patellar eversion or subluxation; a minimally invasive technique requires a lateral approach.

- Make sure the capsular incision does not go above the vastus medialis or lateralis. A Hohmann-type retractor can be used to lever the patella medially or laterally with the knee in flexion to expose the entire femoral condyle.
- To expose the medial compartment, incise the coronary ligament, remove the anterior horn of the medial meniscus, and raise the periosteal sleeve from the anteromedial aspect of the tibia.
- To expose the lateral compartment raise the anterolateral periosteal sleeve to the medial aspect of Gerdy's tubercle.
- Carefully inspect the two compartments being preserved to be sure the patient is a candidate for UKA.

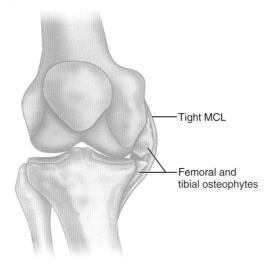

Figure 16-3

- Remove all peripheral osteophytes before the bone cuts are made to allow better exposure especially when a minimally invasive approach is used (Figure 16-3).

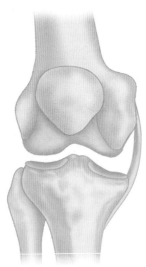

Figure 16-4

- Removal of the tibial peripheral osteophytes should be enough to adequately balance the arthritic compartment. Make certain intercondylar osteophytes also are removed because they can impinge on the cruciate ligaments and damage them (Figure 16-4).
- A need for more extensive soft tissue balancing may indicate inadequate bony resection or a varus deformity that is too severe for UKA.
- With most fixed bearing systems, the matched resection begins with the tibial resection. Use an extramedullary guide to align the proximal tibial cut with the center of the ankle distally and re-create the posterior tibial slope with a 2-mm deep resection, or as otherwise indicated by the implant system. For onlay

tibial implants, use a reciprocating saw to complete the tibial bone cut just medial to the medial tibial eminence.

- With the knee flexed, use a spacer block to make sure the gap is large enough for the smallest tibial resection (this varies according to the implant system used but is usually about 8 mm).
- Move the knee into full extension and use another spacer block to determine the distal femoral resection needed to balance the flexion and extension gaps. Use the implant-specific cutting jig to make the distal femoral cut.

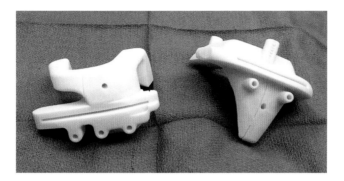

Figure 16-5

- Once the distal femoral cut is made, insert the femoral sizing guide and determine the appropriate sized cutting block. Make the posterior condylar bone resection and chamfer cuts as indicated. Preoperative MR images or CT scans can be used to produce a custom cutting block for the distal femur (Figure 16-5).
- Take care to resect the medial meniscus and remove any loose bodies from the posterior recess of the knee.
- Insert the tibial trial implant and perform a trial reduction to ensure that the joint is stable in extension and flexion and that a full range of motion is possible without overstuffing or excessive laxity.
- Complete bone preparation specific to the implant design and the cementation of the implants as described in Technique 14. Take care to ensure that no loose or excessive amount of bone cement remains in the posterior aspect of the tibia or posterior femoral condyle.
- Close the wound.

CREDITS

Figure 16-1 courtesy Stryker Mako.

See also Video 17-1.

- With the patient supine, place a sandbag under the involved hip to allow easier access to the lateral aspect of the knee. A sandbag taped to the operating table helps maintain 90 degrees of knee flexion during the operation. This position is important because it carries the popliteal vessels and peroneal nerve posteriorly and relaxes the iliotibial band.
- Drape and prepare the limb from the anterior superior iliac spine to the ankle and then apply and inflate a thigh tourniquet.

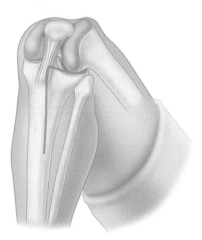

Figure 17-1

- Make an inverted-L–shaped incision for a lateral approach to the proximal tibia. The transverse limb of the incision is at the lateral joint line and extends posteriorly to the fibular head. The vertical limb is midline to the tibia and extends 10 cm distally (Figure 17-1).
- Carefully divide the proximal tibiofibular capsule with a sharp ¾-inch curved osteotome. Use a blunt Hohmann retractor to protect the neurovascular structures throughout the procedure.

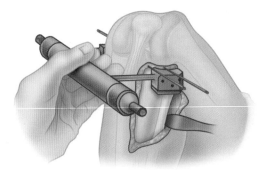

Figure 17-2

- Use Keith needles or small Kirschner wires to identify the joint line and insert the transverse osteotomy jig with the top portion touching the needles or wires (Figure 17-2).
- Stabilize the jig by drilling to the third mark (3 inches) using the 3.2-mm drill bit and fill the hole with a smooth pin (⅛-inch).

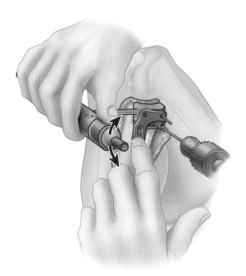

Figure 17-3

- Flex and extend the osteotomy guide to match the patient's posterior slope and to determine proper plate positioning. This can be confirmed by placing the plate over the smooth pin in the jig (Figure 17-3).
- When proper positioning is determined, drill a second hole and fill it with a smooth pin.
- Through the central hole in the transverse osteotomy guide, adjacent to the osteotomy slot, drill completely across the tibia and use a depth gauge to measure the tibial width.
- Insert the calibrated saw blade and make the transverse limb of the osteotomy, keeping a 10-mm bridge of the medial cortex intact.
- Replace the transverse osteotomy jig with the slotted oblique jig; this jig is slotted in 2-mm increments to allow the desired degree of correction (6 degrees to 20 degrees).

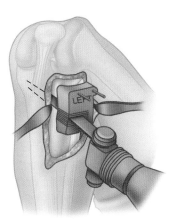

Figure 17-4

- Make the oblique portion of the osteotomy and remove the oblique jig leaving the pins in place (Figure 17-4).
- Remove the wedge of bone and carefully inspect the osteotomy site to ensure no residual bone is left.

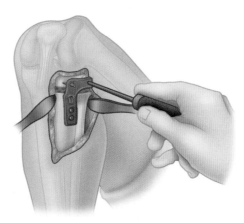

Figure 17-5

- Apply a buttress plate over the two smooth pins. Remove one pin and replace it with a 6.5-mm cancellous screw using the second pin as a parallel alignment marker. Remove the second pin, and replace it with a cancellous screw. Screws 60 to 70 mm long usually are used in men, and screws 50 to 60 mm long usually are used in women. Shorter (50 mm) screws can be used in very young patients to make hardware removal easier when healing is complete. Do not tighten these screws until the distal cortical screws have been inserted (Figure 17-5).

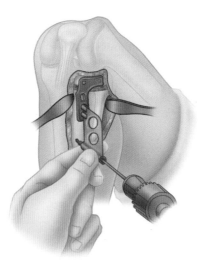

Figure 17-6

- Using the two distal holes in the L-plate as a reference, use the drill alignment guide to place a single-cortex 3.2-mm hole in line with and distal to the plate. Slight toggling of the bit makes application of the compression clamp easier (Figure 17-6).

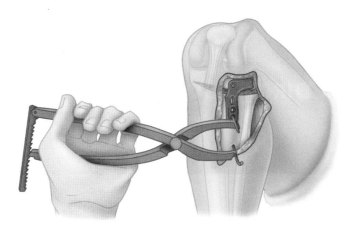

Figure 17-7

- Insert the curved pin at the end of the compression clamp into this hole while placing the straight pin on the end of the clamp into the most distal hole of the L-plate and apply slow compression (Figure 17-7).
- Compression often takes 5 minutes, allowing plastic deformation to occur through the incomplete osteotomy site. If compression is difficult, check that the proximal tibiofibular joint is completely disrupted and that any residual bone wedge has been removed.
- When the osteotomy is closed, evaluate overall alignment with either a long alignment rod or an electrocautery cord. When aligned from the center of the hip to the center of the ankle the plumb line should pass through the lateral compartment of the knee.
- Confirm alignment and placement of the plate with anteroposterior and lateral radiographs or fluoroscopy.

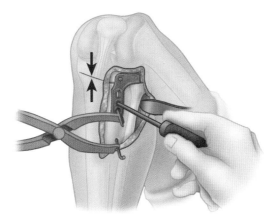

Figure 17-8

- Through the central round hole in the plate, drill a hole with the 3.2-mm drill bit and insert a self-tapping cortical screw (Figure 17-8).
- Remove the compression device and insert a cortical screw in the most distal hole in the plate. Tighten the proximal cancellous screws. Do not apply severe torque when tightening any of the screws, especially the cortical screws. A power screwdriver is not recommended for final tightening.
- Release the tourniquet and obtain hemostasis with electrocautery. Irrigate the wound, insert a small suction drain, and loosely approximate the fascia of the anterior compartment and the iliotibial band with interrupted sutures. Close the subcutaneous tissue with interrupted absorbable sutures, and close the skin with staples and sterile strips. Apply a large compressive Jones dressing.

POSTOPERATIVE CARE 〉

Continuous passive motion is begun immediately after surgery in the recovery room, usually from 0 degrees to 30 degrees of flexion and progressing 10 degrees each day. Ambulation is begun on the second day after surgery and 50% weight bearing is allowed for the first 6 weeks with the use of crutches. Muscle strengthening and active range-of-motion exercises also are begun on postoperative day 2. Full weight bearing is allowed after 6 weeks.

TOTAL ANKLE ARTHROPLASTY

G. Andrew Murphy

TECHNIQUE **18**

Patient Positioning

- Place the patient supine on the operating table with the foot near the end of the table. Place a small bump or lift under the ipsilateral hip to help place the ankle straight and avoid the tendency of the leg to externally rotate.

- After induction of general anesthesia, apply and inflate a thigh tourniquet to control bleeding and improve visualization.

Approach

- Any significant deformity above or below the ankle joint *must* be corrected before placement of the total ankle implants. Placing a total ankle prosthesis into a joint with a malaligned tibia or hindfoot risks early loosening and failure.

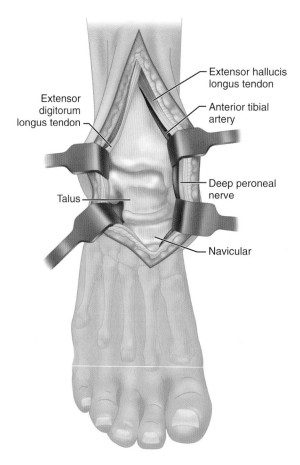

Extensor hallucis longus tendon

Anterior tibial artery

Extensor digitorum longus tendon

Deep peroneal nerve

Talus

Navicular

Figure 18-1

- Most systems require an anterior approach to the ankle. Make an incision from about 10 cm proximal to the ankle joint on the lateral side of the tibialis tendon over the flexor hallucis tendon. This incision is medial to the most medial major branch of the superficial peroneal nerve, the dorsal medial cutaneous nerve. Often a very small medial branch of this nerve crosses the incision just distal to the ankle joint and must be incised for exposure. The patient should be warned before surgery that a small area of numbness may be present just medial to the incision (Figure 18-1).

- Open the flexor hallucis longus sheath and retract the tendon medially. Retract the neurovascular bundle containing the anterior tibial artery, vein, and deep peroneal nerve laterally with the extensor digitorum longus tendons.
- Make a straight incision in line with the skin incision in the ankle capsule and reflect the capsule medially until the medial ankle gutter is exposed and laterally until the lateral gutter is exposed.

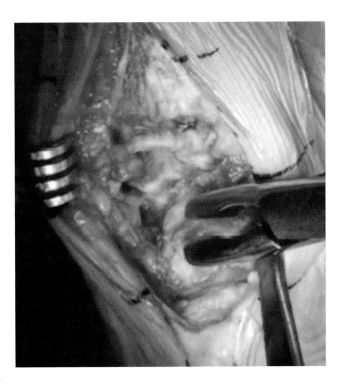

Figure 18-2

- Expose the dorsal talonavicular joint and remove any anterior, medial, or lateral osteophytes. If better exposure of the joint line is needed, use an osteotome to perform a more aggressive removal of the anterior osteophytes (Figure 18-2).

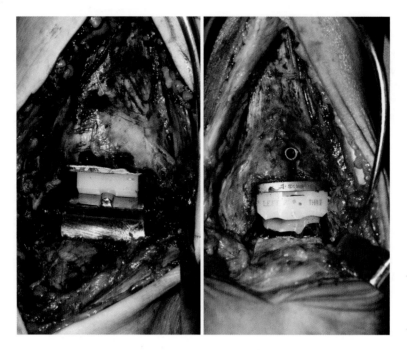

Figure 18-3

- Prepare the bone for implant insertion according to the technique guide specific for the implant selected, taking care to place the implant in proper alignment in all planes and to have sufficient bone coverage of the prosthesis and proper tensioning of the soft tissues and ligamentous support after the final implant. There should be a balance between choosing a thicker polyethylene insert (better for wear characteristics) and excessive bone resection and joint motion and stability (Figure 18-3).

- Close the capsule over the prosthesis and insert a closed suction drain; close the superior extensor retinaculum over the flexor hallucis longus sheath and close the skin in layers.

- A popliteal block is routinely used for postoperative analgesia.

POSTOPERATIVE CARE 〉

At our institution patients are typically kept overnight in the hospital and are seen by a physical therapist the following day for instruction in gait training with touch-down weight bearing. Therapy with antibiotics, binasal cannula oxygen, and deep venous thrombosis prophylaxis with low-molecular-weight heparin is the normal postoperative protocol, although this is not typically continued after discharge unless the patient has risk factors for deep venous thrombosis. Different implants have different recommendations for postoperative care but weight bearing typically delayed for 4 to 6 weeks and active ankle motion begins once the incision is healed, typically 2 weeks after surgery. Gradual progressive weight bearing, calf strengthening, proprioceptive training, and range-of-motion exercises are started at 4 to 6 weeks with the ankle protected in a prefabricated walking boot. A light ankle brace is applied at 8 to 10 weeks and full activities are allowed at 3 months, or when the calf muscles are fully rehabilitated. No restrictions are placed on the patients' activities or sports programs but they are encouraged to avoid impact exercises for conditioning.

This is our preferred technique when coronal plane deformity is minimal (<10 degrees of varus or valgus) and bone quality is satisfactory. The arthroscopic portals are enlarged slightly, the joint is directly observed and prepared, and fixation is inserted. The same benefits of the arthroscopic technique are obtained with a shorter operative time. Miller et al. reported a fusion rate of 98% in two groups of patients using this procedure.

- Place the patient supine on the operating room table with a lift under the ipsilateral hip so that the leg is not externally rotated but the foot is oriented perpendicular to the floor. The foot should be near the end of the table and the table itself able to accept fluoroscopy.

- General anesthesia or a popliteal or ankle block can be used.

- Use a tourniquet to improve visualization and a headlamp and loupe magnification if available. Specialized instruments include Inge lamina spreaders, sharp curets, osteotomes, and a motorized burr.

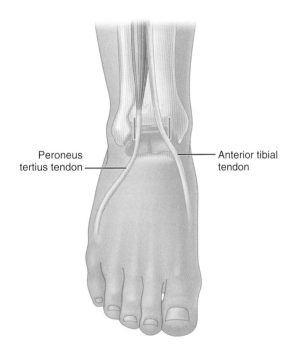

Peroneus tertius tendon —

— Anterior tibial tendon

Figure 19-1

- Make two 1.5-cm incisions one just medial to the tibial tendon and one lateral to the peroneus tertius tendon, taking care to identify the course of the dorsal intermediate cutaneous nerve in the vicinity of the lateral incision. It can usually be seen by inverting the foot and plantar flexing the fourth toe (Figure 19-1).

- Incise the joint capsule in line with the skin and elevate it from the front of the ankle joint with an elevator.

- Inspect the joint and remove any periarticular osteophytes with a rongeur or osteotome to allow placement of the ankle in neutral and to allow evaluation of the joint.

- Place a periosteal elevator in one incision to lever the joint open slightly and place a lamina spreader in the other incision, opening it to allow removal of the remaining cartilage and subchondral bone through the first incision. Use a curet first then a high-speed burr, irrigating through the opposite incision as needed to prevent excessive heat build-up in the bone.

- Prepare the medial gutter in a similar manner, switching the instruments between incisions to complete the preparation.

- Use a small osteotome to "fish scale" the bone and a 2.0-mm drill to penetrate areas that still need to be prepared. There is no consensus regarding whether or not to prepare the lateral gutter for fusion. The extra motion of the fibula may lead to painful nonunion of this joint but even without preparing this joint there is occasionally pain in this area after successful tibiotalar fusion. We generally do not formally prepare this joint and seldom have significant problems with it later.

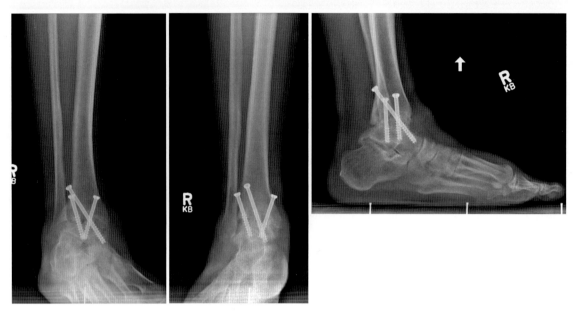

Figure 19-2

- Insert large, partially threaded, cannulated screws (typically 6.5 to 8.0 mm) over guidewires for fixation. Three screws are ideal although sometimes only two are possible. The most desirable position is the so-called "home run" screw placed from the posterolateral tibia into the talar neck/head area distally. A proximal medial screw directed into the posterior body of the talus is usually inserted next, followed by either a proximal lateral to distal medial screw or a distal lateral screw from the lateral process of the talus directed proximal, posterior, and medial (Figure 19-2). Bone graft is typically used. Bone "slurry," created when subchondral bone is resected with a high-speed cutting tool, can be used for local bone graft.
- Close the joint capsule and the skin closed in a routine manner and apply a well-padded short-leg splint with the foot in neutral position.

POSTOPERATIVE CARE 〉

The dressing and sutures are removed at 2 weeks and a short-leg cast is then applied. The patient is instructed to return for a cast change if the cast seems loose and is applying stress to the fusion site. The patient is kept non–weight bearing until the fusion is healed, typically at a minimum of 6 weeks. The use of a rolling walker, on which the patient rests the knee and propels him or herself with the opposite limb dramatically improves quality of life and increases postoperative compliance with the restricted weight-bearing status. Plain radiographs are usually sufficient to assess healing but occasionally computed tomography is necessary. A knee-high walking boot is applied when the fusion is solid, and the patient is allowed to gradually wean from the boot to a shoe. For some patients, a shoe modified with a full-length steel shank and a rocker sole is beneficial for an improved gait pattern.

In certain circumstances arthrodesis of both the ankle and subtalar joints is necessary or advantageous. A lateral approach as just described, with or without the onlay fibular graft, can be used but a posterior approach may be appropriate in some situations. Numerous designs and constructs of intramedullary nails may be employed and a familiarity with the technique associated with the device is essential for a successful outcome.

- After induction of general anesthesia, position the patient supine on the operating table with a small bump under the ipsilateral hip to allow easier access to the fibula. A small lift under the distal leg makes it easier to obtain correct positioning of the ankle for fusion.
- Administer a popliteal block and apply a thigh tourniquet.

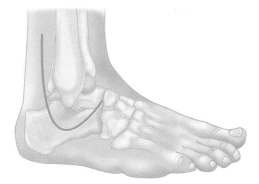

Figure 20-1

- Make an extended approach to the lateral ankle (Figure 20-1), taking care to protect the superficial peroneal nerve. Elevate the periosteum over the anterior half of the fibula and enter the ankle joint capsule by extending the distal approach several centimeters in a J-shaped fashion toward the cuboid. Elevate the periosteum and capsule over the anterior aspect of the tibial plafond.
- Remove any anterior marginal osteophytes from the tibia and talus.

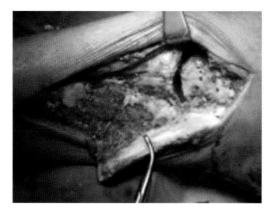

Figure 20-2

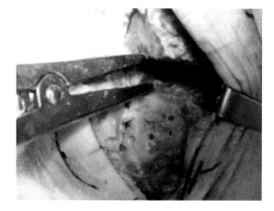

Figure 20-3

- Use a sagittal saw to transect the fibula proximal to the ankle plafond and remove approximately 1 cm with a second parallel cut (Figure 20-2).
- Make a cut in the sagittal plane to remove the medial two thirds of the fibula, preserving the lateral one third with its periosteal attachment.
- Use a laminar spreader to allow removal of residual joint contents (Figure 20-3).

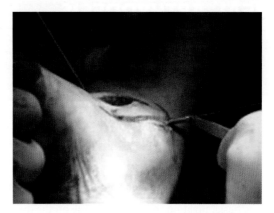

Figure 20-4

- If correction of a valgus deformity is necessary, make a separate medial longitudinal approach to remove the medial malleolus (Figure 20-4); take care to protect the posterior tibial tendon and the neurovascular bundle.
- Preparation of the talotibial joint for fusion varies from "in situ" fusion, in which the normal articular surface topography is maintained for minimal deformity, to flat cuts of the opposing tibial and talar surfaces for more severe deformity. Construct the fusion area to obtain neutral extension, slight external rotation relative to the tibial tubercle, and neutral to slight valgus, depending on the position and flexibility of the rest of the hindfoot and foot. If flat cuts are made, the talus should be slightly translated posteriorly under the tibia. Obtain bleeding, healthy cancellous bone on all fusion surfaces.
- The subtalar joint usually is prepared in situ. Take care not to "overdissect" into the sinus tarsi to avoid disruption of the blood supply to the talus.
- Prepare the lateral tibia and lateral talus in a similar fashion, and manually appose the lateral fibula to this area. Occasionally, a rongeur or "bone biter" can be used to slightly fracture this fibular strut to allow better apposition.
- After the arthrodesis site is prepared, determine the position by holding the patella straight up and placing the foot in neutral dorsiflexion-plantar flexion, 8 degrees to 10 degrees of valgus at the heel, and slight posterior displacement of the calcaneus on the tibia. Hold the foot on the tibia in the proper position (usually with folded towels across the plantar surface of the midfoot).
- Place a guidewire through the heel, pad in line with the center of the tibia. This pin exits the calcaneus just anterior to the posterior facet. Drive the pin into the center of the medullary canal of the tibia under image intensification.

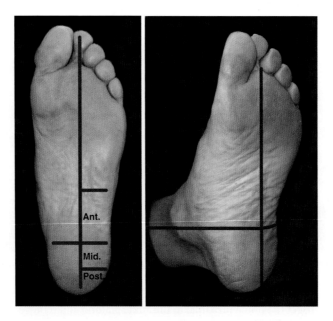

Figure 20-5

- For a simple, reproducible method of determining the correct entry site draw a line from the second toe to the center of the heel in the sagittal plane; in the coronal plane, draw a line at the junction of the anterior and middle thirds of the heel pad. The intersection of these lines indicates the correct entry portal for the nail (Figure 20-5).

- Check the position of the guide pin with image intensification in the anteroposterior plane.
- Drill a hole in the calcaneus through a tissue protector that has been pushed all the way to the bony surface of the calcaneus.

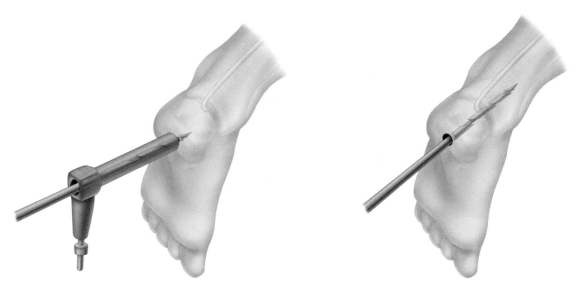

Figure 20-6   Figure 20-7

- Place the guidewire in the center of the medullary canal of the tibia on the anteroposterior and lateral planes, and place an 8- to 9-mm reamer over the guide pin (Figure 20-6).
- Ream the calcaneus and tibia in 1-mm increments, usually 1 mm wider than the nail (13 mm) (Figure 20-7).

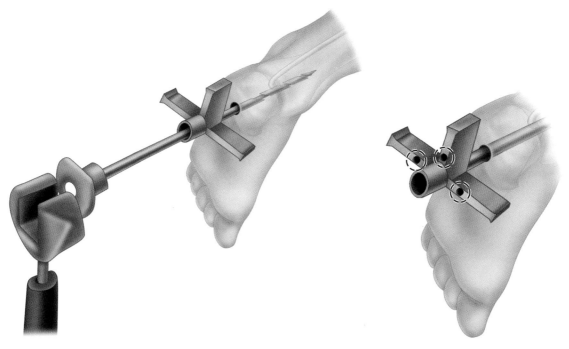

Figure 20-8   Figure 20-9

- After the reaming is completed, load a TRIGEN Hindfoot Fusion Nail (Smith & Nephew, Memphis, TN), which is an intramedullary straight ankle fusion nail, onto a guide. This nail is available in 10- and 11.5-mm diameters and 16-, 20-, and 25-cm lengths (Figure 20-8).
- Place the drill guide sleeves through the drill guide on a back table to ensure that they line up correctly with the holes in the nail. It is essential that the drill passes concentrically through the drill guide and the nail without impinging on the borders of the nail (Figure 20-9).

- Hold the ankle in the proper position, and place the nail over the guidewire with the outrigger guide on the lateral surface of the leg.
- Locking screws generally should be placed sequentially from the calcaneus to the tibia to allow impaction at each joint level.

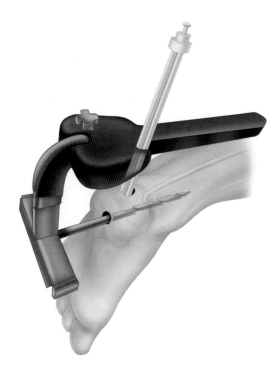

Figure 20-10

- Attach the appropriate drill guide and insert the sleeve assembly through a stab incision so that it rests on the lateral side of the calcaneal tuberosity. If necessary, rotate the nail assembly to keep the screws on the posterior surface. Leave the long pilot drill in the cuboid hole as provisional fixation during insertion of the talar screw (Figure 20-10).

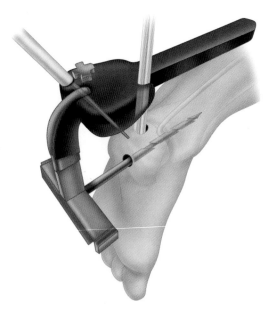

Figure 20-11

- With the appropriate drill sleeves and drill, insert the talar screw from posteroinferior and lateral in the calcaneus to anteromedial in the talar dome, approximately perpendicular to the subtalar joint. Depending on talar height, this screw may engage the anterior tibial plafond (Figure 20-11).
- Insert the cuboid screw oriented posteromedial in the calcaneus to anterolateral in the cuboid.

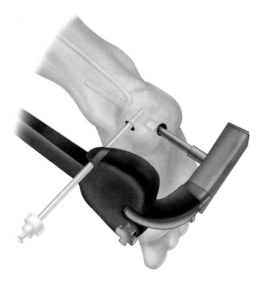

Figure 20-12

- Once the talar and cuboid screws are in place, insert a third transverse distal locking screw (Figure 20-12).

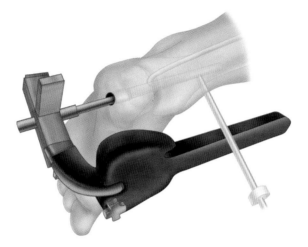

Figure 20-13

- To lock the nail proximally, insert a proximal screw from medial to lateral using the drill guide or a free-hand technique (Figure 20-13).
- Before final seating of the nail, place bone graft from the morselized malleoli in the arthrodesis and in the sinus tarsi area of the calcaneus.

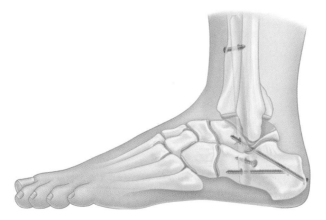

Figure 20-14

- Impact the nail after the bone graft has been applied and before proximal locking. The tip of the nail should rest anywhere from slightly inside the cortex of the calcaneus to approximately 1 cm outside the plantar surface of the calcaneus. Do not allow it to protrude so far that it would impede ambulation (Figure 20-14).

TOTAL SHOULDER ARTHROPLASTY

Thomas W. Throckmorton

TECHNIQUE **21**

See also Video 21-1.

Total shoulder arthroplasty is a well-established procedure with an excellent long-term track record of pain relief and functional improvements. The primary indication for total shoulder arthroplasty is end-stage glenohumeral joint degeneration with an intact rotator cuff.

PREPARATION OF THE HUMERUS ⟩

- Place the patient in the beach chair position using a McConnell headrest (McConnell Orthopaedic Equipment Company, Greenville, TX) to allow positioning of the patient at the top and edge of the table. Pad all bony prominences. The medial border of the scapula should be free and off the table, allowing full adduction to gain access to the intramedullary canal.

- Secure the patient's head to the headrest, holding the head in a position that avoids hyperextension or tilting of the neck, which can cause compression of the cervical roots.

- Prepare the arm and drape it widely. We recommend using occlusive dressings to cover the entire surgical field because of the risk of contamination from the axilla.

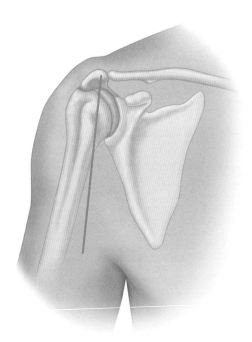

Figure 21-1

- Make an incision anteriorly, approximately halfway between the coracoid and the lateral aspect of the acromion (Figure 21-1). Carry dissection down to the deltoid and raise medial and lateral flaps to mobilize the deltoid.

- Open the deltopectoral interval and allow the cephalic vein to fall medially.

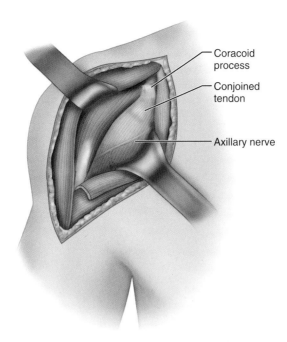

Figure 21-2

- Perform subdeltoid, subcoracoid, and subacromial releases to release the proximal humerus. In the subcoracoid space, locate the axillary nerve by passing the volar surface of the index finger down along the anterior surface of the subscapularis muscle (Figure 21-2). If scarring and adhesions make identification of the nerve difficult, pass an elevator along the anterior surface of the subscapular muscle to create an interval between the muscle and the nerve. Always identify the axillary nerve and carefully retract and hold it out of the way, especially during the crucial steps of releasing and resecting the antero-inferior capsule.

- Incise the subscapularis 1 cm medial to the lesser tuberosity. Place two retention sutures in the subscapularis to be used as traction sutures when freeing the rest of the tendon from the underlying capsule and scar tissue. At closure, use the sutures to repair the tendon.

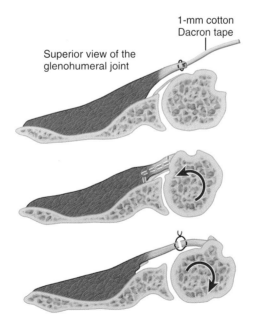

Figure 21-3

- Some authors prefer either a lesser tuberosity osteotomy or a release of the subscapularis directly off of bone. If external rotation is markedly limited, the subscapularis also can be reattached to the proximal humerus more medially to allow increased external rotation. Alternatively, the tendon can be lengthened with a coronal Z-plasty technique (Figure 21-3).

- Incise the rotator interval, directing the cut medially toward the glenoid. Typically, a large amount of synovial fluid escapes as the joint is entered.
- Release the anteroinferior capsule from the humerus and externally rotate the arm to bring the inferior aspect of the shoulder capsule into view. If osteophytes are present inferiorly on the humeral head, remove them to expose the capsule more fully. Take care to stay directly on bone so as not to injure the axillary nerve during the capsular release. The importance of the inferior capsule release cannot be overstated and must be thoroughly carried out to at least the 6 o'clock position to dislocate the humeral head and gain access to the glenoid.

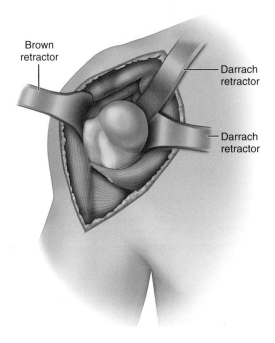

Figure 21-4

- Once the capsule is adequately released, place a large Darrach retractor in the joint and gently externally rotate, adduct, and extend the arm to deliver the humeral head up and out of the glenoid fossa (Figure 21-4). If the humeral head cannot be delivered in this fashion, the inferior capsule must be released further.
- Prepare the humeral canal, using the humeral axis to reference the osteotomy. Initially, open the canal with a high speed burr at the base of the rotator cuff footprint and ream it to a size where appropriate "chatter" is felt in the shaft. Do not use motorized equipment for reaming and be careful not to overream the canal, which could create a stress riser or cause a fracture.
- We prefer to use a cutting guide that employs extramedullary referencing, using the axis of the forearm as the reference point. With the cutting guide pinned into position at 30 degrees of retroversion, recheck the cutting angle and confirm that the height is such that the saw will not violate the rotator cuff or biceps tendon.
- Complete the osteotomy with an oscillating saw. If any inferior humeral head osteophyte remains, remove it with a rongeur.
- After the head cut, broach the humeral canal to the same size as the reamed canal. It is imperative to confirm proper position of the broaches in 30 degrees of retroversion during this step to prevent component malposition.

PREPARATION OF THE GLENOID

- Approach the glenohumeral joint. Once the trial broach is tapped into position remove the retractors from about the humerus.
- Expose the glenoid by placing a Fukuda retractor on the posterior aspect of the glenoid and subluxing the humerus posteriorly.
- Débride the glenoid vault of all remaining labral tissue and articular cartilage.
- If needed for exposure, release the anterior capsule and place a flat Darrach retractor on the anterior glenoid neck to aid exposure.

- The glenoid is not adequately exposed until the anterior, posterior, superior, and inferior aspects of the glenoid can be seen. Once this is accomplished, inspect the glenoid for wear and bone defects.

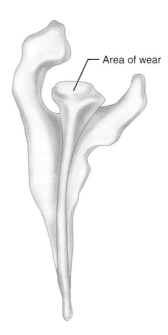

Area of wear

Figure 21-5

- If there is posterior erosion of the glenoid, lower the anterior rim of the glenoid to reestablish the correct version. This can be done by eccentric reaming or with a high-speed burr. A preoperative CT scan can aid in understanding glenoid orientation and morphology (Figure 21-5).

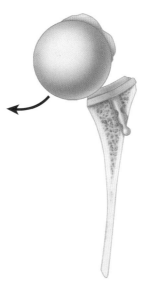

Figure 21-6

- If the glenoid component is inserted without correction of slope the anchoring device passes out of medullary canal; tilt and loss of height also make the implant unstable (Figure 21-6).

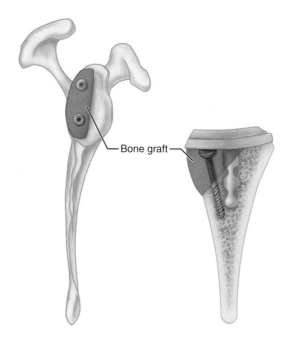

Bone graft

Figure 21-7

- Severe erosion is corrected by bone grafting. A piece of the humeral head is secured to the scapula with a 4-mm AO navicular screw. Lesser erosion can be offset by building up the low side with acrylic cement or lowering the high side. Building up with cement is not recommended because of possible cement loosening. Lowering the high side often requires shortening the holding device of the glenoid component and creates laxity between components, which can make the implant temporarily unstable and requires special postoperative care. A glenoid component with a thick side is available for moderate uneven erosion (Figure 21-7).

- Once the glenoid vault is débrided, make a centering hole typically with a guide. It is often helpful to confirm adequate depth and positioning of the starting hole with a small curet. Once the starting hole is made, proceed with glenoid reaming until the sclerotic bone of the arthritic glenoid is removed and the subchondral plate is seen. With the common posterior wear pattern of osteoarthritis, reaming is typically done in an eccentric fashion so that the anterior lip of the glenoid is planed down. If the posterior rim wear is significant and the anterior rim has not been lowered, the component sits excessively retroverted and anterior glenoid neck perforation is likely. Take care not to ream too aggressively medially and thereby compromise the glenoid bone stock.

- Once reaming is complete, prepare the glenoid for either the pegged or keeled implant. Systems vary in their instrumentation but all involve precise placement of the anchoring pegs or keel. To provide secure fixation and reduce the risk of loosening, the glenoid trial must sit securely against the subchondral bone of the glenoid without any rocking after the glenoid is prepared. Cement cannot be used to adjust for poor seating of the glenoid component.

- Whether using a pegged or keeled component, prepare the glenoid vault for cementing with a pulsed lavage to remove debris and blood. Thoroughly dry the peg holes or keel before cementation.

- Tuberculin syringes are helpful to pressurize the cement. Pack cement into the syringe and then inject it into the peg holes or into the keel.

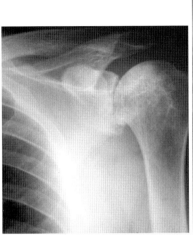
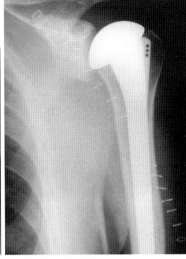

Figure 21-8

- Insert the glenoid component and maintain thumb pressure until the cement has hardened. Most shoulder systems also come with an instrument to hold the glenoid component in place while the cement hardens. This method allows excellent pressurization and interdigitation of the cement into the cancellous bone of the glenoid vault and postoperative radiolucent lines seen with other cementing techniques are minimized. Some systems use a polyethylene or metal ingrowth post to provide a press-fit of the glenoid component. This provides immediate stability so that the component does not rely solely on digital pressure while the cement is curing (Figure 21-8).
- After the cement has hardened, check the broach to ensure that it is still secure within the humeral canal. If so, insert the trial broach and the humeral prosthesis as described in Technique 12-1. Head height, range of motion, and soft tissue balancing are critical to an optimal outcome. Most current systems use modular heads with a variety of diameters and thicknesses.
- Once the appropriate head is selected, dry the Morse taper and tap the head into position. Reduce the glenohumeral joint and close the wound.

POSTOPERATIVE CARE

Patients are instructed in a gentle home exercise program with passive forward elevation to 90 degrees and passive external rotation to neutral. Patients typically are discharged from the hospital 1 or 2 days after surgery and are encouraged to use a pillow behind the elbow while recumbent in the sling to support the extremity. Full-time sling immobilization continues for 6 weeks, followed by 6 weeks of sling use only in unprotected environments. Therapy progresses to full passive range of motion by 6 to 12 weeks and to isometric strengthening at 10 weeks.

See also Video 22-1.

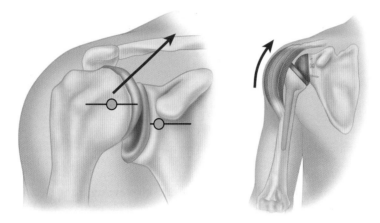

Figure 22-1

The primary indication for reverse total shoulder arthroplasty is a nonfunctional rotator cuff. The reverse prosthesis works by changing the direction of pull of the deltoid muscle. With standard prostheses, absence of the rotator cuff allows the humeral head to subluxate superiorly during deltoid muscle contraction. The reverse prosthesis corrects this by moving the center of rotation of the arm laterally and reestablishing a fulcrum around which the deltoid can pull to restore forward elevation (Figure 22-1).

- Approach the proximal humerus and prepare it for stem implantation as described in Technique 20. Some authors recommend a superior approach but we prefer the deltopectoral approach because of its versatility and extensive nature if exposure is limited. However, there are some important differences in humeral preparation from a total shoulder arthroplasty or hemiarthroplasty. First, because of the common superior subluxation deformity of rotator cuff–deficient shoulders, a larger humeral head cut is required. Second, some authors advocate placing the stem in neutral version to prevent instability in abduction and external rotation We believe, however, that stem placement in 30 degrees of retroversion is not only acceptable but also preferable to prevent the more common instability in adduction and extension seen with the reverse prosthesis. There have been no studies to date that have evaluated this mode of instability with this prosthesis relative to the stem version.

- Once the glenoid vault is adequately débrided and all four borders are visible, identify the centering point. Move the starting point inferiorly 1 to 2 mm to allow inferior placement of the baseplate to prevent scapular notching.

- Place a guide pin through this centering hole using a guide. Take care to place the guide pin in 10 degrees to 15 degrees of inferior tilt, again to prevent scapular notching.

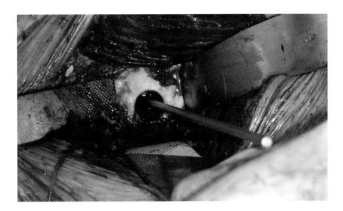

Figure 22-2

- Ream the glenoid until the "smiley face" is achieved with bleeding cancellous bone inferiorly and hard sclerotic bone superiorly. This confirms adequate inferior tilt of the baseplate (Figure 22-2).
- Impact the baseplate and secure it with screws. Dry the Morse taper and impact the glenosphere into position.
- Place the humeral stem using trial components to test for stability and motion. Reduction and dislocation of the glenohumeral joint is typically more difficult than with standard shoulder arthroplasty. Reduction involves a combination of longitudinal traction and forward elevation on the arm. The deltoid tension should be slightly greater than before joint relocation but take care not to overlengthen the deltoid, which can result in dehiscence. The conjoined tendon can also be palpated to confirm slightly increased tension. There should be no more than 2 to 3 mm of gapping in the glenohumeral articulation once the joint is reduced.
- To dislocate the glenohumeral joint, place the dislocation instrument between the bearing surface and glenosphere to disrupt the articulation. Pull the humerus anteriorly (shoulder extension) to deliver the bearing surface.
- Once the proper bearing surface is chosen, dry the Morse taper and impact it into position. Reduce the glenohumeral joint for a final time. Close the wound. Subscapularis repair is especially important in these patients who often have poor tissue around the shoulder for repair. Closure of the subscapularis has been found to correlate with improved stability.

POSTOPERATIVE CARE 〉

Patients are instructed in a gentle home exercise program with passive forward elevation to 90 degrees and passive external rotation to neutral. Patients are typically discharged from the hospital 1 or 2 days after surgery and are encouraged to use a pillow behind the elbow while recumbent in the sling to support the extremity. Full-time sling immobilization continues for 6 weeks followed by 6 weeks of sling use only in unprotected environments. Therapy progresses to a full passive range of motion by 6 to 12 weeks and to isometric strengthening at 10 weeks.

TOTAL ELBOW ARTHROPLASTY
Thomas W. Throckmorton

See also Videos 23-1 and 23-2.

The Coonrad-Morrey prosthesis is a semi-constrained hinged prosthesis with a high-molecular-weight poly-ethylene bushing, and titanium humeral and ulnar components. It was designed with 7 degrees of rotary and side-to-side laxity. Humeral and ulnar stems match the shapes of the medullary canals. The triangular humeral stem is flattened near the base at the inferior flatter and the wider portion of the medullary canal of the humerus. The large medullary stem enhances rigid fixation. Its long stem, contour, and distal anterior flange increase resistance to torque. Careful bone removal in the intercondylar area of the humerus is necessary to allow a tight fit of the humeral prosthesis. The prosthesis is usually inserted with the elbow fully flexed. If necessary it can be disarticulated by removal of the axis pin. The components can also be inserted separately and then joined. Right and left prostheses are available as are trial components. The axis of rotation of this prosthesis is near the anatomical center when the device is properly implanted. It is relatively large, which is a possible disadvantage in smaller patients and occasionally requires manufacture of custom components.

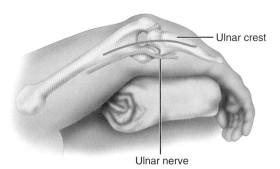

Figure 23-1

- Place the patient supine with the affected arm in front of the chest and with a sandbag beneath the ipsilateral shoulder. When preparing and draping the arm, leave the entire elbow area and forearm exposed so that the prosthesis can be inserted properly. Use a sterile tourniquet and exsanguinate the limb by elevating it for several minutes before inflating the tourniquet (Figure 23-1).
- Use a straight posteromedial incision.
- Identify the ulnar nerve, gently mobilize and protect it, and transpose it anteriorly after the operation.

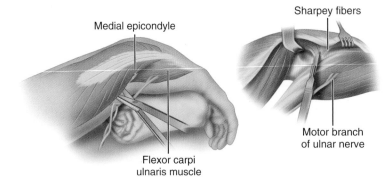

Figure 23-2

- Carefully elevate the triceps mechanism in continuity with the periosteum over the proximal ulna and olecranon to avoid transection or separation of the triceps mechanism (Figure 23-2).

- Reflect the triceps mechanism to the radial side of the olecranon to expose the proximal ulna. The replacement of an intact extensor mechanism is made easier, minimizing the risk of triceps rupture and poor triceps function after surgery.
- Release the collateral ligaments on each side of the elbow.
- Rotate the forearm laterally to dislocate the elbow and allow exposure of the distal humerus.

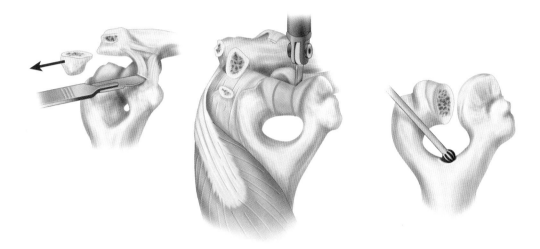

Figure 23-3

- Remove the midportion of the trochlea with an oscillating saw to allow access to the medullary canal of the humerus. Identify the canal with a burr applied to the roof of the olecranon fossa (Figure 23-3) .

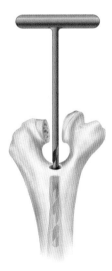

Figure 23-4

- Remove the cortex of the olecranon fossa and open the medullary canal to a size sufficient to allow a twist reamer (Figure 23-4).
- Preserve the medial and lateral portions of the supracondylar columns during the preparation of the distal humerus. Use the medial and lateral supracondylar columns for reference during the bone preparation to ensure satisfactory orientation and alignment.

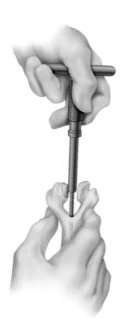

Figure 23-5

- Place the alignment stem down the medullary canal with a T-handle (Figure 23-5).

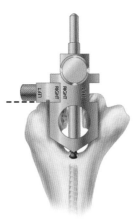

Figure 23-6

- Remove the handle, and apply the cutting block with the appropriate right or left placement of the side arm of the cutting block. Allow the side arm to rest on the capitellum to provide for proper depth of the cut (Figure 23-6).
- Use an oscillating saw to remove the trochlear and capitellar bone to correspond with the size of the appropriate cutting block. If the bone is osteoporotic, score the cortex with electrocautery using the cutting block as a guide.
- Remove any remaining bone after the cut with a rongeur. Avoid injury to the medial and lateral supracondylar columns to avoid fracture. Remove the bone carefully, small amounts at a time, repeatedly inserting the trial prosthesis until the margins of the prosthesis are exactly level with the epicondylar articular surface margins on the capitellar and trochlear sides.

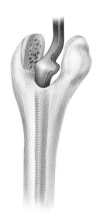

Figure 23-7

- Hollow the flattened areas of the distal humerus to allow a precise fit of the shoulders of the humeral stem by curettage of cancellous bone from the epicondylar and distal flaring portions of the humerus. This should allow satisfactory cement fixation (Figure 23-7).
- Remove the tip of the olecranon.
- Use a high-speed burr and remove subchondral bone to allow identification of the ulnar medullary canal.

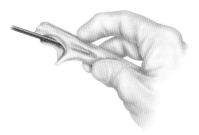

Figure 23-8

- Remove additional bone from the tip of the olecranon to form a notch for placement of the serial reamers down the medullary canal of the ulna. Use the appropriate right or left ulnar rasps as needed (Figure 23-8).

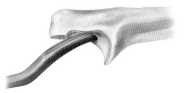

Figure 23-9

- Select the appropriate size rasp and use a burr to remove the subchondral bone gently around the coronoid process (Figure 23-9).
- After the proximal ulna and distal humerus have been prepared, insert a trial prosthesis and evaluate the elbow for complete flexion and extension.
- If there is a limitation to full extension, release the anterior capsule and evaluate the trial components again until the elbow can be straightened.
- Before inserting the final prosthesis with polymethyl methacrylate, use the trial prosthesis to determine if the radial head impinges on the prosthesis. If it is present, resect the radial head.
- Fashion a bone graft from the previously cut trochlea to be placed behind the anterior humeral flange during component implantation. The graft is usually 2 to 3 mm thick, 1.5 cm long, and 1 cm wide. Elevate the brachialis from the anterior humerus to provide a bed for placement of the bone graft.
- Clean the medullary canals of the humerus and ulna with a pulsating lavage irrigating system and dry the canals.
- Place cement restrictors in the humeral and ulnar canals.

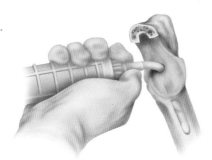

Figure 23-10

- Use a cement gun with flexible tubing to insert the cement into the canals. Inject the cement early in the polymerization process. Inject the cement into the ulna, leaving 1 to 2 cm of medullary canal unfilled to allow for back flow of the cement (Figure 23-10).

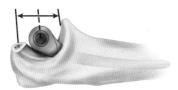

Figure 23-11

- Insert the ulnar component first, as far distally as the coronoid process. Align the center of the ulnar component with the center of the greater sigmoid notch. Remove excess cement from around the ulnar component (Figure 23-11).

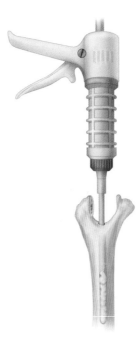

Figure 23-12

- Insert cement into the humeral canal leaving about 1 cm of canal unfilled to allow for back flow of cement (Figure 23-12).

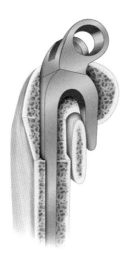

Figure 23-13

- While the cement is still soft, place the humeral component down to a point that allows articulation of the device and placement of the axis pin. Place the bone graft against the distal humerus beneath the soft tissue. At this point the bone graft is partially covered by the anterior flange of the humeral component (Figure 23-13).

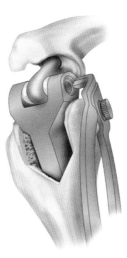

Figure 23-14

- Articulate the humeral device by placing the axis pin through the humerus and ulna. Secure it with a split locking ring. There will be a confirmatory click when the locking device engages (Figure 23-14).

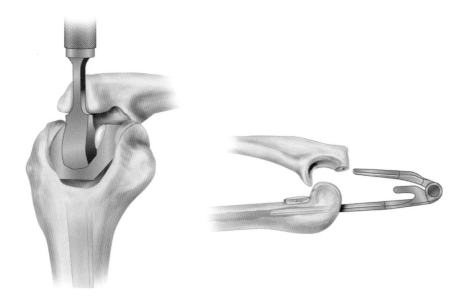

Figure 23-15

- Impact the humeral component into the humerus so that the axis of rotation of the prosthesis is at the level of the normal anatomical axis of rotation. This is usually accomplished when the base of the anterior flange is flush with the anterior bone of the olecranon fossa (Figure 23-15).
- Check the bone graft to ensure that it is still behind the anterior humeral flange and secure between it and the humerus.
- Place the arm in maximal extension while the cement hardens, and while this occurs carefully remove excess cement.
- Deflate the tourniquet and obtain hemostasis. Leave a drain in the depths of the wound.

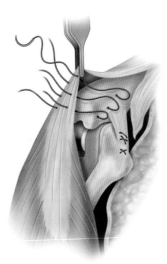

Figure 23-16

- Drill holes in an X configuration through the olecranon to accept the sutures to repair the triceps mechanism with a locking running stitch. Also place a transverse suture through the olecranon and tie it over the top of the approximated triceps to provide additional fixation. Close the remainder of the triceps with an absorbable suture (Figure 23-16).

- Apply a compression dressing with the elbow in full extension and a long anterior splint to minimize pressure on the posterior incision. If immobilization of the elbow in 90 degrees of flexion is preferred, apply a well-padded long-arm splint with extra padding over the posterior surfaces to avoid pressure on the incision.

POSTOPERATIVE CARE

The extremity is elevated overnight with the elbow above the shoulder. The drains and compressive dressing are removed the day after surgery. A light dressing is then applied and passive elbow flexion and extension are allowed as tolerated. A collar and cuff are used, and instructions in the activities of daily living are provided by an occupational therapist. Active elbow extension must be avoided for 3 months until the triceps heals. Strengthening exercises are avoided and the patient is encouraged to avoid lifting more than 5 pounds with the involved arm for the first 3 months after surgery. Thereafter, lifting is restricted to 10 pounds.

POSTERIOR C1-2 FUSION
Keith D. Williams

Posterior fixation of the cervical spine using one of several techniques generally offers biomechanical advantages over anterior fixation but does not allow for preservation of motion at the C1-C2 joint, which is a significant morbidity.

TRANSARTICULAR SCREW FIXATION ⟩

- Careful preoperative planning is needed to assess the safety of the screw placement.
- Shave the patient's head to the level of the inion (posterior occipital protuberance).
- Prepare and drape the posterior head and neck as well as the posterior iliac crest donor site.
- Score the skin sharply from foramen magnum to the C3 level and inject dilute epinephrine solution (1 mg in 500 mL normal saline) through the score incision into the dermis and paraspinal musculature.
- Use lateral image intensification to check the reduction of the C1-C2 complex.
- Perform midline posterior cervical exposure in the routine fashion from C2 to C3. The exposure should be to the lateral edge of the C2 lateral mass.
- Expose the medial wall of the isthmus up to the C1-C2 joint. If possible curet or burr the joint. The area around the greater occipital nerve is highly vascular.
- Place intraarticular bone graft.

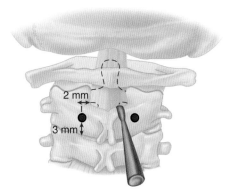

Figure 24-1

- Identify the landmarks for the entry portal of the transarticular screw at the lower medial edge of the inferior articular process of C2. Determine the proper trajectory of the screw and make a stab incision in the skin if needed to attain the correct trajectory, which may be at C7 (Figure 24-1).

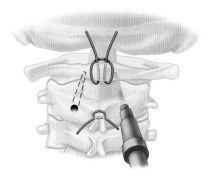

Figure 24-2

- Using a 2-mm bit incrementally drill through the isthmus near its posteromedial surface, exiting from the articular surface of C2 at the posterior aspect of the superior articular surface and entering the lateral mass of the atlas. If the isthmus is oriented too medially the exiting drill will miss the C1 lateral mass or the drill will exit the isthmus laterally and risk injuring the vertebral artery. The drill bit should just perforate the anterior cortex of the lateral mass of C1 (Figure 24-2).

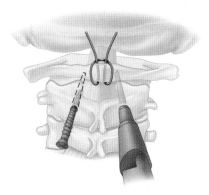

Figure 24-3

- Determine the appropriate screw length. Use a 3.5-mm cortical tap to cut threads in the drill hole and insert the appropriate 3.5-mm cortical screw across the C1-2 joint. Typically screws are 34 to 43 mm in length. Take care not to extend more than 1 mm anterior to the C1 lateral mass. Cannulated screws can be used (Figure 24-3).

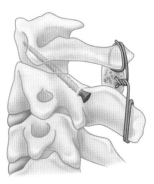

Figure 24-4

- After placing the C1-2 transarticular screws, perform a traditional posterior C1-2 fusion using either the Gallie or the Brooks technique if intraarticular grafting was not possible (Figure 24-4).
- Close the wound in layers over a drain taking care to reattach the fascia to bone at the C2 level. Use a subcuticular skin closure.

POSTOPERATIVE CARE 〉

Because this technique provides excellent rotational stability postoperative immobilization with a halo vest is usually unnecessary. A cervical collar may be worn for 8 to 12 weeks. The drain is removed on the first postoperative day.

TRANSLAMINAR SCREW FIXATION 〉

This technique was described as an alternative technique with less risk for vertebral artery injury, although there are other risks such as dural or spinal cord injuries. When the procedure is done properly these are small risks. Two screws are inserted through the base of the C2 spinous process and contained within the lamina on the contralateral side. The screws must be placed with one slightly more caudal on one side and directed cephalad at a steeper angle than the other screw. The translaminar screws are then connected to the C1 lateral mass screws. If the construct is to extend below C2, rod contouring can be problematic because the translaminar screws are not aligned with the lateral mass screws. Generally, this method is used if anatomical constraints preclude C2 isthmic screw placement with known vertebral artery injuries preoperatively.

- Patient preparation is as described for Transarticular Screw Fixation.
- Use lateral image intensification to check the reduction of the C1-2 complex.
- Perform posterior midline exposure of the cervical spine from the occiput to C2.
- Using a hand drill placed just caudal to the ring of C1 and 3 to 4 mm lateral to the medial edge of the lateral mass, advance the drill at an angle of 10 degrees medially and slightly cephalad to a point just posterior to the anterior margin of the dens on a lateral image intensifier view. This allows for unicortical screw placement and lowers the risk of injury to the internal carotid artery and hypoglossal nerve anterior to the C1 lateral mass.
- Place a polyaxial screw with a 10-mm smooth shank extension to the drilled depth.
- Place a Penfield No. 4 elevator to allow a view of the isthmus medial cortex and determine the line of entry points on the inferior facet of C2 that will allow the medially directed drill to enter the isthmus. Using the lateral image intensifier view select the point on this line that will orient the drill up the center of the isthmus. A high-speed burr is used to penetrate only the cortex at that point. Typically the drill will be directed 25 degrees medially and 20 degrees to 30 degrees cephalad but anatomy varies considerably and careful review of the CT scan is required. Direct the hand drill up the isthmus under fluoroscopic control to a point at the posterior margin of the C2 foramen transversarium as seen on the lateral image intensifier view.
- Place the appropriate length polyaxial screw to stop at the posterior foramen transversarium. In our experience this gives excellent fixation without placing the vertebral artery at risk by crossing the foramen transversarium into the C2 body.
- Cut and contour the rod as desired. Place the rod and tighten the blocker screws securely.
- Fully expose the caudal edge of the C2 lamina at the midline and extend it laterally.
- Use an angled curet to detach the ligamentum flavum from the ventral surface and the cephalad and caudal margin of C2 so that a Penfield No. 4 dissector or other blunt instrument can be used to palpate the anterior C2 lamina during screw placement.
- With a Penfield No. 4 dissector or blunt hook ventral to the lamina, use the drill to penetrate the cortex at the base of the C2 spinous process at the location determined preoperatively to allow room for both screws. Using the Penfield No. 4 as a guide, maintain the drill posterior to the canal and advance it laterally into the C2 inferior articular mass. The drill should not penetrate the posterior or anterior cortex as it is advanced. Screw lengths usually are 25 to 35 mm.
- Place the contralateral screw similarly.
- Contour the rod to engage the C1 lateral mass screws and secure the connections.
- Perform a traditional posterior C1-2 fusion using either the Gallie or the Brooks technique. Alternatively morselized bone graft can be used.
- Close the wound in layers over a drain taking care to reattach the fascia to bone at the C2 level. Use a subcuticular skin closure.

POSTOPERATIVE CARE 〉

Postoperative immobilization with a halo vest usually is unnecessary. A cervical collar may be worn for 8 to 12 weeks. The drain is removed on the first postoperative day.

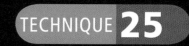
See also Video 25-1.

The primary advantages of anterior cervical spine surgery include decompression of the neural elements and restoration of the axial load-bearing support function with a strut graft and anterior plating, particularly over one or two motion segments.

- If the patient is already in traction maintain traction and alignment. Coordinate with the anesthesiologist for an awake intubation or manually maintain head position and use a GlideScope (Veriathon Inc., Bothell, WA). If the patient has a spinal cord injury maintain a mean arterial pressure of 85 to 90 mm Hg during the procedure.

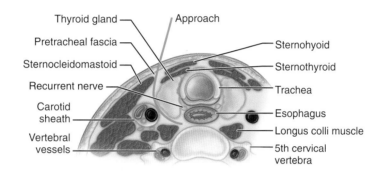

Figure 25-1

- Expose the spine through either a transverse or a longitudinal incision depending on the surgeon's preference. We usually prefer a left-sided transverse incision because of the more constant anatomy of the recurrent laryngeal nerve and the lower risk of inadvertent injury (Figure 25-1).
- Make a 3-cm incision at the cricoid level for the C5 disc or adjust accordingly. A transverse incision can be used even for an extensile exposure. Locate the skin incision with the midpoint on the lateral border of the trachea on the side of the approach.
- Incise the skin and dissect through the subcutaneous layer to the platysma. Sharply dissect the fat off the platysma fascia at least 10 mm in all directions from the incision.
- Incise the platysma muscle vertically in line with its fibers.
- In the lateral portion of the wound identify the medial border of the sternocleidomastoid muscle and bluntly develop the plane to the carotid sheath. At the C5 disc level it will be covered by the omohyoid muscle.
- Sweep the omohyoid superiorly or inferiorly (at the C5 disc level) as needed and sharply incise the pretracheal fascia along the medial border of the carotid sheath.
- With blunt finger dissection develop the plane of the prevertebral space. Use a Kitner dissector to better define the anterior spine that is visible between the longus colli muscles.
- Radiographically identify the injured level with a metallic marker within the injured disc or bone and permanently store the image.
- Using blunt retractors mobilize the trachea and esophagus just enough to safely elevate the longus colli muscles bilaterally from the midbody of the superior end vertebra to the midbody of the inferior end vertebra avoiding unnecessary exposure that may lead to adjacent segment degeneration.

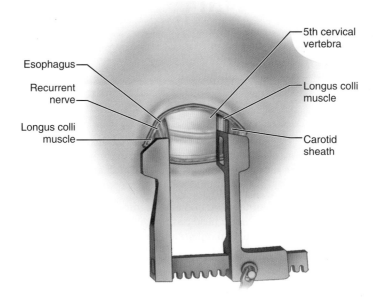

Esophagus

Recurrent nerve

Longus colli muscle

5th cervical vertebra

Longus colli muscle

Carotid sheath

Figure 25-2

- Place a self-retaining retractor with the blade deep to the medial border of the longus colli on each side of the spine at the affected level (Figure 25-2).
- Incise the injured disc widely to the level of the uncinate process bilaterally. Use curets to remove most of the disc and clearly view the uncinate process bilaterally.

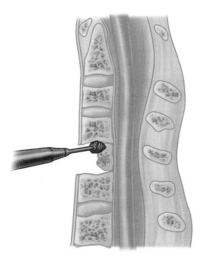

Figure 25-3

- Under the operating microscope use a high-speed burr to remove the anteriormost portion of the inferior body of the cephalad vertebra (Figure 25-3). This bone removal is only to the level of the highest point of the concavity of the inferior endplate. This allows the endplate to be flat and it forms a right angle with the anterior and posterior body walls and preserves the subchondral bone. Remove any anterior osteophyte. With this anterior bone resection, visibility is enhanced and the posterior disc material, posterior longitudinal ligament, and posterior osteophytes can be removed as needed. If the foramina are tight, perform foraminotomies. Contour the superior endplate of the inferior vertebra with a burr preserving the subchondral bone and creating a flat surface with an equal interval between the adjacent endplates left to right and front to back.
- Carefully measure the height of the disc space both with traction applied and without traction. Do not size the graft to maintain the traction interval if there is more than 1 mm difference between the measurements. The graft size should allow for a stable fit without being excessively tight.

- Either harvest tricortical iliac graft or select a composite corticocancellous allograft product. The graft typically is 12 to 13 mm in anterior to posterior dimension so it can be countersunk 2 mm and not intrude into the canal. Tamp the graft into place and verify radiographically or by direct vision that the posterior graft does not enter the canal. With traction removed the graft should be stable enough to resist being pulled easily from the disc space.

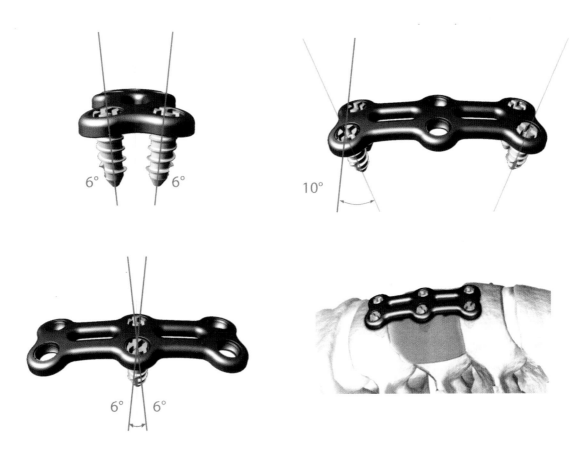

Figure 25-4

- Select the shortest locking plate possible to avoid impingement injury to the adjacent discs. The prepared endplates should be just visible through the screw holes of the plate when it is properly positioned (Figure 25-4).
- Drill and place unicortical screws, which are usually 14 mm in length. Make sure screws are placed at the correct angle to optimize locking of the screw and plate. Engage the anti-backout mechanism of the plate after placing all four screws.
- Achieve meticulous hemostasis and close the platysma over a Blake style drain. Close the remaining layers.

POSTOPERATIVE CARE ⟩

A rigid orthosis is worn for 4 to 6 weeks until there is radiographic evidence of healing at the graft interfaces. Flexion and extension radiographs are obtained to verify stability and to determine if the orthosis can be discontinued.

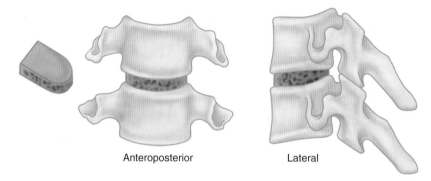

Anteroposterior   Lateral

Figure 26-1

Anterior discectomy and interbody fusion has a wide application, producing excellent results in virtually all forms of cervical disc disease and spondylosis, regardless of objective neurological signs. The Smith-Robinson technique uses a tricortical iliac crest autograft (Figure 26-1).

- Place the patient supine on the operating table with a small roll in the interscapular area.
- Apply a head halter if anterior plate fixation is to be used. Apply 5 to 10 pounds of traction to the head halter if so desired. Otherwise the halter is not necessary because the distraction pins and the retraction set can be used to open the disc space and allow exposure.
- Rotate the patient's head slightly to the side opposite the planned approach.
- Mark the anterior cervical skin, preferably using an existing curved skin crease before placing the adhesive surgical field drape. The hyoid (C3), thyroid cartilage (C4-5), and cricoid cartilage (C6) are useful landmarks. The transverse-type skin incision can be used even for three-level corpectomies if it is well placed, otherwise an incision along the sternocleidomastoid border is useful. Throughout the exposure meticulous hemostasis should be maintained to allow better identification of dissection planes and important anatomic structures.
- After sharply dividing the skin, dissect the subcutaneous layer off the anterior fascia of the platysma to allow mobility of the wound to the desired level.
- Divide the platysma vertically near the midline by lifting it between two pairs of forceps and dividing it sharply in the cephalad and caudal directions. This allows exposure of the sternocleidomastoid border.
- Develop the interval just medial to the sternocleidomastoid to allow palpation and exposure of the carotid sheath and the overlying omohyoid muscle.
- Mobilize the omohyoid and retract caudally for access cephalad to C5 or mobilize cranially for access to C5 or caudal levels.
- Sharply divide the pretracheal fascia medial to the carotid sheath. Take care to avoid any dissection lateral to the carotid sheath that would place the sympathetic chain at risk.
- Once the pretracheal fascia has been incised, adequately develop the prevertebral space using blunt finger dissection directed medially and posteriorly.
- Place blunt hand-held retractors medially to view the paired longus colli muscles. To avoid injury to the midline structures use bipolar cautery and small key-type elevators to subperiosteally elevate the longus colli so that self-retaining retractors can be placed deep to the medial borders of these muscles.
- Obtain a localization radiograph using a prebent spinal needle to mark the disc space before proceeding with disc excision or corpectomy.
- If the superior or inferior thyroid vessels limit exposure ligate and divide the vessels.
- When elevating the longus colli muscles do not extend laterally to the transverse processes to avoid the sympathetic chain and the vertebral artery. This dissection, however, must extend laterally far enough to expose the anterior aspect of the uncovertebral joints bilaterally.

- Place self-retaining retractor blades deep to the longus colli bilaterally and attach to the self-retaining retractor.
- For single-level discectomy distraction pins can be inserted. For multiple-level procedures or if screw fixation is planned the distraction pins are best avoided because of potential microfracture at the pin sites that will compromise screw purchase.
- Once all levels are adequately exposed use a No. 11 blade scalpel to remove the anterior anulus at each level cutting toward the midline from each uncovertebral joint.
- Remove the anulus with pituitary rongeurs and curets to allow exposure of each uncinate process, which appears as a slight upward curve of the endplate of the caudal segment. This marks the safe extent of lateral dissection avoiding the vertebral artery. Remove the anterior one half to two thirds of the disc at each level in this way.
- Use an operating microscope for safe removal of the posterior disc, osteophytes, or posterior longitudinal ligament as needed.

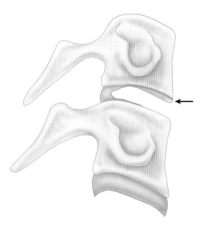

Figure 26-2

- With a high-speed burr remove the anterior lip of the cephalad vertebra to a level matching the subchondral bone at midbody level. This forms a completely flat surface and enhances visibility for removing the remaining disc material and the cartilaginous endplates to the level of the posterior longitudinal ligament (Figure 26-2).
- If preoperative imaging demonstrates a soft disc fragment and this is found without violation of the posterior longitudinal ligament further exploration of the canal is not warranted.
- If necessary perform foraminotomy to remove uncovertebral tissue with small Kerrison rongeurs. If a defect through the posterior longitudinal ligament is found enlarge it and explore the canal for additional fragments.
- If the surgical plan calls for complete removal of the posterior longitudinal ligament complete all corpectomies first.
- To perform the corpectomies use a high-speed burr to create a lateral gutter at the level of the uncinate process bilaterally that extends from one disc space to the next.
- Remove the midline bone to the same depth as the gutters and continue posteriorly until the brisk bleeding of cancellous bone gives way to cortical bone. Usually there will be significant bleeding from the posterior midpoint of the body that can be easily controlled with bipolar cautery once the cortical bone has been drilled away. Do not use unipolar cautery in close proximity to neural tissue.
- Thin the cortical bone with the high-speed burr and remove with angled curets or remove carefully with the burr. If necessary remove the posterior longitudinal ligament by lifting it anteriorly with a small blunt hook and opening the epidural space with a 1-mm Kerrison rongeur. This must be done with excellent visualization and care to avoid dural injury.
- After the epidural space is entered remove the posterior longitudinal ligament entirely if needed. If the canal is significantly compromised carefully free it from the underlying dura with blunt dissection.
- Perform foraminotomies at this time and remove osteophytes if necessary. A small blunt probe should pass easily anterolaterally after foraminotomy. Where possible preserve the posterior longitudinal ligament to enhance construct stability.
- Carefully prepare the adjacent endplates so that all cartilage is removed, subchondral bone is preserved, the entire decompression is the width of the endplate between the uncinate processes, and the endplates are parallel to one another.

- Carefully measure the anterior to posterior dimension at each endplate. The graft depth should be 3 to 4 mm less than the shorter of the two to allow the graft to be recessed 2 mm anteriorly and not compromise the spinal canal posteriorly. Carefully measure the length of graft needed in the cephalad to caudal dimension. Remember to measure with and without traction being applied through the head halter so that the graft will be under proper compression. Make sure at this point that the endplates are parallel to one another.

- Remove the disc laterally to allow visualization of the uncinate process bilaterally, which will appear as a slight upturning of the endplate and marks the safe extent of lateral decompression.

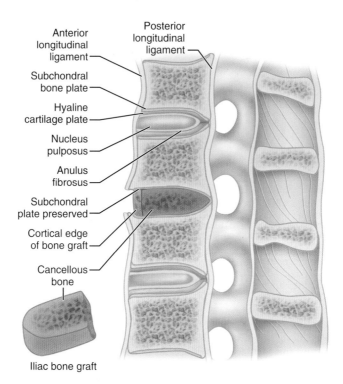

Figure 26-3 Iliac bone graft

- Obtain a tricortical iliac graft using a small oscillating saw (Figure 26-3).
- During preparation of the endplate take care to preserve the anterior cortex of the cephalad and caudal vertebrae.
- Fashion the bone graft to the appropriate depth. Position the graft with the cancellous surface directed posteriorly and bevel the cephalad and caudal posterior margins slightly to facilitate impaction. With traction applied impact the graft into place so that the cortical portion is recessed 1 to 2 mm posterior to the anterior cortex of the vertebral bodies. There should be 2 mm of free space between the posterior margin of the graft and the spinal canal. The graft should fit snugly even when traction is being applied.
- Release traction and check the fit of the graft using a Kocher clamp to grasp it. Repeat this procedure for each additional disc space.
- Apply anterior cervical plate instrumentation if necessary with all traction released. Various systems are available and should be placed according to the manufacturer's recommendations.
- Obtain intraoperative radiographs to verify graft and hardware positions.
- Close the platysmal layer over a soft closed-suction drain and close the skin and subcutaneous layers. Apply a thin dressing. Place the patient in a cervical orthosis before extubation.

POSTOPERATIVE CARE 〉

The patient is allowed to be out of bed later on the day of surgery or the next morning. The drain is removed on the first postoperative day. The cervical orthosis is continued 4 to 6 weeks for discectomy patients and 8 to 12 weeks for patients undergoing corpectomies depending on patient compliance and radiographic appearance of the graft. Occasionally a soft collar is helpful for an additional 1 or 2 weeks. Flexion and extension lateral cervical spine radiographs should reveal no evidence of motion at the fusion site and trabeculation should be present before discontinuation of the rigid cervical orthosis.

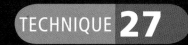
Indications for anterior disc excision and interbody fusion of the lumbar spine include (1) instability causing backache and sciatica, (2) spondylolisthesis of all types, (3) pain after multiple posterior explorations, and (4) failed posterior fusions.

- Administer general anesthesia and place the patient in the Trendelenburg position.
- Develop the retroperitoneal approach to the vertebral bodies and identify the psoas muscle, the iliac artery and vein, and the left ureter. If more than three interspaces are to be fused retract the ureter toward the left.
- Identify the sacral promontory by palpation.
- Inject saline solution under the prevertebral fascia over the lumbar vertebra and lift the sympathetic chain for easier dissection.
- Expose the lumbosacral disc space by retracting the left iliac artery and vein to the left.
- In exposing the fourth lumbar interspace displace the left artery and vein and ureter to the right side.
- Elevate the anterior longitudinal ligament as a flap with the base toward the left.
- Tag the flap with sutures and retract it to give additional protection to the vessels.
- Separate the intervertebral disc and anulus from the cartilaginous endplates of the vertebrae with a thin osteotome and remove them with pituitary rongeurs and large curets.
- Clean the space thoroughly back to the posterior longitudinal ligament without removing bone thereby keeping bleeding to a minimum until the site is ready for grafting.
- Remove the cartilaginous endplates from the vertebral bodies with an osteotome until bleeding bone is encountered.
- Cut shallow notches in the opposing surfaces of the vertebrae and measure the dimensions of the notches carefully with a caliper.

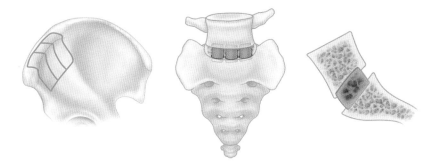

Figure 27-1

- Cut grafts from the iliac wing, making them larger than the notches for later firm impaction (Figure 27-1).
- Hyperextend the spine, insert multiple grafts, and relieve the hyperextension.
- Bipolar electrocautery is useful in obtaining hemostasis but take care not to coagulate the sympathetic fibers over the anterior aspect of the lumbosacral joint. Use of silver clips in this area is preferred.
- After completion of the fusion close all layers with absorbable sutures.
- Estimate the amount of blood lost and replace it.

POSTOPERATIVE CARE

Nasogastric suction may be necessary for gastric decompression for about 36 hours. Attention must be paid to mobilization of the lower extremities to prevent dependency and blood pooling. Thigh-length compression hose, intermittent compression boots, and low-molecular-weight heparin are all used for deep vein thrombosis prophylaxis. In-bed exercises with straight-leg raising are started on the first postoperative day and continued indefinitely. The patient is allowed to sit and walk with a low back corset used for postoperative immobilization as tolerated. Postoperative radiographs are made before discharge from the hospital to serve as a baseline for judging graft appearance. Three months later side-bending and flexion and extension radiographs are made in the standing position to provide information about the success of arthrodesis. Radiographs are then repeated at 6 and 12 months after surgery with the solid fusion not confirmed until 1 year after surgery. Tomograms may be useful in evaluating suspected pseudarthrosis.

MINIMALLY INVASIVE TRANSFORAMINAL LUMBAR INTERBODY FUSION (MITLIF)

Raymond J. Gardocki

Lumbar decompression and fusion is an essential procedure in the treatment of lumbar degenerative conditions such as degenerative spondylolisthesis. The goals of decompression and fusion are to (1) adequately decompress the neural elements and (2) stabilize the spinal segment, and to do so without damage to neural elements or surrounding structures.

Use of the microscope and tubular retractors allows minimally invasive transforaminal lumbar interbody fusions (MITLIF) to achieve decompression and stabilization while safely performing the procedure with less collateral damage to surrounding structures and the posterior dynamic stabilizers of the spine than with open procedures.

Because the surgical corridor required is minimal, the use of tubular retractors eliminates the need for traditional muscle-stripping techniques and preserves the form and function of the paraspinous musculature, which allows more normal physiologic function of the spine and sparing of the dynamic posterior stabilizers. Other advantages include reduced blood loss, less postoperative back pain, shorter time to ambulation, shorter hospital stay, and shorter duration of narcotic usage postoperatively compared to open approaches. Minimally invasive techniques also have been reported to result in significant reductions in total hospital costs compared with standard open techniques, and there is early evidence that adjacent segment degeneration may be decreased compared to open surgery.

- After induction of general endotracheal anesthesia position the patient prone on a radiolucent table. It is beneficial to place the microscope on the primary operative side of the patient and the C-arm on the opposite side of the table. This allows a quick lateral image when necessary during the operative procedure without having to move the microscope base, which adds significant time to the procedure.

- Obtain lateral and anteroposterior C-arm fluoroscopic images to ensure that the pedicles can be adequately imaged. It is helpful to note the three angles necessary for orthogonal views of the cephalad pedicles, disc space, and caudal pedicles for imaging later in the case.

- Insert a spinal needle into the paraspinal musculature with a trajectory that bisects the interspace of interest. The insertion site is typically 40 to 60 mm lateral to the midline depending on patient depth (the larger the patient, the more lateral the starting point) and will follow a trajectory that allows access to the entire disc space. The proper position will allow adequate discectomy and placement of the pedicle screws through the same skin incision. It should be confirmed with lateral fluoroscopy.

- The trajectory should approach the anterior and middle third of the disc space. Infiltrate the operative field (paraspinous muscle, subcutaneous tissue and skin) with 10 mL of 0.25% bupivacaine with epinephrine for preemptive analgesia as well as hemostasis. Remove the needle and make a 25-mm vertical incision at the puncture site.

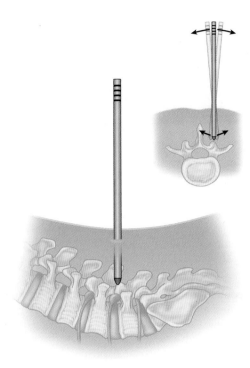

Figure 28-1

- Insert the blunt end of a guidewire through the incision and direct it toward the appropriate anatomy under fluoroscopic guidance. Advance the guidewire only through the lumbodorsal fascia. There is no need to use the sharp end of the guidewire or advance it down to bone because it can inadvertently penetrate the ligamentum flavum and puncture the dura (Figure 28-1).

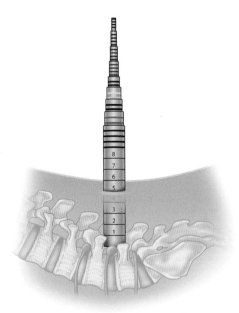

Figure 28-2

- Once the guidewire is through the fascia, advance the first pencil-shaped dilator through the fascia over the guidewire and use it to gently probe for the trailing edge of the cephalad lamina, which should feel like a bump at the end of the dilator. The guidewire can be removed as soon as the lumbodorsal fascia is pierced with the first dilator. Then use progressively larger dilators to create a muscle-sparing surgical corridor down to the appropriate interlaminar space while remaining orthogonal to the disc (Figure 28-2).

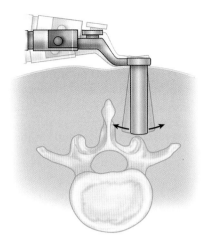

Figure 28-3

- Each dilator can be used as a curet to remove soft tissue attachments from the interlaminar space. The final tubular retractor is then mounted to a stationary arm attached to the table. A final fluoroscopic image confirms the location of the retractor orthogonal with the target disc space before bringing in the microscope and adjusting the field of view. We prefer 18-mm diameter tubular retractors depending on the size of the patient and the surgical level. Tubular retractors in the 20 to 24 mm diameter range can be used when first becoming familiar with this approach. If the interbody implant needed is taller than 12 mm, a 20-mm diameter tube minimum is required for passage of the implant. Dock the appropriate-length 18- or 20-mm tubular retractor on the facet joint complex and interlaminar space and attach it to the table-mounted retractor arm (Figure 28-3).

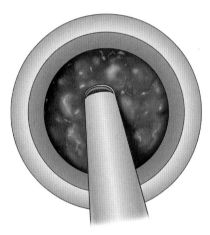

Figure 28-4

- With the use of an operating microscope, perform a total facetectomy with a high-speed drill (preferred) or osteotomes. The osteotomy is L-shaped and should connect the interlaminar space at the base of the spinous process with the pars interarticularis just above the disc space but below the pedicle. The location of the horizontal leg of the L-shaped osteotomy is always confirmed on lateral fluoroscopic image before the osteotomy is completed to ensure adequate exposure of the disc space and to prevent drilling into the cephalad pedicle. Once the facetectomy is complete, a slightly longer tubular retractor can be used for better visualization, since it can be advanced deep to the soft tissue envelope surrounding the facetectomy (Figure 28-4).
- If a contralateral decompression is necessary, perform an undercutting laminoplasty at this point, leaving the ipsilateral ligamentum flavum intact to protect the dura.
- Denude all removed bone of soft tissue and morcellize it for later use as interbody graft material.
- Once the inferior articular process of the cephalad vertebrae is removed and the contralateral decompression is completed as needed, use a curet to release the ipsilateral ligamentum flavum from the cephalad and caudal laminas.
- After the ligamentum flavum has been detached from the caudal edge of the superior lamina and the cephalad edge of the inferior lamina, use a blunt dissector to lift the edge of the ligamentum flavum so

that it can be excised with a Kerrison rongeur. Take care to orient the Kerrison rongeur parallel to the nerve root as much as possible. The goal when resecting the ligamentum flavum should be removal in one piece, which prevents nibbling away at it while trying to grab a mop end with a Kerrison rongeur. En bloc removal is facilitated by using the Kerrison rongeur to remove some bone along with the lateral edge of the ligamentum flavum from caudal to cephalad starting at the critical angle and working up the medial edge of the superior articular process where the ligamentum attaches.

- Amputate the superior articular process above the level of the corresponding pedicle with a drill (preferred) or osteotome, which completes the decompression of the ipsilateral foramen and lateral recess. A lateral fluoroscopic image at this point is helpful to prevent violation of the ipsilateral caudal pedicle.

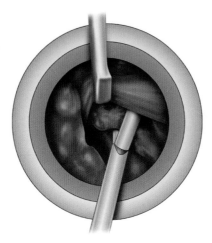

Figure 28-5

- Perform a subtotal discectomy by incising a box-shaped annulotomy with a no. 15 scalpel blade (a bayonet knife handle allows for direct visualization down the tube during the annulotomy) or pituitary rongeur lateral to the dural sac while retracting the traversing nerve root. There is no need to retract the exiting root; retraction can cause a postoperative radiculitis and dysesthesia in the distribution of the retracted dorsal root ganglion (Figure 28-5).

- With a combination of straight and angled instruments, remove all cartilage from the disc space and compressed cancellous bone endplates up to the outer anulus.

- Remove disc material from the cartilaginous endplate covering with shavers and curets. Scrape medially under the midline and gradually work laterally in a sweeping motion until both caudal and cephalad endplates are cleared of cartilage, exposing the compressed cancellous endplates of both vertebrae.

- Once the endplates are denuded, sequentially distract the disc space until adequate disc space height is obtained and the normal foraminal opening is restored. This can be done with endplate shavers, trials, or mechanical distractors depending on the system being used. Simple interbody distraction can reduce a listhesis when the outer annulus is tensioned evenly, analogous to soft tissue balancing in a total knee replacement.

- At this point, place a funnel into the disc space, which facilitates placement of bone graft or equivalent into the disc space without leakage into the epidural space. We always place the autogenous bone from the facet anteriorly into the disc space to allow for easier visualization of a sentinel sign on postoperative radiographs. The autogenous bone from the facet does not provide adequate graft volume for an interbody space and must be supplemented with allograft, autograft, or a bone-graft substitute of the surgeon's choosing.

- Once bone allograft is packed into the disc space, impact a trial one to two sizes smaller than the final interbody implant into the grafted disc space to create a path for the final implant.

- Insert an appropriately sized structural interbody graft/implant based on the distractors or trials. The structural implant material can be bone, polymer, or metal, but we prefer to use structural allograft when using bone allograft chips. Do not place a graft that is too long because it may increase the risk of later posterior displacement. A shorter implant allows the apex to be placed anterior to the midpoint of the disc space, which helps to restore lumbar lordosis.

- Countersink the graft until it is 3 to 5 mm below the posterior margin of the disc space and the apex is anterior to the midpoint of the disc space. Its position should be confirmed on lateral fluoroscopy.

- Probe the extradural space and foramina to ensure adequate decompression of the neural elements and remove any impinging structures. There is no concern for excessive resection of the posterior elements because a fusion is being performed.
- Once the graft is in place, confirm positioning on anteroposterior and lateral fluoroscopic images. If positioned adequately with adequate restoration of disc height and lordosis, place bilateral percutaneous pedicle screws to provide a stable environment for fusion across the disc space.

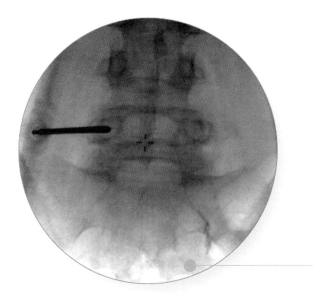

Figure 28-6

- Use anteroposterior and lateral images of the pedicle for cannulation with an appropriately sized Jamshidi needle using a "pencil-in-cup" technique (Figure 28-6). We prefer to use a larger diameter Jamshidi needle (Kyphon, Memphis TN) for pedicle cannulation and guidewire placement, which allows placing cannulated pedicle screws without the need to tap the bone. The slightly larger hole made by the larger diameter needle allows the first threads of self-tapping pedicle screws to grab and advance the screw. Eliminating the need to tap the bone saves surgical time and eliminates a potential source of complication when dealing with the guide-wires. The remaining technique varies depending on the hardware manufacturer.
- Once all hardware is adequately placed, manually palpate the posterior instrumentation and lumbodorsal fascia to confirm there is no fascia or paraspinous musculature trapped beneath the instrumentation, which could cause a paraspinous compartment syndrome. Close the incisions subcutaneously with 2-0 Vicryl and use skin glue for final skin closure. No additional bandages are needed with the skin glue, and patients are allowed to shower on the day of surgery. When a 22-mm or smaller tube is used there is no need for fascial closure

POSTOPERATIVE CARE ⟩

Patients are encouraged to walk as much as possible immediately after surgery. Bending, lifting, and twisting are restricted for 3 months. All activity restrictions are lifted at 3 months if radiographs show appropriate progression of fusion.

In this technique the facets, pars interarticularis, and bases of the transverse processes are fused with chip grafts, and a large graft is placed posterior on the transverse processes. It allows exposure for posterolateral fusion without much need for soft tissue retraction.

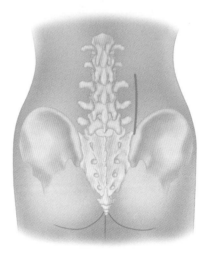

Figure 29-1

- Make a longitudinal skin incision along the lateral border of the paraspinal muscles, curving it medially at the distal end across the posterior crest of the ilium (Figure 29-1). Alternatively, a single midline skin incision can be used with bilateral fascial incisions.

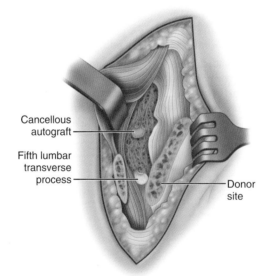

Cancellous autograft

Fifth lumbar transverse process

Donor site

Figure 29-2

- Divide the lumbodorsal fascia and establish the plane of cleavage between the border of the paraspinal muscles and the fascia overlying the transversus abdominis muscle (Figure 29-2). The tips of the transverse processes can now be palpated in the depths of the wound.
- Release the iliac attachment of the muscles with an osteotome, taking a thin layer of ilium. Continue the exposure of the posterior crest of the ilium by subperiosteal dissection, and remove the crest almost flush with the sacroiliac joint, taking enough bone to provide one or two grafts. Removal of the iliac crest increases exposure of the spine.

- Retract the sacrospinalis muscle toward the midline and denude the transverse processes of the dorsal muscle and ligamentous attachments; expose the articular facets by excising the joint capsule.
- Remove the cartilage from the facets with an osteotome and level the area down to allow the graft to fit snugly against the facets, pars interarticularis, and base of the transverse process at each level.
- Comminute the facets with a small gouge or osteotome and turn bone chips up and down from the facet area, upper sacral area, and transverse processes.

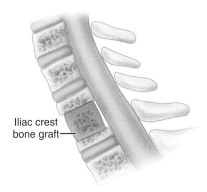

Iliac crest
bone graft

Figure 29-3

- Split the resected iliac crest longitudinally into two grafts. Shape one to fit into the prepared bed, and impact it firmly in place with its cut surface against the spine. Preserve the remaining graft for use on the opposite side with or without additional bone from the other iliac crest (Figure 29-3).
- Pack additional ribbons and chips of cancellous bone from the ilium about the graft.
- Allow the paraspinal muscles to fall in position over the fusion area, and close the wound.

POSTOPERATIVE CARE ⟩

We routinely use closed-wound suction for 12 to 36 hours, with removal of the suction device mandatory by 48 hours. Depending on the level of the arthrodesis, the age of the patient, and the presence or absence of internal fixation, walking is allowed in 24 to 48 hours when pain permits. For obese patients, all types of external fixation or support will probably be inadequate and limitation of activity may be the only reasonable alternative. The appropriateness of bracing remains controversial. Generally, for fusions with marked preoperative instability (e.g., burst fractures), rigid bracing is continued for 12 weeks. For fusions without marked instability (e.g., degenerative spondylolisthesis), bracing if used is generally less rigid and of shorter duration.

MICROSCOPIC LUMBAR DISCECTOMY

Raymond J. Gardocki

See also Video 30-1.

Microscopic lumbar discectomy (MLD) has replaced the standard open laminectomy as the procedure of choice for herniated lumbar discs despite the fact that there is no significant demonstrable difference in long-term outcome. MLD allows better lighting, magnification, and angle of view with a much smaller exposure that causes less soft tissue collateral damage. MLD has become the gold standard because of the limited dissection required, which produces less postoperative pain and a shorter postoperative stay, and it can be reliably performed on an outpatient basis.

- MLD requires a binocular operating microscope, a variety of small-angled Kerrison rongeurs of appropriate length, a high-speed drill, and microinstruments including curets, pituitary rongeurs, dissectors, and preferably a combination suction/nerve root retractor.

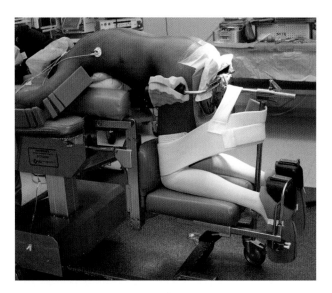

Figure 30-1

- The procedure is performed with the patient prone. A specialized bed such as an Andrews table can be used. There are advantages to using this bed despite the nuisance it causes during positioning: (1) it allows the belly to hang free where venous blood will pool, which results in decreased venous epidural bleeding intraoperatively; (2) the knee-chest position maximizes the lumbar kyphosis, placing the ligamentum flavum on slight tension that allows for easier removal but also opens the interlaminar space, which may provide greater canal access with less bone removal; (3) the small footprint of the bed enables the operating microscope to be placed at the foot, which not only makes access to the ocular lens easier for both the surgeon and assistant standing on opposite sides of the table, but also allows the fluoroscope to be moved into the surgical field for imaging without having to move the microscope base itself (Figure 30-1).

- Alternatively, the patient can be positioned on a Wilson frame or even on chest rolls using a flat top or standard operating room bed. The microscope can be used from skin incision to closure or it can be brought in after the initial dissection is done under direct vision. A lateral radiograph is taken to confirm the level, but fluoroscopy is much quicker when used for localization. Fluoroscopy is essential for localization when using tubular retractors because the field of view is smaller, making the available margin for error in placing the skin incision less.

APPROACH FOR USE OF A MCCULLOCH RETRACTOR ⟩

- Infiltrate the operative field (paraspinous muscle, subcutaneous tissue and skin) with 10 mL of 0.25% bupivacaine with epinephrine for preemptive analgesia as well as hemostasis.

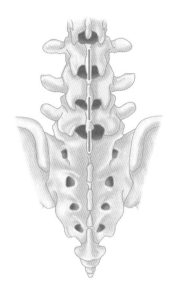

Figure 30-2

- Make the incision from the midspinous process of the upper vertebra to the superior margin of the spinous process of the lower vertebra at the involved level. This usually results in a 1-inch (25 to 30 mm) skin incision. This incision may need to be moved slightly higher for higher lumbar levels (Figure 30-2).
- Maintain meticulous hemostasis with electrocautery as the dissection is carried to the fascia.
- Incise the fascia at the midline using electrocautery. Insert a periosteal elevator in the midline incision. Using gentle lateral movements elevate the deep fascia and muscle subperiosteally from the spinous processes and lamina on the involved side only.
- Obtain a lateral radiograph with a metal clamp attached to the spinous process to verify the level.
- With a Cobb elevator gently sweep the remaining muscular attachments off in a lateral direction to expose the interlaminar space and the edge of each lamina. A sharp elevator makes this task easier. Meticulously cauterize all bleeding points.
- Insert the appropriate length McCullough style retractor with the shorter spike medial and the flat blade lateral into the wound and adjust the microscope. Shaving down the flat blades of the McCullough to produce a narrower retractor can help to minimize the incision size and collateral soft tissue damage.

APPROACH FOR USE OF TUBULAR RETRACTOR

- Alternatively, the approach can be done using a tubular retractor, which further minimizes damage to the paraspinal muscles and prevents detachment of the lumbodorsal fascia from the supraspinous ligament. A curved drill is required for visualization when drilling bone through the tubular retractor because of the narrower operating corridor.
- With fluoroscopic guidance, place an 18-gauge needle through the skin and into the paraspinous muscles with a trajectory toward the target disc space, approximately the radius of the final retractor diameter away from the edge of the spinous process (e.g., 9 mm off the edge of the spinous process if the ultimate tubular retractor diameter will be 18 mm) to prevent conflict between the spinous process and tubular retractor. It is essential that the needle be orthogonal with the target disc space, since it will be used to define the center of the tubular approach. Typically it is best to place the needle in line with the superior endplate of the caudal vertebral body, but that will depend on the type of herniation and its location.
- Infiltrate the operative field (paraspinous muscle, subcutaneous tissue and skin) with 10 mL of 0.25% bupivacaine with epinephrine for preemptive analgesia as well as hemostasis.
- Make a 20-mm long incision centered on the needle stick and place the blunt end of the guidewire just through the lumbodorsal fascia. The younger and more fit the patient, the more force necessary to pop the blunt end of the guidewire through the fascia. There is no need to use the sharp end of the guidewire or to advance the guidewire down to bone, since it is very easy to pierce the interlaminar space and dural sac with the guidewire.
- Once the guidewire is through the fascia, advance the first pencil-shaped dilator through the fascia over the guidewire and use it to gently probe for the trailing edge of the cephalad lamina, which should feel like a bump at the end of the dilator. The guidewire can be removed as soon as the lumbodorsal fascia is pierced with the first dilator.

- Sequentially dilate down to bone with enlarging tubular retractors to expose the interlaminar space. Each dilator can be used as a curet to remove soft tissue attachments from the interlaminar space.
- Mount the final tubular retractor to a stationary arm attached to the table and obtain a final fluoroscopic image to confirm the location of the retractor orthogonal with the target disc space before bringing in the microscope and adjusting the field of view. We prefer 14 to 16 mm diameter tubular retractors for this approach depending on the size of the patient and the level of surgical experience with this technique. Tubular retractors in the 18 to 24 mm diameter range can be used when first becoming familiar with this approach.

From this point on, the surgical technique is essentially the same for both approaches.

- Identify the ligamentum flavum and lamina. Use a curet to elevate the superficial leaf of the ligamentum flavum from the leading edge of the caudal lamina.
- Use a Kerrison rongeur to resect the superficial leaf of the ligamentum flavum to allow identification of the critical angle, which is the junction of the leading edge of the caudal lamina and the medial edge of the superior articular process. Identifying the critical angle is essential in primary MLD because it has a constant relationship to the corresponding pedicle, traversing nerve root, and target disc. The pedicle is always just lateral to the critical angle, the traversing nerve is always just medial to the pedicle, and the disc of interest is always just cephalad to the critical angle and pedicle. It sometimes is necessary to drill the medial aspect of the inferior articular process to allow adequate visualization of the critical angle.
- Use a high-speed drill to remove the trailing edge of the cephalad lamina up to the insertion of the ligamentum flavum to allow easier and more complete removal of the ligament, remembering that the ligament attaches to the lamina more inferiorly as you move medially. This makes initially detaching the ligament from the undersurface of the cephalad lamina with an angled curette much easier toward the midline.

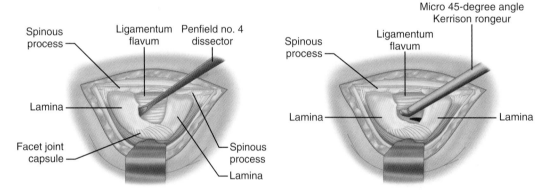

Figure 30-3

- After the lateral portion of the ligamentum flavum has been detached from the caudal edge of the superior lamina and the cephalad edge of the inferior lamina using a curet, use a blunt dissector to lift the edge of the ligamentum flavum so that it can be excised with a Kerrison rongeur. Take care to orient the Kerrison rongeur parallel to the nerve root as much as possible. The goal when resecting the ligamentum flavum should be removal in one piece, which prevents nibbling away at it while trying to grab a mop end with the Kerrison rongeur. En bloc removal is facilitated by using the rongeur to remove some bone along with the lateral edge of the ligamentum flavum from caudal to cephalad, starting at the critical angle and working up the medial edge of the superior articular process where the ligamentum attaches (Figure 30-3).
- Once the ligamentum flavum is removed, the medial wall of the corresponding pedicle should be palpable with a nerve hook or angled dissector. If not, more bone may need to be removed lateral to the critical angle. Once the medial wall of the corresponding pedicle is identified, the traversing nerve can be found just medial to it and the target disc can be found just cephalad to it.
- When the nerve root is identified, carefully mobilize the root medially. Gently dissect the nerve free from the disc fragment to avoid excessive traction on the root. Bipolar cautery for hemostasis is very helpful. When mobilized, retract the root medially. If the root is difficult to mobilize consider that a conjoined root may be present.
- Make a gentle extradural exploration beneath the nerve using a 90-degree blunt hook taking care not to tear the dura. The small opening and magnification can make the edge of the dural sac appear to be the nerve root.

- When using bipolar cautery ensure that only one side is in contact with the nerve root to avoid thermal injury to the nerve. Epidural fat is not removed in this procedure.
- Insert the suction/nerve root retractor with its tip turned medially under the nerve root and hold the manifold between the thumb and index finger. With the nerve root retracted the disc now is visible as a white, fibrous, avascular structure. Small tears may be visible in the anulus under magnification.

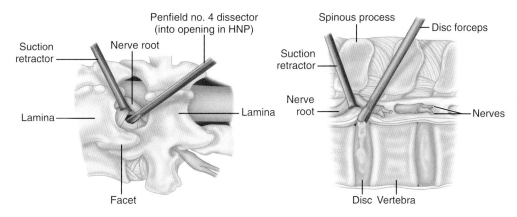

Figure 30-4

- Enlarge the annular tear with a Penfield no. 4 dissector and remove the disc material with the appropriate sized pituitary rongeur. Do not insert the instrument into the disc space beyond the angle of the jaws, usually about 15 mm, to minimize the risk of anterior perforation and vascular injury. Downward pressure on the adjacent intact annulus can sometimes help express loose disc fragment from the sub-annular space (Figure 30-4).
- Remove the exposed disc material. Remove additional loose disc or cartilage fragments. Inspect the root and adjacent dura for disc fragments. Forcefully irrigate the disc space using a Luer-Lok syringe and an unused #8 suction tip inserted into the disc space. Maintain meticulous hemostasis.
- The discectomy is complete when (1) the lateral recess is adequately decompressed; (2) the 90-degree dissector can be probed to the back of the cephalad vertebral body, the disc space, and the back of the caudal vertebral body out to the midline without any protrusions into the canal; (3) the 90-degree dissector can be spun (helicopter maneuver) beneath the traversing nerve root without any restrictions; and (4) the traversing nerve root is freely retractable both medially and laterally. It is comforting to see the dura pulsate with the heartbeat and expand and contract with respiration but these findings alone do not indicate an adequate discectomy and decompression.
- If the expected pathological process is not found, review preoperative imaging studies for the correct level and side. Also obtain a repeat radiograph or fluoroscopic image with a metallic marker at the disc level to verify the level. Be aware of bony anomalies that may alter the numbering of the vertebrae on imaging studies.
- Close the fascia and the skin in the usual fashion using absorbable sutures if using the McCullough retractor. When using a tubular retractor, it can simply be removed and the skin closed subcutaneously because the lumbodorsal fascia will seal itself like Chinese finger cuffs when the paraspinous muscles contract, since the lumbodorsal fascia was only dilated between its fibers and not incised.

POSTOPERATIVE CARE 〉

Postoperative care is similar to that after standard open disc surgery. Typically this procedure is done on an outpatient basis. Injecting the paraspinal muscles on the involved side with bupivacaine 0.25% with epinephrine at the beginning of the procedure and additional bupivacaine at the conclusion aids patient mobilization immediately postoperatively. We prefer to use a skin glue product for final skin closure without the use of a dressing and allow the patient to shower the day of the surgery. Activity can be allowed as tolerated once the skin incision is healed (typically 2 weeks).

Raymond J. Gardocki • Ashley L. Park

Information obtained from epidural injections in the cervical, thoracic, and lumbosacral spine can be helpful in confirming pain generators that are responsible for a patient's discomfort; they also can help manage pain and alleviate or decrease the need for oral analgesics. We perform epidural injections in a fluoroscopy suite equipped with resuscitative and monitoring equipment. Fluoroscopic guidance is essential to avoid needle misplacement.

INTERLAMINAR CERVICAL EPIDURAL INJECTION 〉

- Place the patient prone on a pain management table. We use a low-attenuated carbon fiber tabletop that allows better imaging and permits unobstructed C-arm viewing. For optimal placement and comfort place the patient's face in a cervical prone cutout cushion.

- Cervical epidural injections using a paramedian approach should be done routinely at the C7-T1 interspace unless previous surgery of the posterior cervical spine has been done at that level, in which case the C6-7 or T1-2 level is injected. Aseptically prepare the skin area with isopropyl alcohol and povidone-iodine several segments above and below the laminar interspace to be injected. If the patient is allergic to povidone-iodine use chlorhexidine gluconate (Hibiclens).

- Drape the area in sterile fashion.

- Using anteroposterior fluoroscopic imaging identify the target laminar interspace. With the use of a 27-gauge, $\frac{1}{4}$-inch needle, anesthetize the skin so that a skin wheal is raised over the target interspace on the side of the patient's pain with 1 to 2 mL of 1% preservative-free lidocaine without epinephrine. To diminish the burning discomfort of the anesthetic mix 3 mL of 8.4% sodium bicarbonate in a 30-mL bottle of 1% preservative-free lidocaine without epinephrine. Nick the skin with an 18-gauge hypodermic needle. Under fluoroscopic control insert and advance a 22-gauge, $3\frac{1}{2}$-inch spinal needle in a vertical fashion until contact is made with the upper edge of the T1 lamina 1 to 2 mm lateral to the midline.

- Anesthetize the lamina with 1 to 2 mL of 1% preservative-free lidocaine without epinephrine. Anesthetize the soft tissues with 2 mL of 1% preservative-free lidocaine without epinephrine as the spinal needle is withdrawn.

- Insert an 18-gauge, $3\frac{1}{2}$-inch Tuohy epidural needle and advance it vertically within the anesthetized soft tissue track until contact is made with the T1 lamina under fluoroscopy.

- "Walk off" the lamina with the Tuohy needle onto the ligamentum flavum. Remove the stylet from the Tuohy needle and attach a 10-mL syringe filled halfway with air and sterile saline. Advance the Tuohy needle into the epidural space using the loss-of-resistance technique. When loss of resistance has been achieved, aspirate to check for blood or cerebral spinal fluid (CSF). If neither blood nor CSF is evident remove the syringe from the Tuohy needle and attach a 5-mL syringe containing 1.5 mL of nonionic contrast dye.

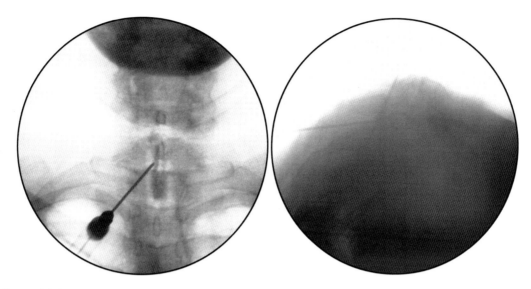

Figure 31-1

- Confirm epidural placement by producing an epidurogram with the nonionic contrast agent. To confirm proper placement further, adjust the C-arm to view the area from a lateral perspective. A spot radiograph can be obtained to document placement (Figure 31-1).

- Inject a test dose of 1 to 2 mL of 1% preservative-free lidocaine without epinephrine and wait 3 minutes. If the patient does not complain of warmth, burning, or significant paresthesias, or show signs of apnea, place a 10-mL syringe on the Tuohy needle and slowly inject 2 mL of 1% preservative-free lidocaine without epinephrine and 2 mL of 6 mg/mL Celestone Soluspan slowly into the epidural space. If Celestone Soluspan cannot be obtained 40 mg/mL of triamcinolone is a good substitute.

INTERLAMINAR THORACIC EPIDURAL INJECTION 〉

- A paramedian rather than a midline approach is used because of the angulation of the spinous processes.

- Place the patient prone on a pain management table. The preparation of the patient and equipment are identical to that used for interlaminar cervical epidural injections. Aseptically prepare the skin area several segments above and below the interspace to be injected. Drape the area in sterile fashion.

- Identify the target laminar interspace using anteroposterior fluoroscopic guidance.

- Anesthetize the skin over the target interspace on the side of the patient's pain. Under fluoroscopic control, insert and advance a 22-gauge, $3\frac{1}{2}$-inch spinal needle to the superior edge of the target lamina. Anesthetize the lamina and the soft tissues as the spinal needle is withdrawn.

- Mark the skin with an 18-gauge hypodermic needle and insert an 18-gauge, $3\frac{1}{2}$-inch Tuohy epidural needle, advancing it at a 50- to 60-degree angle to the axis of the spine and a 15- to 30-degree angle toward the midline until contact with the lamina is made. To view the thoracic interspace better, position the C-arm so that the fluoroscopy beam is in the same plane as the Tuohy epidural needle.

- "Walk off" the lamina with the Tuohy needle into the ligamentum flavum. Remove the stylet from the Tuohy needle and using the loss-of-resistance technique, advance it into the epidural space. When loss of resistance has been achieved aspirate to check for blood or CSF. If neither blood nor CSF is evident, inject 1.5 mL of nonionic contrast dye to confirm epidural placement.

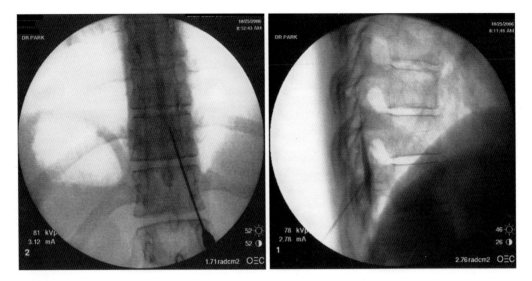

Figure 31-2

- To confirm proper placement further, adjust the C-arm to view the area from a lateral projection. A spot radiograph or epidurogram can be obtained. Inject 2 mL of 1% preservative-free lidocaine without epinephrine and 2 mL of 6 mg/mL Celestone Soluspan slowly into the epidural space (Figure 31-2).

INTERLAMINAR LUMBAR EPIDURAL INJECTION ⟩

- Place the patient prone on a pain management table. Aseptically prepare the skin area with isopropyl alcohol and povidone-iodine several segments above and below the laminar interspace to be injected. Drape the area in a sterile fashion.
- Under anteroposterior fluoroscopy guidance identify the target laminar interspace. Using a 27-gauge, $\frac{1}{4}$-inch needle anesthetize the skin over the target interspace on the side of the patient's pain with 1 to 2 mL of 1% preservative-free lidocaine without epinephrine.
- Insert a 22-gauge, $3\frac{1}{2}$-inch spinal needle vertically until contact is made with the upper edge of the inferior lamina at the target interspace 1 to 2 cm lateral to the caudal tip of the inferior spinous process under fluoroscopy. Anesthetize the lamina with 2 mL of 1% preservative-free lidocaine without epinephrine. Anesthetize the soft tissue with 2 mL of 1% lidocaine as the spinal needle is withdrawn.
- Nick the skin with an 18-gauge hypodermic needle, and insert a 17-gauge, $3\frac{1}{2}$-inch Tuohy epidural needle and advance it vertically within the anesthetized soft tissue track until contact with the lamina has been made under fluoroscopy.
- "Walk off" the lamina with the Tuohy needle onto the ligamentum flavum. Remove the stylet from the Tuohy needle, and attach a 10-mL syringe filled halfway with air and sterile saline to the Tuohy needle. Advance the Tuohy needle into the epidural space using the loss-of-resistance technique. Avoid lateral needle placement to decrease the likelihood of encountering an epidural vein or adjacent nerve root. Remove the stylet when loss of resistance has been achieved. Aspirate to check for blood or CSF. If neither blood nor CSF is present remove the syringe from the Tuohy needle and attach a 5-mL syringe containing 2 mL of nonionic contrast dye.

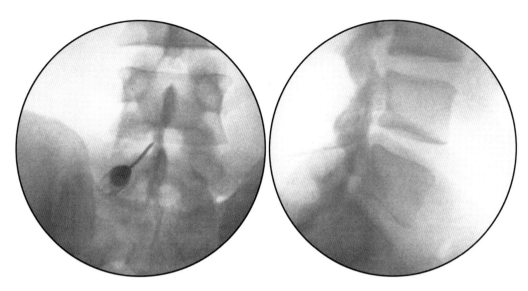

Figure 31-3

- Confirm epidural placement by producing an epidurogram with the nonionic contrast agent. A spot radiograph can be taken to document placement (Figure 31-3).
- Remove the 5-mL syringe and place on the Tuohy needle a 10-mL syringe containing 2 mL of 1% preservative-free lidocaine and 2 mL of 6 mg/mL Celestone Soluspan. Inject the corticosteroid preparation slowly into the epidural space.

TRANSFORAMINAL LUMBAR AND SACRAL EPIDURAL INJECTION 〉

- Place the patient prone on a pain management table. Aseptically prepare the skin area with isopropyl alcohol and povidone-iodine several segments above and below the interspace to be injected. Drape the area in sterile fashion.
- Under anteroposterior fluoroscopic guidance identify the target interspace. Anesthetize the soft tissues over the lateral border and midway between the two adjacent transverse processes at the target interspace.
- Insert a 22-gauge, 4¾-inch spinal needle and advance it within the anesthetized soft tissue track under fluoroscopy until contact is made with the lower edge of the superior transverse process near its junction with the superior articular process.
- Retract the spinal needle 2 to 3 mm and redirect it toward the base of the appropriate pedicle. Advance it slowly to the 6-o'clock position of the pedicle under fluoroscopy. Adjust the C-arm to a lateral projection to confirm the position and then return the C-arm to the anteroposterior view.

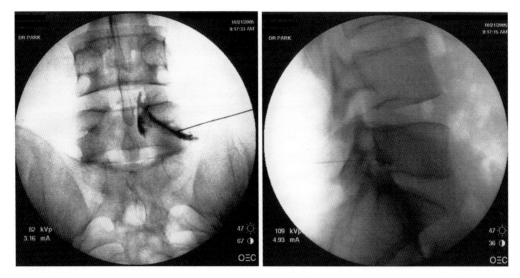

Figure 31-4

- Remove the stylet. Inject 1 mL of nonionic contrast agent slowly to produce a perineurosheathogram. After an adequate dye pattern is observed, inject slowly a 2-mL volume containing 1 mL of 0.75% preservative-free bupivacaine and 1 mL of 6 mg/mL Celestone Soluspan (Figure 31-4).
- The S1 nerve root also can be injected using the transforaminal approach.
- Place the patient prone on the pain management table.
- After appropriate aseptic preparation direct the C-arm so that the fluoroscopy beam is in a cephalocaudad and lateral-to-medial direction so that the anterior and posterior S1 foramina are aligned.
- Anesthetize the soft tissues and the dorsal aspect of the sacrum with 2 to 3 mL of 1% preservative-free lidocaine without epinephrine. Insert a 22-gauge, $3\frac{1}{2}$-inch spinal needle and advance it within the anesthetized soft tissue track under fluoroscopy until contact is made with posterior sacral bone slightly lateral and inferior to the S1 pedicle. "Walk" the spinal needle off the sacrum into the posterior S1 foramen to the medial edge of the pedicle.

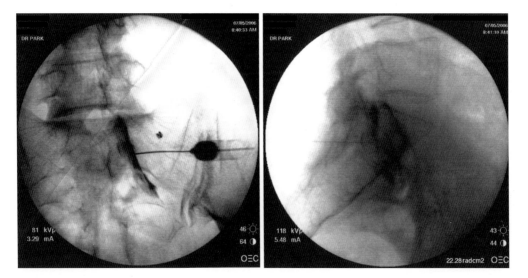

Figure 31-5

- Adjust the C-arm to a lateral projection to confirm the position and return it to the anteroposterior view.
- Remove the stylet. Inject 1 mL of nonionic contrast slowly to produce a perineurosheathogram. After an adequate dye pattern of the S1 nerve root is obtained insert a 2-mL volume containing 1 mL of 0.75% preservative-free bupivacaine and 1 mL of 6 mg/mL Celestone Soluspan (Figure 31-5).

CAUDAL SACRAL EPIDURAL INJECTION

- Place the patient prone on a pain management table. Aseptically prepare the skin area from the lumbosacral junction to the coccyx with isopropyl alcohol and povidone-iodine. Drape the area in sterile fashion.

- Try to identify by palpation the sacral hiatus, which is located between the two horns of the sacral cornua. The sacral hiatus can be best observed by directing the fluoroscopic beam laterally.

- Anesthetize the soft tissues and the dorsal aspect of the sacrum with 2 to 3 mL of 1% preservative-free lidocaine without epinephrine. Keep the C-arm positioned so that the fluoroscopic beam remains lateral.

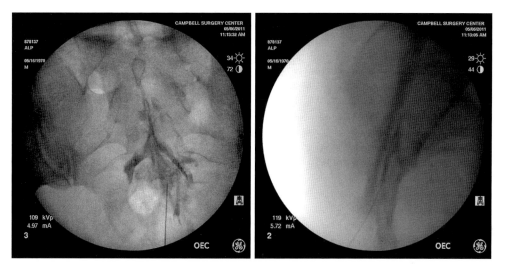

Figure 31-6

- Insert a 22-gauge, 3½-inch spinal needle between the sacral cornua at about 45 degrees with the bevel of the spinal needle facing ventrally until contact with the sacrum is made. Using fluoroscopic guidance redirect the spinal needle more cephalad, horizontal and parallel to the table advancing it into the sacral canal through the sacrococcygeal ligament and into the epidural space (Figure 31-6).

- Remove the stylet. Aspirate to check for blood or CSF. If neither blood nor CSF is evident inject 2 mL of nonionic contrast dye to confirm placement. Move the C-arm into the anteroposterior position and look for the characteristic "Christmas tree" pattern of epidural flow. If a vascular pattern is seen reposition the spinal needle and confirm epidural placement with nonionic contrast dye.

- When the correct contrast pattern is obtained slowly inject a 10-mL volume containing 3 mL of 1% preservative-free lidocaine without epinephrine, 3 mL of 6 mg/mL Celestone Soluspan, and 4 mL of sterile normal saline.

FACET BLOCK INJECTIONS: CERVICAL, LUMBAR, SACROILIAC JOINT

 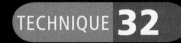

Raymond J. Gardocki • Ashley L. Park

Fluoroscopically guided facet joint injections are commonly considered the gold standard for isolating or excluding the facet joint as a source of spine or extremity pain. They also may help focus treatment on a specific spinal segment and provide adequate pain relief to allow progression in therapy.

CERVICAL MEDIAL BRANCH BLOCK INJECTION 〉

- Place the patient prone on the pain management table. Rotate the patient's neck so that the symptomatic side is down. This allows the vertebral artery to be positioned farther beneath the articular pillar, creates greater accentuation of the cervical waists, and prevents the jaw from being superimposed. Aseptically prepare and drape the side to be injected.

- Identify the target location using anteroposteriorly directed fluoroscopy. Each cervical facet joint from C3-4 to C7-T1 is supplied from the medial nerve branch above and below the joint that curves consistently around the "waist" of the articular pillar of the same numbered vertebrae. To block the C6 facet joint nerve supply anesthetize the C6 and C7 medial branches.

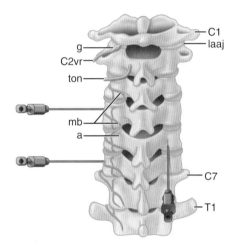

Figure 32-1

- Proper needle placement for a posterior approach to C4 and C6 medial branch blocks (Figure 32-1). Second cervical ganglion (g), third occipital nerve (ton), C2 ventral ramus (C2vr), and lateral atlantoaxial joint (laaj) are noted. a, articular facet; mb, medial branch.

- Insert a 22- or 25-gauge, 3½-inch spinal needle perpendicular to the pain management table and advance it under fluoroscopic control ventrally and medially until contact is made with periosteum. Direct the spinal needle laterally until the needle tip reaches the lateral margin of the waist of the articular pillar and then direct the needle until it rests at the deepest point of the articular pillar's concavity under fluoroscopy.

- Remove the stylet. If there is a negative aspirate inject 0.5 mL of 0.75% preservative-free bupivacaine.

LUMBAR INTRAARTICULAR INJECTION 〉

- Place the patient prone on a pain management table. Aseptically prepare and drape the patient.

- Under fluoroscopic guidance identify the target segment to be injected. Upper lumbar facet joints are oriented in the sagittal (vertical) plane and often can be seen on direct anteroposterior views whereas the lower lumbar facet joints, especially at L5-S1, are obliquely oriented and require an ipsilateral oblique rotation of the C-arm to be seen.

- Position the C-arm under fluoroscopy until the joint silhouette first appears. Insert and advance a 22- or 25-gauge, 3½-inch spinal needle toward the target joint along the axis of the fluoroscopy beam until contact is made with the articular processes of the joint. Enter the joint cavity through the softer capsule, and advance the needle only a few millimeters. Capsular penetration is perceived as a subtle change of resistance. If midpoint needle entry is difficult redirect the spinal needle to the superior or inferior joint recesses.

- Confirm placement with less than 0.1 mL of nonionic contrast dye with a 3-mL syringe to minimize injection pressure under fluoroscopic guidance. When intraarticular placement has been verified inject a total volume of 1 mL of injectant (local anesthetic with or without corticosteroids) into the joint.

LUMBAR MEDIAL BRANCH BLOCK INJECTION 〉

- Place the patient prone on a pain management table. Aseptically prepare and drape the area to be injected.
- Because there is dual innervation of each lumbar facet joint two medial branch blocks are required. The medial branches cross the transverse processes below their origin. The L4-5 facet joint is anesthetized by blocking the L3 medial branch at the transverse process of L4 and the L4 medial branch at the transverse process of L5. In the case of the L5-S1 facet joint anesthetize the L4 medial branch as it passes over the L5 transverse process and the L5 medial branch as it passes across the sacral ala.

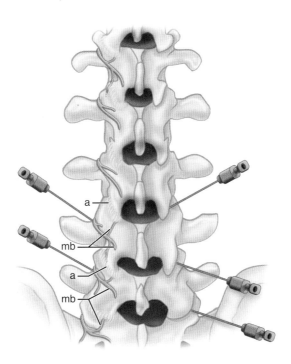

Figure 32-2

- Posterior view of lumbar spine (Figure 32-2) shows the location of the medial branches (mb) of the dorsal rami, which innervate lumbar facet joints (a). Needle position for L3 and L4 medial branch blocks shown on left half of diagram would be used to anesthetize the L4-5 facet joint. Right half of diagram shows L3-4, L4-5, and L5-S1 intraarticular facet joint injection positions.
- Using anteroposterior fluoroscopic imaging identify the target transverse process. For L1 through L4 medial branch blocks penetrate the skin using a 22- or 25-gauge, 3½-inch spinal needle lateral and superior to the target location.
- Under fluoroscopic guidance advance the spinal needle until contact is made with the dorsal superior and medial aspects of the base of the transverse process so that the needle rests against the periosteum. To ensure optimal spinal needle placement reposition the C-arm so that the fluoroscopy beam is ipsilateral oblique and the "Scotty dog" is seen. Position the spinal needle in the middle of the "eye" of the Scotty dog. Slowly inject (over 30 seconds) 0.5 mL of 0.75% bupivacaine.
- To inject the L5 medial branch (more correctly, the L5 dorsal ramus) position the patient prone on the pain management table with the fluoroscopic beam in the anteroposterior projection.
- Identify the sacral ala. Rotate the C-arm 15 to 20 degrees ipsilateral obliquely to maximize exposure between the junction of the sacral ala and the superior process of S1. Insert a 22- or 25-gauge, 3½-inch

spinal needle directly into the osseous landmarks approximately 5 mm below the superior junction of the sacral ala with the superior articular process of the sacrum under fluoroscopy. Rest the spinal needle on the periosteum and position the bevel of the spinal needle medial and away from the foramen to minimize flow through the L5 or S1 foramen. Slowly inject 0.5 mL of 0.75% bupivacaine.

SACROILIAC JOINT INJECTION 〉

- Place the patient prone on a pain management table. Aseptically prepare and drape the side to be injected. Rotate the C-arm until the medial (posterior) joint line is seen.
- Use a 27-gauge, ¼-inch needle to anesthetize the skin of the buttock 1 to 3 cm inferior to the lowest aspect of the joint. Using fluoroscopy, insert a 22-gauge, 3½-inch spinal needle until the needle rests 1 cm above the most posteroinferior aspect of the joint (Fig. 32-3). A larger spinal needle may be required with obese patients. Advance the spinal needle into the sacroiliac joint until capsular penetration occurs.

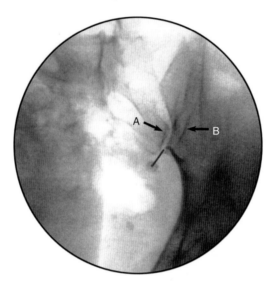

Figure 32-3

- Sacroiliac joint injection showing medial (*A*) and lateral (*B*) joint planes (silhouettes) (Figure 32-3).

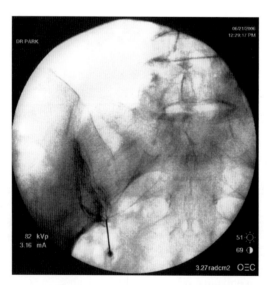

Figure 32-4

- Confirm intraarticular placement under fluoroscopy with 0.5 mL of nonionic contrast dye. A spot radiograph can be taken to document placement. Inject a 2-mL volume containing 1 mL of 0.75% preservative-free bupivacaine and 1 mL of 6 mg/mL Celestone Soluspan into the joint (Figure 32-4).

ANKLE ARTHROSCOPY
Susan N. Ishikawa

The current most common indications for ankle arthroscopy include soft tissue or bony impingement and treatment of osteochondral lesions of the talus; it also has been used to treat ankle instability, septic arthritis, arthrofibrosis, and loose bodies.

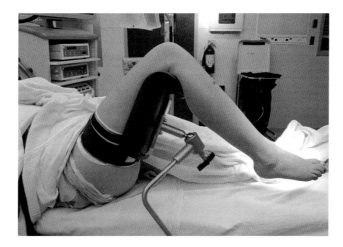

Figure 33-1

- For routine ankle arthroscopy place the patient supine with the operative extremity in a leg holder such that the hip and knee are flexed with the foot hanging free resulting in gravity-assisted distraction. This also allows free ankle range of motion, which can assist in access to different parts of the ankle (Figure 33-1).

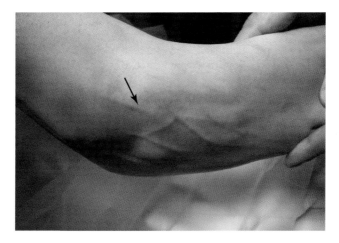

Figure 33-2

- Mark portal placement after establishing the path of the superficial peroneal nerve, which can be seen subcutaneously after plantar flexion and inversion of the foot (Figure 33-2).

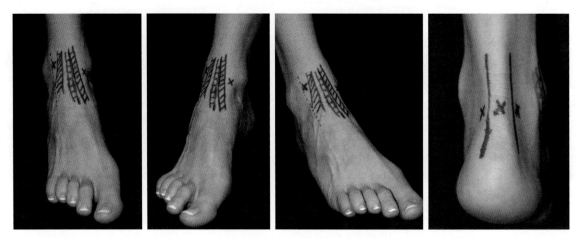

Figure 33-3

- Mark anterolateral and anteromedial portals at the joint line, which can be palpated, staying away from the peroneal nerve (Figure 33-3).

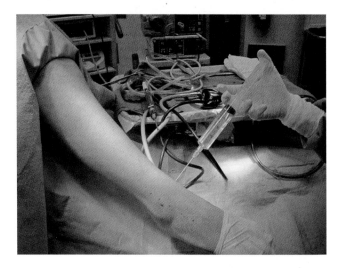

Figure 33-4

- After Esmarch exsanguination of the extremity and inflation of the thigh tourniquet establish the antero-medial portal by inserting an 18-gauge spinal needle at the marked site and insufflating the joint with saline to ensure intraarticular placement and to provide more space for introduction of the blunt trocar. Successful insufflation occurs when there is minimal resistance to the introduction of saline, when the foot dorsiflexes as the joint capsule becomes tight, and when there is backflow of the saline into the syringe after the joint is maximally distended. The anteromedial portal is established first because there are fewer structures at risk than with the anterolateral portal (Figure 33-4).
- After localization of the anteromedial portal with the spinal needle make a skin incision just large enough to insert the cannula. A large incision allows more extravasation of fluid into the surrounding soft tissues and can make the procedure more difficult.
- Further penetrate the joint with a blunt straight hemostat to avoid damage to the saphenous nerve, which is at risk in this area.
- Place a 2.7-mm 30-degree arthroscope into the anteromedial portal, and establish the anterolateral portal by direct visualization of a spinal needle introduced at the site of the anticipated portal placement.

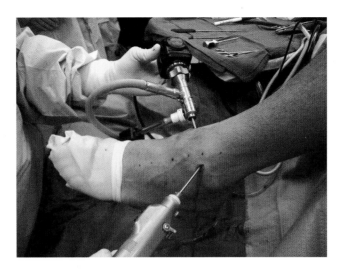

Figure 33-5

- When appropriate needle placement is seen make the skin incision for the anterolateral portal and penetrate the joint with a blunt instrument. Next introduce the arthroscopic shaver in this portal (Figure 33-5).

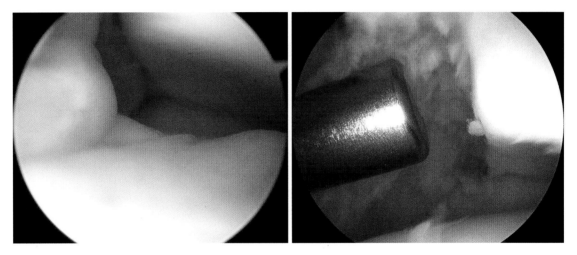

Figure 33-6

- Inspect the lateral aspect of the joint with use of instruments in the anterolateral portal as needed for débridement (Figure 33-6),

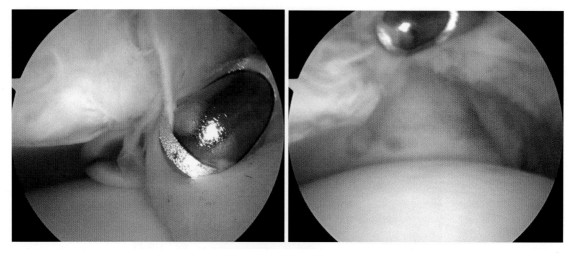

Figure 33-7

- Switch portals (arthroscope in the anterolateral portal and instruments in the anteromedial portal) for treatment of the medial side of the joint (Figure 33-7).

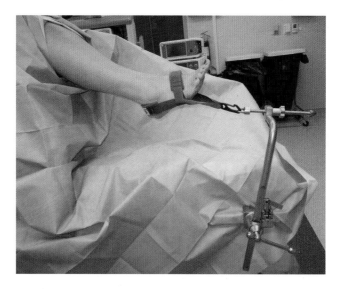

Figure 33-8

- Noninvasive distraction can be used if needed to access the deeper aspects of the joint. Occasionally a posterolateral portal is needed to treat pathological processes in the posterior aspect of the ankle that cannot be reached even after distraction is applied (Figure 33-8).
- After the procedure is completed close the portals with suture to avoid the development of a fistula, which is a reported complication of ankle arthroscopy.

POSTOPERATIVE CARE

Patients are placed in a walking boot and can bear weight as tolerated but should be cautioned against excessive activity because this could cause the ankle to become inflamed. Physical therapy should be started once the wounds have healed and postoperative pain is minimal.

Barry B. Phillips • Marc J. Mihalko

DRILLING OF AN INTACT LESION 〉

Intact osteochondral lesions with only a minor irregularity of the articular surface and no break in the continuity of the surface can be treated by drilling multiple holes through the articular surface and into the subchondral fragment and underlying vascular bone.

- Perform a complete and systematic diagnostic arthroscopy with the 30-degree viewing arthroscope in the anterolateral portal.

- Inspect carefully the articular surface of the medial femoral condyle varying the degree of flexion of the knee between 20 and 90 degrees to view the posterior extent of the lesion. The articular surfaces appear smooth except for a slightly raised irregularity at the borders of the lesion.

- Insert a probe through the anteromedial portal and carefully probe this irregular line to ensure there is no break in the continuity of the articular surface overlying the subchondral bone lesion.

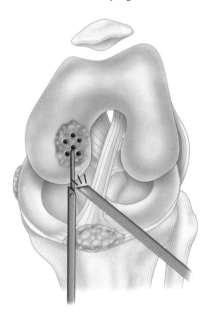

Figure 34-1

- If the lesion is intact perforate it with multiple holes using a 0.045-inch Kirschner wire (Figure 34-1). Position the Kirschner wire perpendicular to the articular surface with the soft tissues protected by a sleeve or cannula over the wire. Access for drilling inferocentral lesions of the medial femoral condyle is usually through the anteromedial portal; laterocentral lesions may be approached better by bringing the Kirschner wire through the anterolateral portal while viewing through the anteromedial portal. If the patient is not fully skeletally mature and the physis is open, take care not to penetrate too deeply and injure the physis. A radiographic image may be used to pass a 0.045-inch Kirschner wire starting distal to the growth plate and ending just proximal to the articular suture thus preserving the cartilage. Passing one wire through the cartilage to exit laterally can act as a guide for the wires to be passed from proximal to the lesion.

- Thoroughly lavage and suction the joint, and remove the instruments.

POSTOPERATIVE CARE 〉

Postoperative management consists of immobilization in a restricted motion brace with the arc of motion controlled to prevent contact of the tibial articular surface with the lesion. Use of crutches with partial weight bearing is encouraged until early healing is noted radiographically. Between 4 and 6 weeks of immobilization for young patients is common, whereas older patients with larger lesions should continue the immobilization and avoid weight bearing until definite radiographic evidence of healing is noted. Range-of-motion exercises should be performed for 15 to 20 minutes two to three times daily.

OSTEOCHONDRAL AUTOGRAFT TRANSFER 〉

Osteochondral autograft transfer is indicated for patients younger than 45 years of age who have a sharply defined defect with normal-appearing hyaline cartilage surrounding the borders of the defect. Lesions should be unipolar and generally no more than 2.0 to 2.5 cm. Normal mechanical alignment and a stable knee are necessary for the best long-term results.

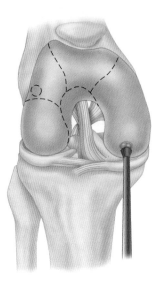

Figure 34-2

- Inspect the osteochondral defect arthroscopically and measure the size of the lesion. Use a set of OATS sizer/tamps with heads of 5 to 10 mm to determine precisely the diameter of the defect. The color-coded tamps correspond in size with the diameter of the tube harvesters (Figure 34-2).

- Assemble the tube harvester driver/extractor.

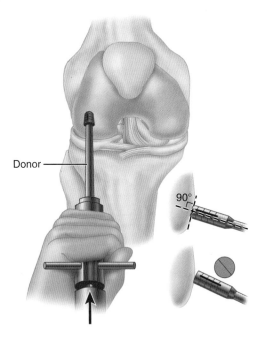

Figure 34-3

- Load the donor tube harvester with the collared pin into the base of the driver and tighten the chuck. Screw a cartilage protector cap onto the back of the driver. When seated the collared pin protrudes a few millimeters past the sharp cutting tip of the harvester to protect articular surfaces (Figure 34-3).

- When an acceptable position is established drive the donor harvester with a mallet into subchondral bone or to a depth of approximately 15 mm. Avoid rotating the harvester during impaction.

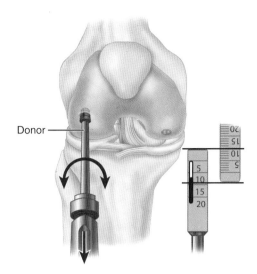

Figure 34-4

- Remove the harvester and bone core by axially loading the harvester and rotating the driver 90 degrees clockwise and then 90 degrees counterclockwise (Figure 34-4).

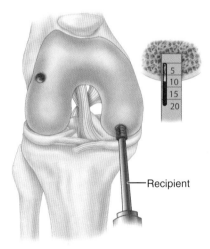

Figure 34-5

- Fully insert the recipient harvester into the driver and insert the protector caps in a similar fashion. During socket creation maintain a 90-degree angle to the articular surface to end up with a flush transfer. Rotate the harvester so that the depth markings are seen. Maintain a constant knee flexion angle during harvesting (Figure 34-5).

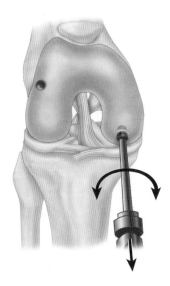

Figure 34-6

- After using a mallet to drive the tube harvester into subchondral bone to a depth of approximately 13 mm (2 mm less than the length of the donor core), extract the recipient bone core in the same manner as the donor bone core and measure and record the depth of the core (Figure 34-6).

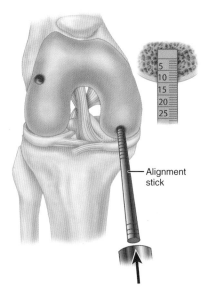

Alignment stick

Figure 34-7

- Use the calibrated OATS alignment stick of the appropriate diameter to measure the recipient socket depth and align the angle of the recipient socket correctly in relation to the position of the insertion portal when using an arthroscopic approach (Figure 34-7).
- Reinsert the donor harvester, collared pin, and autograft core into the driver. Unscrew the cap and remove the T-handled midsection. This exposes the end of the collared pin that is used to advance the bone into the recipient socket.

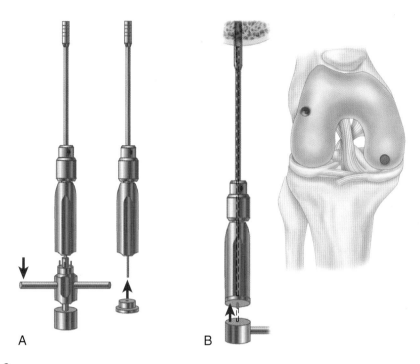

A   B

Figure 34-8

- Insert the pin calibrator over the guide pin, and press into the open back of the driver (Figure 34-8 , **A**). Insert the donor tube harvester's beveled edge fully into the recipient socket. Stabilize the harvester during autograft impaction. Use a mallet to tap the end of the collared pin lightly and drive the bone core into the recipient socket (**B**).

- Maintain a stable knee flexion angle and position of the harvester during this step. Carefully advance the collared pin until the end of the pin is flush with the pin calibrator on the back of the driver/extractor. This provides exact mechanical control to ensure proper bone core insertion depth. The predetermined length of the collared pin is designed to advance the bone core so that 1 mm of graft is exposed from the recipient socket when the pin is driven flush with the end of the pin calibrator. One can see the core insertion as it is occurring by viewing the core and the collared pin advancement through the slots in the side of the harvester.

- An alternative to the core extruder is the option of using the mallet to insert the bone core into the recipient socket. Place the donor harvester into the chuck of the fully assembled tube harvester driver/extractor. As described previously insert the beveled edge of the donor tube harvester into the recipient socket. While keeping the donor tube harvester firmly in position, slowly screw the core extruder into the rear of the fully assembled driver/extractor. Advance the core extruder by turning it in a clockwise motion forcing the bone core from the donor tube harvester into the recipient socket. When the core extruder is fully seated the bone core should remain slightly proud.

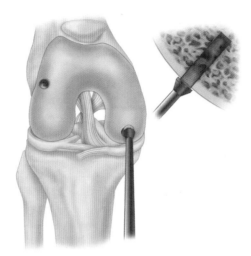

Figure 34-9

- Remove the donor tube harvester and position a sizer tamp, measuring at least 1 mm in diameter larger than the diameter of the bone core, over the bone core. Final seating of the bone core flush with surrounding cartilage is achieved by tapping the tamp lightly with the mallet (Figure 34-9).

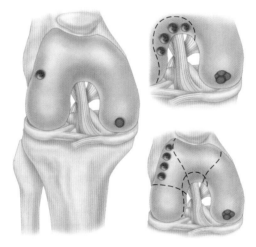

Figure 34-10

- When multiple cores of various diameters are elected to be harvested and transferred into specific quadrants of the defect each core transfer should be completed before proceeding with further recipient socket creation. This prevents potential recipient tunnel wall fracture and allows subsequent cores to be placed directly adjacent to previously inserted bone cores (Figure 34-10).

Most techniques described for reconstruction of the medial patellofemoral ligament (MPFL) use autogenous doubled semitendinosus-hamstring grafts placed in a physiometric position confirmed by palpation of landmarks and imaging and tested for isometry. This technique has low recurrence rates and a low risk of producing patellofemoral arthrosis or loss of motion from overconstraint.

- With the patient supine, place a tourniquet on the upper thigh. Use a lateral post on the operating table to assist with arthroscopic examination.
- After sterile preparation and draping arthroscopically examine the knee through standard medial and lateral portals to evaluate patellar tracking and look for intraarticular damage and chondral damage to the patella. This evaluation is essential for determining appropriate treatment.
- Make a 3-cm incision 3 cm medial to the inferior portion of the patellar tuberosity and harvest the semitendinosus tendon in standard fashion. Size the graft so that the appropriately sized tunnel can be reamed later.
- Depending on the size of the patient and the pathology present use one 4-cm longitudinal incision centered between the patella and the femoral medial epicondyle or two smaller incisions one just off the superior portion of the patella and another starting at the adductor tubercle and extending just distal to the medial epicondyle of the femur, to expose the patellofemoral ligament.
- Dissect subcutaneously to expose the proximal medial retinaculum at its insertion into the proximal portion of the patella. Make a 1.5-cm incision in the retinaculum.
- Use blunt dissection to spread between layers 2 and 3 (between the MPFL and the capsular layer) staying extrasynovial and developing the plane with a curved Kelly clamp directed toward the medial epicondyle and spreading between the layers to create a soft tissue tunnel.
- If two incisions are to be used, make the second 3-cm incision in the area of the tip of the Kelly clamp, which is in the saddle area between the adductor tubercle and the medial epicondyle.

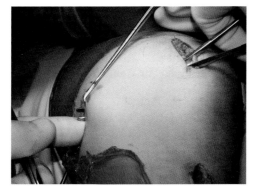

Figure 35-1

- Use a rongeur to make a superficial trough along the medial aspect of the patella in the proximal half. Center the trough between the cortex and the articular surface (Figure 35-1).
- Place two double-loaded suture anchors in the trough with the knee flexed 45 degrees to help stabilize the patella during insertion. Place one anchor just proximal to the midpatella and the other distal to the superior tip of the patella, making sure that both are angled so that they enter strong cancellous bone.

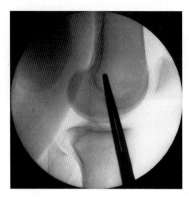

Figure 35-2

- Select the site for the femoral tunnel approximately 1 cm distal and 5 mm posterior to the adductor tubercle slightly proximal to the epicondyle. Confirm correct position with imaging (Figure 35-2).

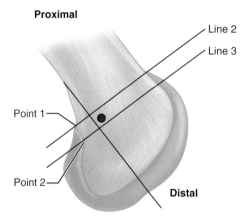

Figure 35-3

- Schöttle et al.'s radiographic landmark for femoral tunnel placement in medial patellofemoral ligament reconstruction. Two perpendicular lines to line 1 are drawn intersecting the contact point of the medial condyle and posterior cortex (point 1, line 2) and intersecting the most posterior point of the Blumensaat line (point 2, line 3). For determination of vertical position the distance between line 2 and the lead ball center is measured as is the distance between line 2 and line 3 (Figure 35-3).
- Place a Beath-tip guidewire at the chosen spot and pass two suture tails from the suture anchor through the soft tissue trough to the area of the wire. Mark the sutures so that pistoning of the sutures can be identified with range of motion of the knee.
- Move the knee through a range of motion and observe the sutures, which should have minimal motion between 0 and 70 degrees of flexion and slight laxity above 70 degrees. If tension increases with flexion the femoral tunnel site is too far proximal (most commonly) or possibly too far anterior. If the sutures tighten excessively in extension, the tunnel is too far distal or too far posterior. If necessary correct the guidewire position and repeat the evaluation.

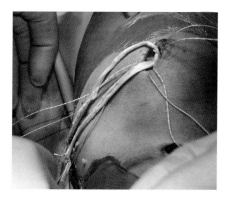

Figure 35-4

- Measure at least 16 cm of the harvested semitendinosus and remove any excess length; place a whip stitch in each tail of the graft (Figure 35-4).
- With the graft loop placed in the patellar trough secure the graft to the patella with one of the paired sutures in each of the anchors in the superior part of the patella. Leave the second set of sutures for later repair of the retinaculum over the graft.
- At the selected femoral tunnel site ream a 22-mm tunnel the diameter of the doubled tendon.

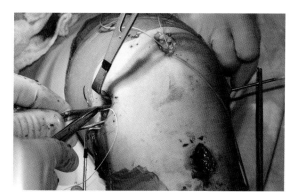

Figure 35-5

- Pass the graft tails through the soft tissue tunnel to the level of the femoral tunnel. Pull the graft taut and stress the patella so as to allow for one to two quadrants of lateral passive glide. When the physiological amount of tension on the graft is determined make a mark on the graft, which will correspond to the aperture of the femoral tunnel (Figure 35-5).
- Cut the graft 20 mm distal to this mark to allow 17 to 20 mm of graft to be placed into the tunnel.
- Place absorbable whip sutures in the tails of the graft, place them into the tip of a Beath pin, and pull them out laterally.
- Before fixation with a biocomposite screw move the knee through a range of motion, once again making sure that the tendons do not become taut in flexion and that the tendon length is appropriate to allow one to two quadrants of passive glide at 30 degrees of flexion so as not to overconstrain the patella.
- Maintain this graft length while it is secured with a biocomposite screw 1 mm smaller than the tunnel size chosen. Again move the knee through a range of motion to make sure motion is not inhibited.

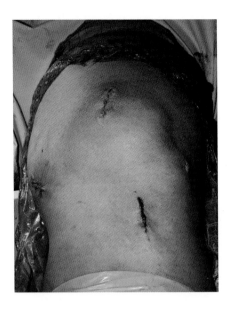

Figure 35-6

- Repair the retinaculum over the reconstructed patellofemoral ligament with the second set of sutures from each anchor. Close the subcutaneous tissues with 2-0 Vicryl and the skin with Monocryl. Apply a postoperative dressing and a knee brace (Figure 35-6).

POSTOPERATIVE CARE ⟩

The knee joint is immobilized in extension with a simple knee brace for 3 days after surgery. Range-of-motion exercises and gait with weight bearing on two crutches are started and gradually progressed. Weight bearing is allowed as tolerated immediately after surgery. Walking with full weight bearing usually is possible 2 or 3 weeks after surgery. Extension during walking is maintained with a knee brace for 6 weeks. Achieving at least 90 degrees knee flexion by the end of postoperative week 3 is encouraged. Jogging is allowed after 3 months and participation in the original sporting activity is allowed 6 months after surgery depending on the patient.

Indications for distal realignment include patellar instability secondary to malalignment indicated by a Q angle of more than 20 degrees and anterior tibial tuberosity-to-trochlear groove distance of more than 25 mm and patellar instability with inferior and lateral chondromalacia.

MODIFIED ELMSLIE-TRILLAT OPERATION

- Make a 6-cm lateral parapatellar incision approximately 1 cm lateral to the patellar tendon.
- Perform a lateral release from the tibial tubercle to the level of the insertion of the vastus lateralis tendon on the proximal patella. The release is considered adequate when the patellar articular surface can be everted 90 degrees laterally.
- Approach the tibial tubercle through the same parapatellar incision and identify the patellar tendon insertion. Using a 2.5-cm flat osteotome raise a flat 6-cm long, 7-mm thick osteoperiosteal flap tapering anteriorly and hinged distally with periosteum. Do not violate the soft tissues.
- Rotate the bone flap medially, cracking the cortex distally, and hold it in place with a Kirschner wire while the knee is moved through a full passive range of motion to evaluate patellar tracking.
- If tracking is acceptable and the transferred tubercle fits flush with the underlying tibia fix it with one or two AO 4-mm cancellous lag screws. Use a 2.7-mm bit to drill through the tubercle and tibia. Angle the drill toward the joint and advance it until the posterior cortex is felt. Angling the drill proximally allows fixation to be placed in cancellous bone near the proximal tibia. Bicortical fixation is not used, and the screw should be long enough (usually 40 to 50 mm) to come near, but not penetrate, the posterior cortex.

POSTOPERATIVE CARE

Weight bearing is allowed to tolerance using a straight-leg splint for ambulation for the first 6 weeks after surgery. At 1 week after surgery closed chain kinetic strengthening is begun with a goal of achieving 70% strength by 6 weeks. A functional progression program that allows the patient to return to unrestricted sports is begun 8 to 12 weeks after surgery.

FULKERSON OSTEOTOMY

The Fulkerson osteotomy is a slightly oblique osteotomy of the tuberosity that transfers the tuberosity anteriorly and medially. It is indicated when grade 3 or 4 chondromalacia is associated with recurrent patellar dislocations. It generally is not indicated for athletes and should be reserved for patients with severe patellofemoral degenerative changes.

- Make a 9-cm lateral parapatellar incision extending from the inferior pole of the patella distally. Exposure is similar to the Elmslie-Trillat procedure with the difference being in the oblique osteotomy of the tuberosity.
- Extend the cut distally about 6 cm with the medial tip of the cut being more superficial.
- Drill holes to perforate the cortex distally so that the fragment can be hinged.
- Using an osteotome complete the osteotomy deep and just proximal to the insertion of the patellar tendon and pry the tuberosity medially so that the Q angle is corrected to between 10 and 15 degrees. This usually requires moving the tuberosity anteriorly 8 to 10 mm.
- Secure the transferred tuberosity by placing a drill bit proximally through the tuberosity and tibia with the knee in 90 degrees of flexion to decrease risk to neurovascular structures.
- Move the knee through a range of motion and evaluate patellar tracking.

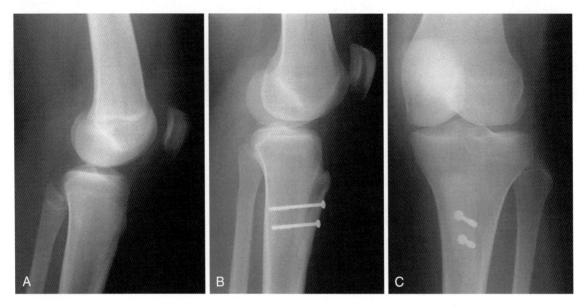

Figure 36-1

- If tracking is satisfactory secure the tuberosity with two countersunk, low-profile, cancellous screws (Figure 36-1, **A,** Preoperative lateral radiograph. **B,** Postoperative lateral radiograph. **C,** Anteroposterior radiograph).
- Close the medial retinaculum in a pants-over-vest fashion plicating the medial side. Do no close the lateral retinaculum.

POSTOPERATIVE CARE ⟩

Weight bearing is allowed as tolerated after surgery. Immobilization is continued 4 to 6 weeks, at which time range-of-motion and strengthening exercises are instituted. Return to sports usually is allowed at 6 to 9 months after surgery. In our opinion there is some long-term risk of fracture after this procedure.

ANTERIOR CRUCIATE LIGAMENT RECONSTRUCTION: ANATOMICAL SINGLE-BUNDLE ENDOSCOPIC RECONSTRUCTION USING BONE–PATELLAR TENDON–BONE GRAFT

Barry B. Phillips • Marc J. Mihalko

Most ACL reconstructions currently are done arthroscopically because of the advantages of smaller skin and capsular incisions, less extensor mechanism trauma, improved viewing of the intercondylar notch for placement of the tunnel and attachment sites, less postoperative pain, fewer adhesions, earlier motion, and easier rehabilitation.

- Place the patient supine on the operating table.
- After general endotracheal anesthesia has been administered examine the uninjured knee to obtain a reference examination for ligamentous laxity. Examine the injured knee and record Lachman and pivot shift instability.

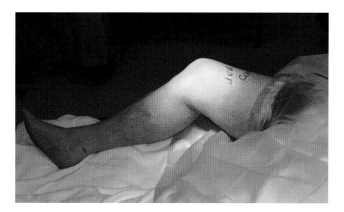

Figure 37-1

- Apply a tourniquet around the upper thigh and use a well-padded lateral post. Secure a 5-L intravenous saline bag to the table to act as a stop to maintain 90 degrees of knee flexion (Figure 37-1).
- Prepare and drape the extremity with standard arthroscopy drapes and use an Esmarch wrap for exsanguination. Inflate the tourniquet to 100 mm Hg above the patient's systolic pressure.
- If preoperative examination revealed significant laxity proceed with patellar tendon harvesting.
- Arthroscopic joint portals can be made through this initial skin incision. If the status of the anterior cruciate ligament is in question, or if more than 90 minutes of tourniquet time is anticipated for completion of the procedure, arthroscopy portals should be made for joint evaluation and notch débridement before inflating the tourniquet and making the skin incision for harvest of the patellar tendon.
- Inject the portals with lidocaine and epinephrine to help control bleeding and maintain hypotensive anesthesia. An arthroscopy pump can be used to maintain proper joint distention and reduce bone bleeding.
- Unless contraindicated administer antibiotics and ketorolac (Toradol) before tourniquet inflation (30 mg intravenously in patients younger than 65 years; 15 mg in patients older than 65 years or in those weighing less than 50 kg). Two additional doses can be given postoperatively, not to exceed 120 mg or 60 mg, respectively.

Graft Harvest

- With the knee held in 90 degrees of flexion make a 4- to 6-cm medial parapatellar incision starting inferior to the patella and extending distally medial to the tibial tuberosity. The length of this incision depends on the size of the patient.
- Expose the patella and tendon by subcutaneous dissection.
- Make a straight midline incision through the peritenon and dissect the peritenon from the patellar tendon, taking the flaps medially and laterally.
- With the knee held flexed to maintain some tension on the patellar tendon measure the width of the tendon.

- Harvest a 10-mm-wide graft or one third of the tendon, whichever is smaller, from the central portion of the tendon extending distally from the palpable inferior tip of the patella. Maintain straight single-fiber plane incisions while harvesting the tendon. The size of the graft is individualized. For a large football lineman an 11-mm graft or double-bundle graft may be indicated. For a small patient a 9-mm or possibly an 8-mm graft and tunnels may be indicated.
- Use an oscillating saw with a 1-cm-wide blade to make the bone cuts. Run the saw blade 15 degrees oblique to a line perpendicular to the anterior cortex of the patella keeping 2 mm of the saw blade visible and making a cut 8 mm in depth. This cut should be about 10 mm wide × 20 mm long measured from the bony tip of the patella.
- Make 25-mm-long cuts distally and free the tibial graft with a curved osteotome.
- Flip the plug and place it back into the harvest site. Drill a 2-mm hole 3 mm from the distal tip of the plug and pass a no. 5 Tevdek suture (Deknatel OSP, Fall River, MA). An assistant should hold this at all times to ensure that the graft is not contaminated.
- Complete the patellar cut with the saw or an osteotome placed at the inferior pole of the patella 7 to 8 mm deep and parallel to the anterior cortex.

Graft Preparation

- Secure the graft to the top drape on a previously prepared table that holds appropriate-sized bone plug trials, rongeurs, a 2-mm drill bit, a Silastic block, a skin marker, no. 5 Tevdek sutures on Keith needles, and an 18-gauge steel wire.
- Commercially available graft preparation boards make tensioning and graft preparation much easier.
- Contour the graft with the rongeurs so that it fits through the 10-mm trial ensuring that the complete graft would pass through the trial.
- Drill a single hole in the patellar plug about 3 mm from the end.
- Bullet the end of the bone plug to make passage easier.
- Drill a hole in the tibial bone plug. This plug should be 20 mm.
- Place a no. 5 nonabsorbable suture through the better bone plug to be placed into the femoral tunnel and an 18-gauge wire through the other plug, which is placed into the tibial tunnel. The use of a wire prevents cut-out before firm fixation is obtained.
- Mark the bone-tendon junction on the cancellous side of the graft at both ends with a methylene blue pencil and measure the total graft length. Wrap it in a sterile saline-soaked sponge and place it in a safe holding location.
- Use electrocautery to make an inverted L-shaped flap through the tibial periosteum starting about 2.5 cm distal to the joint line and extending distally 1 cm medial to the tibial tuberosity.
- Reflect the flap medially with a periosteal elevator to expose the proximal tibia for later placement of the tibial tunnel.
- Make standard anteromedial and anterolateral arthroscopy portals taking care not to damage the remaining portion of the patellar tendon. If a separate inflow is being used for the arthroscopy pump, make a portal just medial to the inferior pole of the patella so that the cannula can be placed just superior to the notch for an unobstructed flow.
- Systematically examine the knee and evaluate and treat any associated intraarticular pathological condition.
- Perform meniscal suturing before securing the anterior cruciate ligament graft.
- Tie the meniscal sutures after completing the anterior cruciate ligament reconstruction.
- With the arthroscope in the anterolateral portal and a 5.5-mm full-radius resector in the anteromedial portal, release the ligamentum mucosum and partially resect the fat pad to allow full exposure of the joint during the procedure.
- Resect the soft tissue from the intercondylar notch and from the tibial stump by sliding the resector between the remaining stump of the anterior cruciate ligament and the posterior cruciate ligament. The opening of the blade should always be pointed superiorly or laterally to avoid damage to the posterior cruciate ligament.

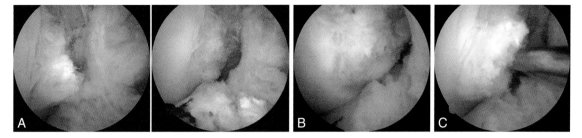

Figure 37-2

- Leave the outline of the tibial and femoral footprint intact as a reference guide (Figure 37-2, **A,** ACL footprint through lateral parapatellar portal; **B,** from medial parapatellar portal). Visualize the lateral intercondylar ridge, the lateral bifurcate ridge, and the extent of the footprint that covers the lower third of the notch wall. Use an awl to make a hole slightly posterior to the center of the footprint so that the tunnel will have a 3-mm posterior wall and be about 3 mm superior to the articular cartilage (**C**). After properly marking the footprint while visualizing from the anteromedial portal the scope may be changed to the anterolateral portal and a small internal notchplasty can be performed to aid with graft placement.

- With the knee in 30 degrees of flexion to expose the opening of the notch evaluate the available space between the posterior cruciate ligament and lateral wall and the architecture of the roof. Use a 5.5-mm burr to enlarge the notch as indicated. The notch should be opened to look like an inverted U. Do not extend the notchplasty too far medially or superiorly, which would interfere with the patellofemoral articulation. Often the opening needs to be enlarged only 2 to 3 mm superiorly and laterally. The burr can be placed in reverse to remove the articular fringe and smooth the initial notchplasty.

- As the notchplasty proceeds posteriorly flex the knee from 45 to 60 degrees; when the notchplasty is complete the knee should be at 90 degrees of flexion. Use controlled strokes with the burr from posterior to anterior. Posteriorly open the notch enough to accommodate the 10-mm endoscopic reamer. Smooth the edges of the tunnel by placing the burr in reverse or by using an arthroscopic rasp.

Tibial Tunnel Preparation and Determining Appropriate Length

- If transosseous drilling of the femoral tunnel is planned the tibial tunnel will need to be placed at a 45-degree sagittal angle, starting just lateral to the medial collateral ligament. More acute angles tend to undercut the tibial articular suture and result in an oblique nonanatomical aperture. This does allow for a longer tibial tunnel and the anatomical femoral footprint can be successfully reamed about 60% of the time through the tibial tunnel. A low medial portal may be preferable to independently ream the femur so that the tibial tunnel can be placed vertical as described later.

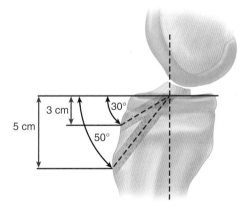

Figure 37-3

- When placing the tibial guide intraarticularly be aware of the intended tunnel length and direction so that the graft can be secured in an anatomical impingement-free position. Proper length and direction of the tunnel require a starting point approximately 1 cm proximal to the pes anserinus and about 1.5 cm medial to the tibial tuberosity to form a 30- to 40-degree angle with the shaft of the tibia. One should see this wire being directed to approach the femoral pilot (Figure 37-3).

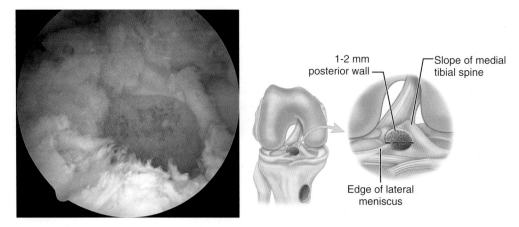

1-2 mm
posterior wall

Slope of medial
tibial spine

Edge of lateral
meniscus

Figure 37-4

- When evaluating pin placement in a two-dimensional picture in the anteroposterior plane, ensure that the guidewire exits just anterior to a reference line extended medially from the inner edge of the lateral meniscus. This point should be approximately 7 mm anterior to the posterior cruciate ligament and 2 to 3 mm anterior to the peak of the medial spine just anterior to the center of the anterior cruciate ligament footprint. In the mediolateral plane ensure that the wire enters at the base of the medial spine or just slightly medial to the center of the anterior cruciate ligament footprint (Figure 37-4).

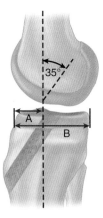

35°

A

B

Figure 37-5

- The unaltered roof of the intercondylar notch normally forms an angle of 35 to 40 degrees with the long axis of the femur. To prevent impingement an internal notchplasty, as previously described, may be necessary as is appropriate tunnel placement. Use the tibial and femoral landmarks described earlier and place the guide at 55 to 60 degrees to the tibial plateau surface to obtain sufficient tunnel length and an angle that allows the graft angle to approximate that of the original. Measure the tibial tunnel length directly off the guide calibrations and approximate the length of the tendinous portion of the graft. The tunnel length should be sufficient to allow at least 20 mm of bone to be secured in the tibial tunnel for stable fixation (Figure 37-5).
- If the tendinous portion of the graft is 50 mm long or less increase the guide angle to produce a longer tibial tunnel. The tunnel can be easily increased to 45 to 50 mm long to accommodate the longer graft. Recessing the graft into the femoral tunnel can take up more slack. Recess the graft as necessary into the femoral tunnel and fix the graft and the tunnel aperture with a screw long enough to securely engage the bone plug.
- Using the guide, advance the wire approximately 10 mm into the knee while observing through the arthroscope.

- Place a clamp over the intraarticular end of the Kirschner wire to prevent advancement. Ream over the wire with a reamer 2 mm smaller than the intended final tunnel.
- Leave the protruding end of the reamer in the tunnel and examine the tunnel for appropriate impingement-free position as the knee is moved through a full range of motion.
- Make necessary adjustments with the 8-mm reamer.
- Prevent bowstringing of the anterior cruciate ligament graft over the posterior cruciate ligament by leaving a 2-mm posterior wall between the tibial tunnel and the posterior cruciate ligament. By directing the tunnel just lateral to the posterior cruciate ligament the graft lies on the posterior cruciate ligament without bowing around the ligament.
- Ream the tunnel with a reamer the size of the graft and use the full-radius resector to contour the edges of the tunnel and resect any remaining soft tissue that might block extension.
- Place a rasp through the tunnel to complete contouring and ensure that the external portion of the tunnel is free of soft tissue.

Femoral Tunnel Preparation

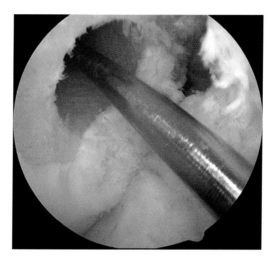

Figure 37-6

- Use a spinal needle to identify the best position for a low medial portal about 2.5 cm medial to the patellar tendon and just above the meniscus. A guide is placed to ensure that the tunnel is just anterior to the anteromedial bundle, that is, leaving a 3-mm posterior wall and about 3 mm from the femoral articular surface. Flex the knee 120 degrees, and use a hemispherical reamer to avoid articular damage. Advance the reamer 1 mm and recheck the tunnel location. If it is in the desired location ream a 30-mm tunnel if possible (Figure 37-6).
- Carefully retract the reamer and remove it from the joint being careful not to enlarge the tunnel and ream out the posterior wall of the femur.
- Smooth the edges of the femoral tunnel with a full-radius resector.
- Use the tunnel notcher to make a 25-mm-long slot per the guidewire.

Graft Passage

- Use the eyelet guidewire to pass a suture loop with tails through the femoral tunnel and out through the lateral thigh. Retrieve the loop through the femoral tunnel. Use this loop to pass the graft up through the tibial tunnel and then guide it into the femoral tunnel using a probe. The cancellous surface of the femoral bone plug is positioned to face anteriorly.
- When the graft is in the femoral tunnel, pass a flexible screw guidewire through the medial portal and with the wire parallel to the graft advance both up into the tunnel. Ensure that at least 2 cm of bone plug remains in the tibial tunnel for later fixation; if necessary, recess the graft into the femoral tunnel and choose a longer interference screw to fix the graft at the femoral aperture.

Graft Fixation

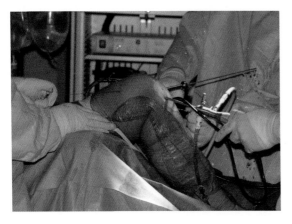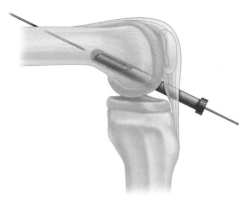

Figure 37-7

- Secure the graft with an interference screw with a sheath passed through the low medial portal to form a straight line with the tunnel. The screw should firmly engage the bone and be flush with the femoral aperture. Visualization is aided by placing the scope into the top of the notch and looking down on the tunnel (Figure 37-7).
- Move the knee through a range of motion while holding tension distally on the graft to ensure that there is no impingement or pistoning of the graft. If the graft tightens more than 2 mm with knee flexion remove the graft and move the femoral tunnel or both tunnels slightly posterior using a convex arthroscopic rasp. Slight tightening during knee extension is normal.
- Rotate the tibial bone plug counter clockwise (right knee) so that the cancellous plug faces laterally thus replicating the anterior cruciate ligament fiber orientation.
- If no graft pistoning or impingement is evident hold the tension on the graft for approximately 3 minutes while cycling the knee to allow for collagen fiber stress relaxation. If the graft tends to impinge in one direction use the screw to push the bone graft in the opposite direction.
- Tension the graft with 8 to 10 lb of pull. Overtensioning of the graft can cause failure because of joint capture or graft necrosis.
- Secure the graft with a screw equal to the gap size plus 5 mm.
- If the tendon is so long that the bone plug is completely out of the tibial tunnel, as may be the case with an allograft mismatch, then a biocomposite or noncutting screw 1 mm smaller than the tunnel may be used for soft tissue fixation of the patellar tendon and bone construct.
- Move the knee through a full range of motion and ensure there is no evidence of capture of the knee joint. Observe and probe the graft arthroscopically to ensure that it is taut. The graft should be slightly tighter than a normal anterior cruciate ligament. Also ensure that there is no impingement and that no bone or screw protrudes into the joint from the tibial or femoral tunnel.
- Check the stability of the knee by Lachman and pivot shift maneuvers. The knee should be just slightly tighter than the uninjured knee.
- If fixation is secure remove the 18-gauge wire and the tension sutures.

Closure

- Loosely approximate the patellar tendon with simple interrupted absorbable sutures through the anterior portion of the fiber of the tendon.
- Place bone saved from contouring of the bone plugs into the patellar defect and close the peritenon.
- Remove the sutures from the thigh proximally (femoral bone plug) and from the tibial bone plug distally.
- Remove any protruding bone leaving a smooth surface distally.
- Close the periosteal flap back over the tunnel.
- Close the subcutaneous tissues with interrupted 2-0 Vicryl suture and approximate the skin with a running subcuticular 4-0 Monocryl suture.
- Apply adhesive strips loosely over the closure and apply a sterile dressing, a cooling sleeve, and an elastic wrap.

POSTOPERATIVE CARE

BOX	37-1	Anterior Cruciate Ligament Rehabilitation Protocol

Stage I: 0 to 2 Weeks
- Patellar mobilizations (emphasize superior/inferior glides)
- MCB 0 to 90 degrees
- Quadriceps sets/SLR all planes (emphasize SLR without extension lag)
- Prone/standing hamstring curls
- Passive extension (emphasize full extension)
- Prone hangs
- Pillow under heel
- Passive, active, and active-assisted ROM knee flexion
- Wall slides
- Sitting slides
- Prone towel pulls
- Edema control—compression pump
- Electrical stimulation for muscle re-education if poor QS
- PWB 50% to 75% with crutches or WBTT without crutches if MCB locked in full extension
- Sleep in brace locked in extension

Goals
- Full knee extension ROM
- 90-degree knee flexion ROM
- Good QS
- Emphasize normal gait pattern

Stage II: 2 to 4 Weeks
- MCB full ROM
- Progress ROM to 120 degrees by week 4
- Progress SLR and prone/standing hamstring curls with weights
- Bike for ROM, begin low-resistance program when ROM adequate
- Stool scoots
- FWB with crutches; discontinue crutches when ambulating without limp
- Begin double-leg BAPS, progress to single leg
- Begin double-leg press with light weight/high repetitions
- Wall sits at 45-degree angle with tibia vertical, progress time
- Lateral step-ups (4 inches) when able to perform single-leg quarter squat
- Hip machine and hamstring machine when able to perform SLR with 10 lb
- Treadmill (forward and backward) with emphasis on normal gait
- Knee extension 90 to 60 degrees (submaximal) with manual resistance by therapist

Goals
- ROM 0 to 120 degrees
- FWB without crutches, no limp

Continued

BOX	37-1	Anterior Cruciate Ligament Rehabilitation Protocol—cont'd

Stage II: 4 to 6 Weeks
- Progress to full ROM by 6 weeks
- Begin Kin-Com isokinetic hamstring progression (isotonic/isokinetic)
- Begin Kin-Com dynamometer quadriceps work 90 to 40 degrees isotonics with antishear pad
- StairMaster (forward and backward)
- Progress closed chain exercises
- At 6 weeks, begin Kin-Com dynamometer quadriceps work 90 to 40 degrees isokinetics (start with higher speed and work on endurance)
- Aquatic exercises

Stage II: 8 to 10 Weeks
- Progress above-listed exercises
- Slow-form running with sport cord (forward and backward)
- Isokinetic quadriceps work at different speeds (60, 90, 120 degrees per second)
- Begin lunges
- At 10 weeks, begin Fitter, slide board

Stage III: 12 to 16 Weeks
- Full range isotonics on Kin-Com dynamometer (begin moving antishear pad down)
- Knee extension machine with low weight/high repetitions
- Lateral sport cord drills (slow, controlled)
- Kin-Com dynamometer test hamstrings, discontinue isokinetic hamstrings if 90%
- Progress isokinetic quadriceps to full extension by 16 weeks

Stage IV: 16 to 18 Weeks
- Kin-Com dynamometer test for quadriceps, retest hamstrings if necessary
- Begin plyometric program with shuttle, minitrampoline, jump rope if quadriceps strength 65%, no effusion, full ROM, stable knee
- Begin jogging program if quadriceps strength is 65%

Stage V: 5 to 6 Months
- Agility training
- Sport-specific drills (e.g., carioca, 45 cutting, figure-of-eight)
- Retest quadriceps if necessary

Stage VI: 6 Months
- Return to sport if:
  - Motion > 130 degrees
  - Hamstrings > 90%
  - Quadriceps > 85%
  - Sport-specific agility training completed
- Maintenance exercises two to three times per week

BAPS, Biomechanical ankle platform system; *FWB,* full weight bearing; *MCB,* motion control brace; *PWB,* partial weight bearing; *QS,* quadriceps setting; *ROM,* range of motion; *SLR,* straight-leg raises; *WBTT,* weight bearing to tolerance.

Barry B. Phillips • Marc J. Mihalko

Graft selection for ACL reconstruction depends on the surgeon's preference and the tissues available. Currently, the most frequently used autogenous grafts are central-third patellar tendon, quadrupled hamstring, and, less commonly, quadriceps tendon grafts. Some studies have found patellar tendon grafts to be slightly more stable than hamstring grafts; kneeling pain is more frequent with patellar tendon grafts.

GRAFT HARVEST 〉

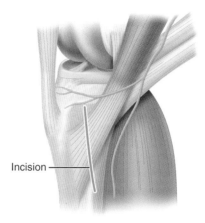

Incision

Figure 38-1

- Make a 4-cm incision anteromedially on the tibia starting approximately 4 cm distal to the joint line and 3 cm medial to the tibial tuberosity (Figure 38-1).
- Expose the pes anserinus insertion with subcutaneous dissection.

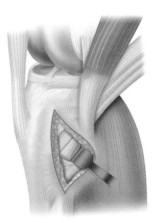

Figure 38-2

- Palpate the upper and lower borders of the sartorius tendon and identify the palpable gracilis and semitendinosus tendons 3 to 4 cm medial to the tendinous insertion (Figure 38-2).
- Make a short incision in line with the upper border of the gracilis tendon and carry the incision just through the first layer, taking care not to injure the underlying medial collateral ligament.
- With Metzenbaum scissors carry the dissection proximally up the thigh. Stay in the same plane, and maintain adequate exposure by using properly placed retractors. Careful observation of structures is necessary to avoid injuring the saphenous vein or nerve by straying from the plane of dissection.
- With a curved hemostat dissect the gracilis and semitendinosus tendons from the surrounding soft tissues about 3 cm medial to their insertion onto the tibia.

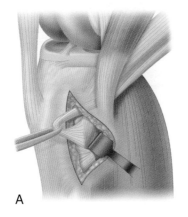
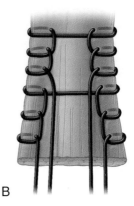

Figure 38-3 A B

- After carefully identifying each tendon use a right-angle vascular clamp to pass a Penrose drain around the gracilis tendon and release its fibrous extensions to the gastrocnemius and semimembranosus muscles (Figure 38-3, **A**). These fibrous extensions come off the hamstring tendons at 6 to 7 cm proximal to their distal attachment. Subperiosteally dissect the tendons medially to the insertion and release them sharply. Do not damage or release the sartorius tendon. Place a nonabsorbable Krackow stitch on the tendon ends using different colored sutures to differentiate the two tendons (**B**). Use a tendon tube sizer to accurately measure the give of the quadrupled tendon.

- Palpate all sides of the tendon to ensure there are no fibrous extensions before releasing it with an open-end tendon stripper. If firm resistance is felt redissect around the tendons with a periosteal elevator and Metzenbaum scissors. Release the tendon proximally by controlled tension on the tendon while advancing the stripper proximally. The muscle should slide off the tendon as the stripper is advanced proximally.

- Use the same procedure to release the semitendinosus tendon.

- At a separate table separate the muscle from the tendon with a no. 10 blade.

- Place a Krackow-type whipstitch in both ends of each tendon with no. 2 nonabsorbable sutures. Fold both tendons in half to form four strands of tendon.

- Perform a limited notchplasty and tunnel placement as described for the endoscopic bone-tendon-bone technique.

- Ream the tibial tunnel at 50 degrees to the tibial articular surface. The tunnel is reamed 2 mm smaller than the graft size and serially dilated to produce a snug fit. Cain, Phillips, and Azar have shown that dilating the tibial tunnel significantly increases the pull-out strength. The tunnel length should be 30 to 35 mm to allow fixation near the articular surface.

- A low anteromedial portal is used for reaming the femoral tunnel. Use an EndoButton or similar type device to secure 20 to 25 mm of tendon in the femoral tunnel. After tensioning the graft for 3 minutes while cycling the knee use a biocompatible screw 1 mm smaller than the tunnel for tibial fixation and use secondary suture and post fixation. A screw sheath, soft tissue fixation device may also be used to secure the tibial end of the graft.

POSTOPERATIVE CARE 〉

See Technique 37 for postoperative anterior cruciate ligament rehabilitation. We generally proceed more slowly with rehabilitation when a hamstring graft has been used. The patient is generally allowed to return to full activity at around 9 months.

Anatomical double-bundle anterior cruciate ligament reconstruction places the femoral graft into the femoral footprint of the native anterior cruciate ligament, which has been shown to result in closer knee joint kinematics than the original isometric femoral position. A three-portal technique adds an accessory medial portal to create the femoral tunnel.

- A three-portal approach, using standard anterolateral and central medial portals and an accessory anteromedial portal, allows for a complete view of the entire anterior cruciate ligament and its femoral and tibial insertion sites.

- After creation of a standard anterolateral portal, use a spinal needle to create the central portal while viewing through the anterolateral portal. The spinal needle should be in the center of the notch in a proximal to distal direction.

- Create the accessory anteromedial portal superior to the medial joint line, approximately 2 cm medial to the medial border of the patellar tendon. The femoral tunnels can be drilled through the accessory medial portal.

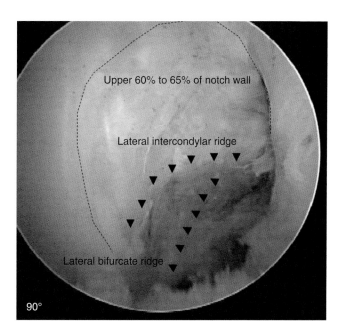

Figure 39-1

- Locate the ideal anterior cruciate ligament insertion sites for anatomical tunnel placement. Anterior cruciate ligament remnants can be used to determine this site. On the femoral side the bony landmarks, such as the lateral intercondylar ridge and lateral bifurcate ridge, may be used as well as posterior cartilage border. With the knee flexed 90 degrees the femoral insertion site encompasses the lower 30% to 35% of the notch wall (Figure 39-1).

- Mark the tibial and femoral insertion sites of the anterior cruciate ligament and measure to determine the tunnel location and size. If the insertion site is smaller than 14 mm in diameter a double-bundle reconstruction may become challenging. The width of the notch entrance and its shape will determine if a double-bundle technique can be used, but generally a notch width no smaller than 12 mm is the minimum size required.

- Create the femoral posterolateral tunnel first, through the accessory anteromedial portal, followed by the tibial anteromedial and posterolateral tunnels. Place the anteromedial and posterolateral tunnels in the center of the native anteromedial and posterolateral tibial and femoral insertion sites.
- Drill the femoral anteromedial tunnel through the accessory medial portal or through the tibial anteromedial or posterolateral tunnel if this allows for the native femoral insertion site to be reached.
- In determining the size of the tunnels, aim to restore as much of the native insertion site as possible while maintaining an approximately 2-mm bony bridge between the bundles.
- After the tunnels have been drilled prepare the grafts. The graft size should be equal to the tunnel diameter. Tension the anteromedial and posterolateral grafts separately, tensioning the anteromedial graft with the knee in approximately 45 degrees of knee flexion and the posterolateral graft with the knee in full extension.
- For fixation use suspensory fixation on the femoral side to avoid disruption of the insertion site, which can occur with aperture interference screw fixation. Use interference screw fixation on the cortical tibial side.

TRANSEPIPHYSEAL REPLACEMENT OF ANTERIOR CRUCIATE LIGAMENT USING QUADRUPLE HAMSTRING GRAFTS

The transepiphyseal reconstruction of the anterior cruciate ligament using quadruple hamstring grafts procedure described by Anderson is indicated in patients in Tanner stage I, II, or III of development. The procedure is contraindicated in patients in Tanner stage IV of development, who can have conventional anterior cruciate ligament reconstruction. Pitfalls of this procedure include suboptimal graft placement, incorrect diameter of transepiphyseal drill holes, failure of fixation, and graft slippage with suture post fixation.

BOX	40-1	Avoiding Pitfalls of Transepiphyseal ACL Reconstruction in Skeletally Immature Patients

Suboptimal Graft Placement

- Avoid placing the femoral or tibial drill hole anterior; correct positioning of the drill hole is crucial in preventing graft impingement.
- Surgery should not proceed without clearly seeing the physes on anteroposterior and lateral planes using a C-arm.
- Guidewires should be inserted under real-time C-arm viewing.
- Confirm arthroscopically that the guidewires enter the joint in the center of the footprint of the anterior cruciate ligament on the femur and in the posterior footprint of the anterior cruciate ligament on the tibia.

Incorrect Diameter of Transepiphyseal Drill Holes

- A drill bit corresponding to the smallest size through which the tendon would easily pass should be used to make transepiphyseal holes.
- A small-diameter drill bit is less likely to damage the physes, and a snug fit promotes healing of the graft to bone.
- The graft passage can be eased by chamfering the femoral hole and pushing the graft into the hole using a blunt instrument through an anteromedial portal while pulling a no. 5 FiberWire suture tied to an EndoButton.

Failure of Fixation

- Load to failure in this technique exceeds normal tensile loads on the anterior cruciate ligament.
- In the early phase of healing, failure of fixation can lead to instability.
- Check the femoral side fixation with the C-arm to confirm that the EndoButton washer is flush on the lateral femoral condyle.

Graft Slippage Associated with Suture Post Fixation

- Minimize slippage by meticulous placement of whipstitches in tendon ends with tight loops placed in close proximity.
- Pretension graft using Graftmaster (Smith & Nephew Endoscopy, Andover, MA).
- When the tendon graft extends through the tibial hole, augment the tibial fixation by suturing the tendons through the periosteum.

Data from Anderson AF: Transepiphyseal replacement of the anterior cruciate ligament using quadruple hamstring grafts in skeletally immature patients, *J Bone Joint Surg* 86A:201, 2004.

- Place the injured lower limb in an arthroscopic leg holder with the hip flexed to 20 degrees to facilitate C-arm fluoroscopic viewing of the knee in the lateral plane.
- Position the C-arm on the side of the table opposite the injured knee, and place the monitor at the head of the table. View the tibial and femoral physes in the anteroposterior and lateral planes before the limb is prepared and draped. When the distal part of the femur is viewed, adjust the C-arm so that the medial and lateral femoral condyles line up perfectly with the lateral plane. Rotate the C-arm to see the extension of the tibial physis into the tibial tubercle on the lateral view of the tibia.
- Make an oblique 4-cm incision over the semitendinosus and gracilis tendons. Dissect these tendons free, and transect at the musculotendinous junction with use of a standard tendon stripper, and detach distally.
- Double the tendons, and place a no. 5 FiberWire suture (Arthrex, Naples, FL) in the ends of the tendons with a whipstitch.
- Place the doubled tendons under 4.5 kg (10 lb) of tension on the back table with the use of the Graftmaster device (Acufex-Smith Nephew, Andover, MA).
- Insert the arthroscope into the anterolateral portal, and insert a probe through the anteromedial portal.
- Perform intraarticular examination in the usual manner.
- Remove debris in the intercondylar notch and perform a notchplasty to see the anatomical footprint of the anterior cruciate ligament on the femur.
- Repair any substantial meniscal tears found.
- With the C-arm in the lateral position, adjust the limb to show a perfect lateral view.

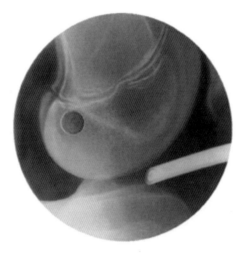

Figure 40-1

- Place the point of the guidewire over the lateral femoral condyle, corresponding with the location of the footprint of the anterior cruciate ligament on the femur. This point is approximately one fourth of the distance from posterior to anterior along the Blumensaat line and one fourth of the distance down from the Blumensaat line. Make a 2-cm lateral incision at this point (Figure 40-1).
- Incise the iliotibial tract longitudinally, and strip the periosteum from a small area of the lateral femoral condyle.
- Use the C-arm to view the entry point of the guidewire in the anteroposterior and the lateral planes. With the C-arm in the lateral plane and with the use of a free-hand technique, introduce the point of the guidewire 2 to 3 mm into the femoral epiphysis. Do not angulate the pin anteriorly or posteriorly, but rather keep it perpendicular to the femur in the coronal plane. Rotate the C-arm to the anteroposterior plane to ensure that the guidewire is not angulated superiorly or inferiorly.
- Drive the guidewire across the femoral epiphysis, perpendicular to the femur and distal to the physis. Through the arthroscope, view the entrance of the guidewire into the intercondylar notch. The guidewire should enter the joint 1 mm posterior and superior to the center of the anatomical footprint of the anterior cruciate ligament on the femur.

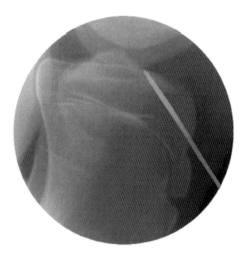

Figure 40-2

- Leave the femoral guidewire in place, and insert a second guidewire into the anteromedial aspect of the tibia, through the epiphysis, with the aid of a tibial drill guide. From the direct lateral position, rotate the C-arm externally approximately 30 degrees to show the physis clearly extending into the tibial tubercle. Drill the guidewire into the tibial epiphysis under real-time fluoroscopic imaging. The handle of the drill guide must be lifted for the wire to clear the anterior part of the tibial physis. The wire should enter the joint at the level of the free edge of the lateral meniscus and in the posterior footprint of the anterior cruciate ligament on the tibia (Figure 40-2).
- Arthroscopically confirm the appropriate position of both guidewires at this point.
- Use tendon sizers to measure the diameter of the quadruple tendon graft (which typically is 6 to 8 mm). A tight fit is important; consequently, use the smallest appropriate drill to ream over both guidewires.
- Chamfer the edge of the femoral hole intraarticularly, and measure the width of the lateral femoral condyle. Choose the appropriate EndoButton continuous loop (Acufex-Smith Nephew, Memphis, TN) (2 to 3 cm) so that approximately 2 cm of the quadruple hamstring tendon graft remains within the lateral femoral condyle.

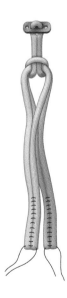

Figure 40-3

- Pass the EndoButton continuous loop around the middle of the double tendons, and loop the inside of itself to secure the tendons proximally (Figure 40-3). Alternatively, the tendons can be placed through the continuous loop before the tendon ends are sutured together. However, this requires drilling and measuring the length of the femoral hole before graft preparation. Otherwise, it is difficult to determine the appropriate length of the EndoButton continuous loop necessary to leave 2 cm of the tendon graft within the lateral femoral condyle.

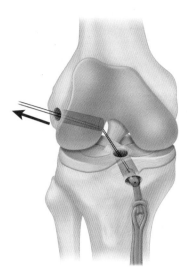

Figure 40-4

- Place a no. 5 FiberWire suture in one end of the EndoButton, and pass a suture passer from anterior to posterior through the tibia and out of the lateral femoral condyle. Pull the EndoButton and tendons up through the tibia and out of the femoral hole with the use of the no. 5 suture (Figure 40-4).

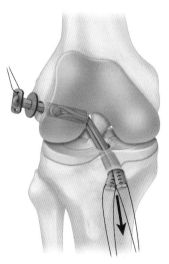

Figure 40-5

- Place an EndoButton washer (Smith & Nephew, Memphis, TN), 3 to 4 mm larger than the femoral hole, over the EndoButton. Apply tension to the tendons distally, pulling the EndoButton and washer to the surface of the lateral femoral condyle. The washer is necessary to anchor the graft proximally because the hole in the femoral condyle is larger than the EndoButton (Figure 40-5).
- Place the graft under tension, and extend the knee to determine arthroscopically if there is impingement of the graft on the intercondylar notch.
- An anterior notchplasty usually is unnecessary when this technique is used; however, if the anterior outlet of the intercondylar notch touches or indents the graft in terminal extension, remove a small portion of the anterior outlet.

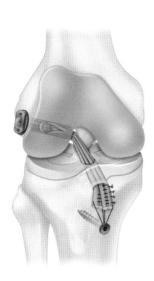
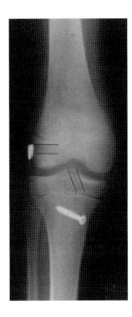

Figure 40-6

- With the knee in 10 degrees of flexion, secure the quadruple hamstring graft distally by tying the no. 5 FiberWire sutures over a tibial screw and post that is placed medial to the tibial tubercle apophysis and distal to the proximal tibial physis (Figure 40-6).

- If the tendon graft extends through the tibial drill hole, secure it to the periosteum of the anterior tibia with multiple no. 1 Ethibond sutures with use of figure-of-eight stitches. Close the subcutaneous tissue and skin in a routine fashion, and apply a hinged brace.

PHYSEAL-SPARING RECONSTRUCTION OF THE ANTERIOR CRUCIATE LIGAMENT ⟩

The procedure of Kocher, Garg, and Micheli consists of arthroscopically assisted, physeal-sparing, combined intraarticular and extraarticular reconstruction of the anterior cruciate ligament with use of an autogenous iliotibial band graft. This is a modification of the combined intraarticular and extraarticular reconstruction described by MacIntosh and Darby (Figure 40-7). Modifications include application in skeletally immature patients, arthroscopic assistance, graft fixation, and accelerated rehabilitation. Rehabilitation must be geared to the age of the young patient.

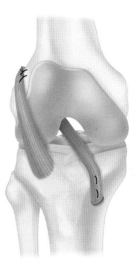

Figure 40-7

- The procedure is done with the patient under general anesthesia as an overnight observation procedure.

- Position the child supine on the operating table with a pneumatic tourniquet around the proximal aspect of the thigh.

- With the patient under anesthesia, confirm anterior cruciate ligament insufficiency.
- Make an incision of approximately 6 cm obliquely from the lateral joint line to the superior border of the iliotibial band. Separate the iliotibial band proximally from the subcutaneous tissue with the use of a periosteal elevator under the skin of the lateral part of the thigh.
- Incise the anterior and posterior borders of the iliotibial band, and carry the incisions proximally under the skin with the use of a curved meniscotome.
- Detach the iliotibial band proximally under the skin with the use of a curved meniscotome or an open tendon stripper.
- Leave the iliotibial band attached distally at Gerdy's tubercle.
- Dissect distally to separate the iliotibial band from the joint capsule and from the lateral patellar retinaculum.
- Tubularize the free proximal end of the iliotibial band with a whipstitch using a no. 5 Ethibond suture (Ethicon, Johnson & Johnson, Somerville, NJ).
- Examine the knee with the arthroscope through standard anterolateral and anteromedial portals, treat any meniscal injury or chondral injury, and excise the anterior cruciate ligament remnant.
- Identify the over-the-top position on the femur and the over-the-front position under the intermeniscal ligament.
- Perform a minimal notchplasty to avoid iatrogenic injury to the perichondral ring of the distal femoral physis, which is in close proximity to the over-the-top position.
- Bring the free end of the iliotibial band graft through the over-the-top position with the use of a full-length clamp or a two-incision, rear-entry guide and out through the anteromedial portal.
- Make a second incision of approximately 4.5 cm over the proximal medial aspect of the tibia in the region of the pes anserinus. Carry the dissection through the subcutaneous tissue to the periosteum.
- Place a curved clamp from this incision into the joint under the intermeniscal ligament.
- Make a small groove in the anteromedial aspect of the proximal tibial epiphysis under the intermeniscal ligament with the use of a curved rat-tail rasp to bring the tibial graft placement more posterior.
- Bring the free end of the graft through the joint, under the intermeniscal ligament in the anteromedial epiphyseal groove, and out through the medial tibial incision.
- Place the knee in 90 degrees of flexion and 15 degrees of external rotation. For extraarticular reconstruction, fix the graft on the femoral side through the lateral incision using mattress sutures on the lateral femoral condyle at the insertion of the lateral intermuscular septum.
- Fix the tibial side through the medial incision with the knee flexed 20 degrees and tension applied to the graft.
- Make a periosteal incision distal to the proximal tibial physis as confirmed fluoroscopically.
- Make a trough in the proximal medial tibial metaphyseal cortex, and suture the graft to the periosteum at the rough margins with mattress sutures.

POSTOPERATIVE CARE 〉

Postoperatively, the patient is permitted touch-down weight bearing for 6 weeks. Immediate mobilization from 0 to 90 degrees is allowed for the first 2 weeks, followed by progression to full range of motion. Continuous passive motion from 0 to 90 degrees is used for the first 2 weeks postoperatively to initiate motion and overcome the anxiety associated with postoperative movement in young children. A protective hinged knee brace is used for 6 weeks after surgery with motion limits of 0 to 90 degrees for the first 2 weeks. Progressive rehabilitation consists of range-of-motion exercises, patellar mobilization, electrical stimulation, pool therapy (if available), proprioception exercises, and closed-chain strengthening exercises during the first 3 months postoperatively followed by straight-line jogging, plyometric exercises, sport cord exercises, and sport-specific exercises. Return to full activity, including sports that involve cutting, usually is allowed 6 months postoperatively. A custom-made knee brace is used routinely during cutting and pivoting activities for the first 2 years after return to sports.

OPEN RECONSTRUCTION OF POSTERIOR CRUCIATE LIGAMENT WITH PATELLAR TENDON GRAFT

Robert H. Miller III • Frederick M. Azar

CLANCY TECHNIQUE ⟩

Any of the commercial drill guides or systems can be used to determine the tunnel locations. Interference screw fixation of the bone plugs in the femoral and tibial tunnels is preferred by most surgeons, although it may be more difficult than with anterior cruciate ligament reconstructions. In particular the length of the tibial tunnel for posterior cruciate ligament reconstruction is greater than that for anterior cruciate ligament reconstruction; therefore, the distal bone plug can be more difficult to see in the tunnel for interference screw fixation. A longer plug of bone from the tibial tuberosity is advised. However, a long fragment of bone on the proximal end of the graft can make its entrance into the femoral tunnel more difficult. An anterolateral rather than anteromedial tibial tunnel starting point has been recommended to avoid the "killer turn" as the graft emerges from the tibia. This position was found to be associated with improved objective outcomes, but clinical results were not significantly correlated to a specific graft position.

If no femoral stump is present for reference to the most isometric point, the most isometric region is located toward the roof of the intercondylar notch and on average is 11 mm from the junction of the notch and the trochlear groove. This isometric attachment area extends approximately 1 cm from the roof in a posterior and slightly distal direction. A strong suture or wire should be passed through holes drilled in the selected tibial and femoral condyles and attached to an isometer device. Length change of 2 mm or less is acceptable; if more, the femoral site should be adjusted. If length increases with flexion during isometric testing, the selected site is distal to the most isometric region; the opposite is true if length decreases with flexion.

- Prepare and drape the leg in the standard fashion and inflate the tourniquet.
- Make a standard medial parapatellar incision, curved posteriorly at the superior aspect in line with the medial femoral epicondyle but approximately two fingerbreadths proximal. Incise the subcutaneous tissue in a similar fashion.
- Make a medial arthrotomy close to the medial aspect of the patellar tendon. Inspect the knee joint and excise and repair any meniscal tears or excise the meniscus if necessary. If the tear of the posterior cruciate ligament is acute, place sutures through the larger remnant.
- In an isolated posterior cruciate ligament injury, the ligament of Humphry usually is intact and can be mistaken for an intact posterior cruciate ligament. However, careful dissection shows that its most anterior fibers follow a lateral course to the posterior horn of the lateral meniscus.
- The ligament of Wrisberg also may be present; it is composed of fibers attaching to the posterior cruciate ligament and also travels in a lateral direction toward the posterior horn of the lateral meniscus.
- If either of these ligaments is intact, the tibia will move only slightly backward when it is held in marked internal rotation and a posterior drawer maneuver is done. These ligaments decrease the expected excessive internal rotation and posterior translation of the tibia and can lead to a mistaken diagnosis of pure posterolateral rotary instability. If neither ligament is intact, the tibia will have significant posterior and internal rotational excursions on the femur.
- Now direct attention to the posteromedial aspect of the knee.
- With the knee flexed to 90 degrees, sharply dissect the subcutaneous tissue and overlying skin to expose the anteromedial aspect of the medial gastrocnemius and semimembranosus tendons.
- Make a posterior incision in the capsule just anterior to the medial gastrocnemius tendon. Make the incision through the synovium and posterior capsule, keeping it posteromedially from the medial meniscus so that the meniscus can be preserved if it is intact.
- If necessary for exposure, release the medial third of the medial gastrocnemius tendon just distal to its insertion onto the femur.
- With the knee flexed to 90 degrees, use a curved retractor to retract the posterior capsule and synovium, exposing the old insertion of the posterior cruciate ligament onto the tibia.

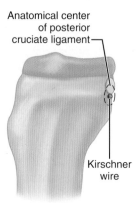

Anatomical center
of posterior
cruciate ligament

Kirschner
wire

Figure 41-1

- Place a drill guide or a gloved finger posterolateral to the anatomical center of the posterior cruciate ligament attachment on the tibia (Figure 41-1).

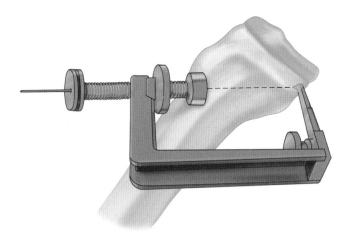

Figure 41-2

- Place the anterior part of the drill guide or a Kirschner wire distal and medial to the tibial insertion of the patellar tendon (Figure 41-2).

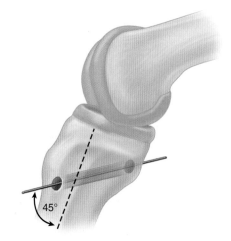

45°

Figure 41-3

- Drill a tunnel from distal to proximal through the tibia at an angle of approximately 45 degrees (Figure 41-3).

- Place the Kirschner wire, with or without the drill guide, at the anterior site so that it will exit posterolaterally to the anatomical center of the posterior cruciate ligament insertion. Then overdrill the Kirschner wire with a 10-mm drill bit.

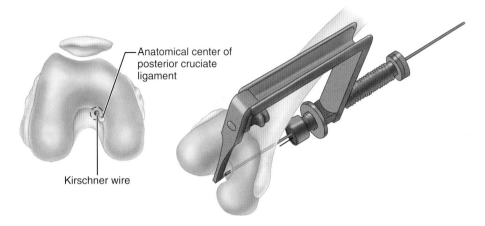

Figure 41-4

- Use the drill guide to insert the Kirschner wire through the medial femoral condyle so that it exits anterosuperior to the anatomical center of the original posterior cruciate ligament attachment, usually at the edge of the osteochondral junction (Figure 41-4).
- Drill it to enter posterosuperior to the femoral epicondyle and then overdrill the wire with a 10-mm reamer.
- Undermine the vastus medialis inferiorly and retract it to expose the exit tunnel.
- Now harvest the graft. Free the medial third of the patellar tendon (leaving a 5-mm intact border) from the remaining patellar tendon.
- Use power instruments to remove a patellar bone block 10 mm wide, 4 mm deep, and 25 mm long; do not take any quadriceps tendon with the bone block.
- Drill three holes through the bone block with a 0.062-inch Kirschner wire and place a no. 5 nonabsorbable suture through each hole.

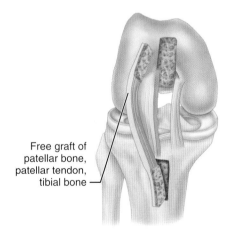

Free graft of
patellar bone,
patellar tendon,
tibial bone —

Figure 41-5

- Remove a bone block the same size as the patellar bone block from the tibial tuberosity insertion of the patellar tendon (Figure 41-5).

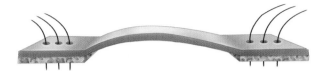

Figure 41-6

- Drill three holes through this block and place a no. 5 nonabsorbable suture through each hole (Figure 41-6).

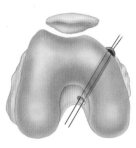

Figure 41-7

- Place the patellar bone block in the femoral tunnel so that it lies entirely within the medial femoral condyle (Figure 41-7).

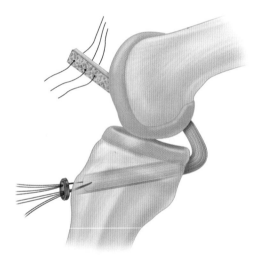

Figure 41-8

- Tie the femoral sutures loosely over a button placed over the exit of the femoral tunnel (Figure 41-8).
- Pass a suture passer into the posteromedial capsular incision and then into the intercondylar notch.
- Place the sutures into the tibial graft and pull them out through the posteromedial capsular incision, pulling the tibial graft gently through the intercondylar notch.
- Pass the suture passer into the tibial tunnel anteriorly and curve it out through the posteromedial capsular incision.
- Pass the tibial graft sutures through the suture passer and bring them out anteriorly. Tilt the tibial bone graft so that its inferior tip is angled anteriorly to allow easy passage into the tibial tunnel posteriorly.
- If the graft is difficult to place in the tunnel, soft tissue may be blocking the tunnel entrance, the tibial graft may be too long to be angled sufficiently to enter the tunnel, or the tunnel may be too low. If the tunnel is too low, enlarge it by reaming with gentle anterosuperior pressure on the reamer.
- Insert an AO malleolar screw and washer 5 mm longer than measured by the depth gauge at the inferior edge of the tibial tunnel.
- At the femoral tunnel, tie the patellar bone sutures over a button.
- Then, with the knee in 90 degrees of flexion, pull forward on the tibia and tie the tibial bone sutures over the AO screw and washer.

- Tighten one suture with the knee in 90 degrees of flexion; bring the knee to 30 degrees of flexion and retighten the suture while maintaining the anterior drawer.
- Secure the remaining ties and tighten the screw.
- Perform a posterior drawer test and examine the knee for the normal step-off of the medial and lateral femoral condyles. Place the knee through a full range of motion and perform a posterior drawer test.
- Close the capsular arthrotomies in the standard fashion and place a drain in the medial side.
- Close the subcutaneous tissue and skin in the standard fashion.

If a central-third autogenous patellar tendon is chosen as the graft source, a limited incision placed anteriorly of the patellar tendon can be made for graft harvest. The intraarticular portion of the procedure can be done arthroscopically, or the menisci and intercondylar notch can be exposed through the defect in the patellar tendon after graft harvest.

SALLAY AND MCCARROLL TECHNIQUE 〉

- Carefully identify the plane between the scarred posterior cruciate ligament and the anterior cruciate ligament to prevent damage to the anterior cruciate ligament while excising remnants of the posterior cruciate ligament. Preserve a minimal amount of tissue at the femoral attachment site to identify the anatomical footprint.
- Make a second incision to identify the tibial insertion of the posterior cruciate ligament to safely drill the tibial tunnel and to facilitate graft passage. Many surgeons elect to make a small posteromedial incision, identical to the exposure for a medial meniscal repair, regardless of the basic technique chosen for posterior cruciate ligament reconstruction (including arthroscopic), to protect the neurovascular structures and to facilitate graft passage. Sallay and McCarroll based the site of their incision on the need to treat associated medial or lateral injury. In the absence of injury to the lateral side, the standard approach has been a 4-cm posteromedial incision.

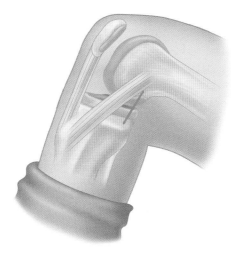

Figure 41-9

- Begin the proximal portion of the incision below and posterior to the medial femoral epicondyle, extending it vertically downward, parallel to the lines of skin cleavage (Figure 41-9).
- Incise the investing fascia (layer I) in line with the skin incision superior to the leading edge of the sartorius muscle. Protect the infrapatellar branch of the saphenous nerve in the inferior aspect of the wound.
- Retract the pes tendons posteriorly, exposing the medial collateral ligament and the posterior oblique ligament.
- Make a vertical arthrotomy between the posterior oblique ligament and the medial head of the gastrocnemius tendon.
- Sharply dissect the capsule off its tibial attachment, leaving the meniscotibial ligament intact. In chronic tears, this plane may be obscured by scarring of the posterior capsule to the posterior cruciate ligament. To prevent injury to the popliteal contents, carefully mobilize the scar tissue by blunt dissection to reflect the capsule off the tibial insertion of the posterior cruciate ligament.
- Now identify the posterior tibial sulcus by palpation and observation.

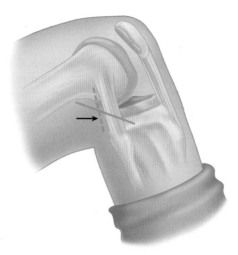

Figure 41-10

- If there is an associated injury to the posterolateral corner, a lateral approach is preferred. Make a short, oblique incision, 6 cm long, just posterior to the lateral collateral ligament (Figure 41-10).
- Incise the iliotibial band (layer I) in line with its fibers.
- The lateral collateral ligament lies beneath a superficial lamina (layer II). Divide this layer posterior to the lateral collateral ligament, exposing the deep capsular lamina (layer III).
- Divide the capsule in line with the posterior aspect of the lateral collateral ligament, exposing the postero-lateral joint space. Protect the popliteal tendon in the inferior aspect of the wound.
- Release the capsule and its attachment to the popliteus and meniscotibial ligament as described for the medial approach. In patients with acute injury of the posterior cruciate ligament and the posterolateral corner, much of the exposure and dissection has been done by the disruption.
- To create the tibial tunnel, make an L-shaped periosteal flap 1 cm medial to the distal portion of the tibial tubercle just proximal to the pes tendon group insertion.
- With use of a commercially available drill guide, advance a guide pin from this site in a posterolateral and proximal direction, exiting at the inferior and lateral quadrant of the posterior tibial sulcus.
- Confirm and document the proper position of the guide pin with an intraoperative radiograph.
- Bone guides allow calculation of the distance of the tibial tunnel, and the guide pin can be "chucked down" to the proper length to prevent overpenetration; placing a finger through the posteromedial incision to palpate the tibial fovea also protects the neurovascular structures from overpenetration. Some surgeons prefer to perform this step under imaging guidance to ensure proper placement of the guidewire.
- Overream the pin with the 10-mm reamer, again using a finger to protect the neurovascular structures. Some surgeons remove the power source and complete the last portion of the reaming by hand because certain reamers pull tissue toward the reamer as they advance along a guidewire. Paulos et al. used an oscillating reamer and drill stop to prevent vascular complications. Sallay and McCarroll used a reamer with a conical profile because the standard square profile reamers have been shown to cut out the posterior tibial cortex as far as 2 cm inferior to the intended exit site.
- Be careful not to apply counterpressure at the level of the popliteal fossa because this could compress the popliteal structures against the posterior tibia during the reaming process.
- By use of an angled curet or sharp dissection over the tip of the reamer while it is still in the tunnel, debride the edge of the tunnel of residual soft tissue to avoid entrapment of the bone plug during later passage of the graft.
- Chamfer the edges of the tunnel with a rasp.
- The femoral tunnel can be prepared by one of two methods. The standard method begins with exposure of the anteromedial femoral cortex, using the superior portion of the medial incision.
- Elevate the vastus medialis proximally to allow access to the anteromedial aspect of the distal femur.
- Use a commercial drill guide to advance a guide pin from a point just proximal to the medial femoral epicondyle into the intercondylar notch. Pin entry should be at the junction of the anterior and middle thirds of the intercondylar notch (roughly 10 mm proximal to the articular surface) and at the 2-o'clock position for the right knee (10-o'clock position for the left knee), corresponding to the center of the ana-tomical insertion of the anterolateral fibers.

- Overream the pin with a 10-mm reamer and chamfer the tunnel edges with a rasp.
- The second technique for preparation of the femoral tunnel does not require dissection of the medial femoral cortex.
- Advance a long Beath pin through the capsule lateral to the patellar tendon to obtain the appropriate tunnel trajectory. The point of entry should correspond to the anatomical insertion of the anterior fibers.
- Advance the pin through the vastus medialis muscle and skin.

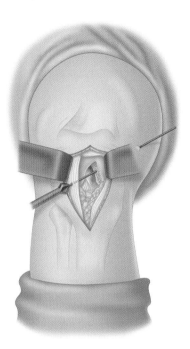

Figure 41-11

- Ream over the guide pin from the intercondylar side with a 10-mm reamer, stopping short of the medial femoral cortex (Figure 41-11).
- Withdraw the reamer, leaving the Beath pin in place. This creates a blind-end tunnel from inside to out.
- The graft can be passed in two ways, depending on the preference of the surgeon.
- The first technique begins by passing the smaller, bullet-shaped bone plug through the tibial tunnel from anterior to posterior.
- Use a suture passer to retrieve the traction sutures into the posteromedial (lateral) wound.

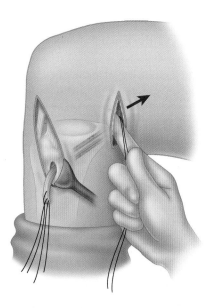

Figure 41-12

- With constant tension applied parallel to the direction of the tibial tunnel, deliver the bone plug into the posterior recess. Avoid pulling at an angle oblique to the tunnel because this causes the bone plug to bend at the posterior tunnel opening (Figure 41-12).
- Use the suture passer to retrieve the bone plug into the intercondylar notch.
- Direct the graft into the femoral tunnel with the traction suture.
- The second technique uses the Beath pin to assist in passage of the femoral bone plug.
- Thread the traction sutures of the bone plug through the eyelet at the end of the guide pin.
- Withdraw the pin from the medial aspect of the knee, leaving the traction sutures in the tunnel exiting the medial soft tissues.
- Advance the bone plug into the tunnel with the tendon portion facing the articular surface until the end of the bone plug is flush with the wall of the intercondylar notch. Abrasion of the graft is minimized because the tendon does not rest against the edge of the femoral tunnel.
- Thread the sutures of the other bone plug through a DePuy graft passer (DePuy, Warsaw, IN). Advance the free end of the graft passer through the patellar tendon defect and the notch into the posterior recess. Apply gentle tension to the sutures to seat the end of the bone plug firmly in the mount of the graft passer.
- Thread the free end of the graft passer through the tibial tunnel from posterior to anterior, using an arthroscopic clamp.
- Place a heavy clamp on the end of the graft passer, preventing relative motion between the passer and the graft. Apply firm tension to the graft passer to deliver the graft through the notch and into the tibial tunnel. Maintaining an anterior drawer force on the tibia also aids graft passage into the tunnel.
- Fixation can be achieved by tying the sutures over ligament buttons, interference screws, or both.
- Fix the femoral bone plug first.
- Move the knee through a full range of motion to evaluate relative motion of the tibial bone plug with respect to the tibial tunnel. An appropriately placed graft should have no more than 2 mm of relative motion.
- Fix the tibial side with the knee flexed to 90 degrees with an anterior drawer force applied to re-create the normal femoral-tibial relationship. Secure the bone plug with a 9 × 20-mm cannulated interference screw. If the end of the graft is difficult to see, place the arthroscope into the tibial tunnel to allow more accurate screw fixation. As an alternative, tie the sutures over a ligament button.
- Perform a posterior drawer test to ensure adequate stability. Residual laxity should be grade I or less.
- Close in routine fashion over a drain.

POSTOPERATIVE CARE ⟩

Restoring motion and reducing swelling take priority within the first week. Patients are encouraged to perform active range-of-motion exercises, quadriceps training, and full weight bearing in an extension brace in the immediate postoperative period. Immobilization is continued in extension for 3 weeks in patients in whom medial or lateral capsuloligamentous structures were repaired. Strengthening and functional activities are introduced in a stepwise program.

ARTHROSCOPIC-ASSISTED POSTERIOR CRUCIATE LIGAMENT RECONSTRUCTION — SINGLE AND DOUBLE TUNNEL

Barry B. Phillips • Marc J. Mihalko

For most high-impact knee injuries, we perform a posterolateral corner repair or reconstruction using a figure-of-eight tendon reconstruction technique. The femoral tunnel can be single or double; the double-tunnel technique practically and biomechanically provides better stability. The single-tunnel technique is used primarily in reconstruction of multiple knee ligaments in knee dislocations; the double-tunnel technique is used primarily for isolated PCL reconstruction.

SINGLE-TUNNEL POSTERIOR CRUCIATE LIGAMENT RECONSTRUCTION 》

- Place the patient supine and apply a tourniquet high around the thigh. Use a padded lateral post to assist with valgus stress. Tape a 3-L saline bag to the table before draping to use as a foot bolster to help maintain 80 to 90 degrees of knee flexion during the procedure.

- Perform a routine systematic arthroscopic examination of the knee and repair any associated intraarticular abnormalities as necessary. If a meniscal repair is performed, the sutures should be tied after the ligament reconstruction is completed.

- Using standard anterolateral and anteromedial portals, débride the soft tissue and remaining cruciate ligament from the intercondylar notch.

- Perform an internal bony notchplasty as necessary.

- Viewing of the tibial attachment site of the posterior cruciate ligament is improved by using a 70-degree viewing arthroscope in the anterolateral portal or by placing the 30-degree viewing arthroscope through a posteromedial portal.

- Using a full-radius resector, remove the remaining stump of the posterior cruciate ligament. Specially designed back-cutting knives, curets, and rasps also are available to assist in removing the remnants.

- Elevate the posterior capsule from its attachment to the posterior flat spot on the tibia using a curved curet or periosteal elevator passed through the intercondylar notch or the posteromedial portal.

- Contour an Achilles tendon allograft to make a bone plug 11 mm wide × 20 mm long.

- Place the tendinous part of the graft under tension and roll the graft with a running Vicryl suture. Place a no. 5 tension suture in the distal 5 cm of the graft using a running interlocking suture. Place the graft on a graft tension board, maintained with 10 lb of tension for 15 minutes.

- If an autogenous patellar tendon is chosen as a graft, make a 7-cm midline incision starting at the inferior patella and extending distally over the tibial tuberosity.

- Harvest the central third of the patellar tendon—10 to 11 mm wide and 25 mm long—with 8-mm-thick bone plugs.

- Contour the graft to pass through a 10- or 11-mm trial. The bone plug to be secured in the femoral tunnel should be shortened to approximately 20 mm to make intraarticular passage easier.

- For making the tibial tunnel, we prefer to use the Arthrex drill guide system. With the 70-degree arthroscope in the anterolateral portal, insert the guide through the anteromedial portal and pass it through the notch.

- Place the guide tip 10 to 12 mm below the joint line in the posterior cruciate ligament facet.

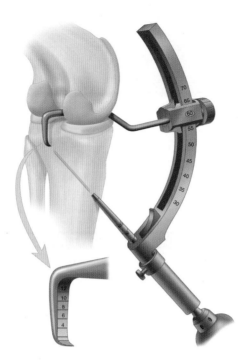

Figure 42-1

- Orient the drill guide approximately 60 degrees to the articular surface of the tibia starting just inferior and medial to the tibial tuberosity. A more perpendicular angle would create too much of an acute angle at the posterior tibia that may abrade the graft. A tibial tunnel that is started too distally may ream out the posterior tibial shelf. The simultaneous use of image intensification and arthroscopy aids in proper positioning of the drill guide before and during drilling. Calibrations on the tibial guide accurately measure the distance from the anterior tibial cortex to the tip of the guide (Figure 42-1).

- Adjust the guide pin so that it is protruding from the tip of the drill 1 cm less than the distance measured on the guide system to help prevent overdrilling. The guide pin should exit posteriorly at the physeal scar area.

- Tap the pin in the final 1 cm to help prevent penetration. While tapping the pin in, place a curet through the posteromedial portal to protect the neurovascular structures from pin penetration during advancement and reaming. If adequate soft tissue débridement has been performed, the guide pin can be observed arthroscopically as it exits the tibia. An image intensifier is used to confirm appropriate guidewire placement.

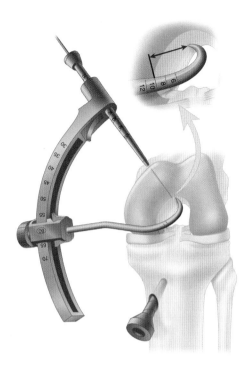

Figure 42-2

- The femoral physiometric point is 8 mm proximal to the articular cartilage at the 1-o'clock position on the right knee and at the 11-o'clock position on the left knee. Place the tip of the posterior cruciate ligament femoral guide through the anteromedial portal while viewing with the arthroscope in the anterolateral portal (Figure 42-2).
- Expose the femoral cortex through the 3-cm longitudinal incision and elevate the vastus medialis obliquus superiorly.
- Insert the guide pin midway between the articular margin of the medial femoral condyle and the medial epicondyle.
- Use the appropriate size reamer for the available graft leaving 1 to 2 mm of distal bone at the articular margin.

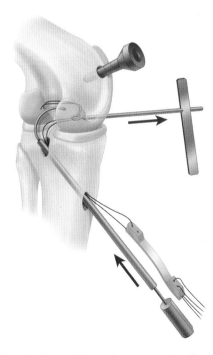

Figure 42-3

- Pass a Gore smoother through the tibial tunnel into the joint and pull it through the central fat pad portal. The smoother is used to smooth and remove the posterior soft-tissue remnants. Do not enlarge the tibial tunnel excessively (Figure 42-3).

- When the smoother passes without undue resistance, attach the graft to the end of the smoother, and pull the graft sutures and bone plug into the joint.
- Extreme flexion of the knee sometimes aids passage of the patellar bone plug from the posterior tibial aperture into the joint. Placing a switching stick through the posteromedial portal allows the guide sutures to be redirected over the stick to assist in passing the graft.
- Place a grasper through the femoral tunnel to grab the sutures. Use a probe or Allis clamp to assist the graft into the femoral tunnel.
- Place the cancellous portion of the bone plug posteriorly to reduce graft abrasion.
- Before tibial fixation ensure that the femoral bone plug would fit appropriately at the aperture of the femoral tunnel.
- Put the knee through a range of motion and ensure there is no more than 3 mm of graft pistoning through range of motion from 0 to 100 degrees. If excessive pistoning is encountered, rasp the femoral tunnel proximal wall.
- Secure the femoral bone plug with a metal interference screw.
- Maintain graft tension and put the knee through a range of motion for 20 cycles to allow stress relaxation of the graft.
- Secure the graft with an interference screw. If a soft tissue graft is used, back-up fixation over a post is indicated.

POSTOPERATIVE CARE 〉

Rehabilitation depends on the graft material selected, the size of the patient, and any other surgery done. After isolated posterior cruciate ligament reconstruction, the knee can be immobilized in extension in a removable knee immobilizer for 4 weeks. Early range-of-motion and quadriceps exercises are encouraged but flexion is limited to 90 degrees for the first 4 weeks. Hamstring strengthening is begun at 3 months. During motion and strengthening therapy care is taken to prevent posterior tibial stress. Return to sports is allowed at 9 months.

DOUBLE-TUNNEL POSTERIOR CRUCIATE LIGAMENT RECONSTRUCTION 〉

- Harvest a patellar tendon bone plug 10 mm wide × 10 to 20 mm long from the patella and tibial tubercle or a quadriceps tendon through a separate small incision above the patella (8 mm wide × 10 to 20 mm long).
- Place three no. 5 Ethibond sutures in each end of the graft for later fixation.
- Alternatively the semitendinosus tendon can be harvested through the inferior incision and doubled over itself to form a double-strength graft.
- After débridement of the posterior cruciate ligament remnant from the femur and débridement of the tibial insertion side of the posterior cruciate ligament, create the tibial tunnel.
- When the site of insertion of the posterior cruciate ligament has been fully identified, drive a guide pin from the anterior tibia (12 to 15 mm distal to the site of graft harvest from the tibial tubercle) into the center of the insertion of the posterior cruciate ligament. The entry point of the guide pin into the tibia is important because it creates a vertical tunnel (which eases graft passage into the tibia and facilitates tensioning of the graft) and avoids creating an oblique hole at the exit site of the tunnel in the fovea. Drilling a hole that enters medial or lateral to the tibial tubercle creates an oblique exit hole in the tibial fovea and can result in excessive medial or lateral placement of the graft.
- Drive a 10-mm reamer over the guidewire and then a 12-mm reamer. Leave the arthroscope in the posteromedial portal to ensure that neither the guide pin nor the reamers penetrate the knee joint during reaming.
- When the tibial tunnel has been reamed, débride the foveal site of any remaining tissue.
- Pass a no. 5 Ethibond suture through the tibial drill hole and out the central fat pad portal. This suture is used during passage of the graft into the tibial tunnel.
- To create the femoral tunnels, use the remaining fibers of the posterior cruciate ligament on the medial femoral condyle as a guide.
- Drill a 10-mm anterior proximal tunnel and an 8-mm posterior distal tunnel, keeping them separated by a 3- to 4-mm bony bridge.

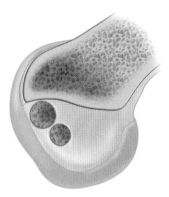

Figure 42-4

- A small (00) curet is used to make marks in the medial femoral condyle at the desired tunnel sites. The anterior proximal tunnel guide pin should enter the intracondylar notch at the 10:30-o'clock position in the left knee (1:30-o'clock position in the right knee) approximately 6 mm posterior to the articular surface of the medial femoral condyle (Figure 42-4).

- Place the posterior distal tunnel approximately 5 mm posterior and 5 mm distal to the anterior proximal tunnel making sure that the tunnel sites remain within the anatomical site of origin of the posterior cruciate ligament and that both tunnels are entirely anterior to the ridge in the medial femoral condyle. Noyes suggested 1-o'clock and 3-o'clock positions and 6 mm and 8 mm off the articular surface. He uses a two-limb quadriceps graft.

- Make an incision over the vastus medialis muscle at the level of the adductor tubercle and elevate the fibers of the vastus medialis anteriorly.

- Use a vector guide to place a pin from the region of the adductor tubercle into the desired position of the anterior proximal tunnel and drive a 10-mm reamer over this guide.

- Drive a second guide pin from a separate site in the medial femoral condyle into the desired site of the posterior distal tunnel and drive an 8-mm reamer over this guide pin. Ensure that an adequate bony bridge separates these two tunnels.

- Pass two no. 5 Ethibond sutures, which will be used later for graft passage, through these tunnels and exit out the central fat pad portal.

- If using the endoscopic technique a specially designed custom guide, flexible guide pins, and reamers are used to ream the two tunnels from the inside of the notch.

- Each tunnel is reamed to a depth of 25 to 30 mm with the appropriate-sized reamer and a 4.5-mm drill is used to drill out the medial femoral cortex.

- The grafts are fixed using an EndoButton device allowing an entirely endoscopic reconstruction.

- Pass the grafts into the femoral tunnels using the previously placed sutures through the central fat pad portal and the femoral tunnels.

- Place the quadriceps or semitendinosus graft first and fix it at the medial femoral condyle using either a simple button (open technique) or an EndoButton (endoscopic technique).

- After femoral fixation of this graft, pass the patellar tendon into the femur and fix in a similar fashion.

- When both grafts have been fixed at the medial femoral condyle, pass them through the central fat pad portal and into the tibia using the previously placed suture through the tibial tunnel. This step can be facilitated with the use of a specialized graft passer, which encloses the grafts and provides a smooth surface to slide through the tibial tunnel. The application of an anterior drawer maneuver at the time of graft passage into the tibia helps the graft to turn the corner at the proximal part of the tibial tunnel.

- The final step in the procedure is fixation of the grafts to the tibia.

- Fix the patellar tendon graft first and tension it at 90 degrees of flexion with an anterior drawer maneuver.

- Tie the sutures from the patellar bone plug over a screw and washer and tighten at the end of the procedure.

- Tighten the quadriceps or hamstring graft at 30 degrees of flexion and tie these sutures over the same screw as those from the patellar tendon graft. Irrigate the wounds and close in routine fashion.

POSTOPERATIVE CARE 〉

The rehabilitation protocol should begin on the first postoperative day. In the immediate postoperative phase the patient is encouraged to bear 50% of weight as tolerated using two crutches to do ankle and hip exercises and to perform knee extensions from 60 to 0 degrees.

Full weight bearing is allowed 2 to 6 weeks after surgery. Multiangle quadriceps and isometric exercises at 60, 40, and 20 degrees are performed. Leg presses and squats from 0 to 60 degrees are introduced and well-leg bicycling is performed. By week 4, range of motion should be to 90 degrees and bicycling can be encouraged for range of motion and endurance. Exercises in the pool are initiated at week 5.

Swimming, closed kinetic chain rehabilitation, and a stretching program are begun at 6 to 12 weeks to increase quadriceps strength. By week 12 the patient can begin lateral step-ups, cycling for endurance (30 minutes), hamstring curls from 0 to 60 degrees with low weight, and a walking program. These exercises should be continued to week 16. By 5 to 6 months after surgery the patient should be performing plyometric exercises and agility and balance drills. The patient can return to sports when KT-2000, isokinetic testing, and functional testing yield satisfactory results.

Open repair of acute Achilles tendon ruptures remains the gold standard of operative treatment, especially for athletic individuals, because of the historically low rate of reruptures, high rate of return to sports, and decreased complication rates with newer techniques. Advocates of open repair argue that Achilles tendon injuries often result in complex obliquely oriented tears that cannot be adequately apposed and repaired with percutaneous of mini-invasive techniques.

OPEN REPAIR OF ACHILLES TENDON RUPTURE — KRACKOW ET AL. 〉

- With the patient prone, make a posteromedial incision approximately 10 cm long about 1 cm medial to the tendon and ending proximal to where the shoe counter strikes the heel.
- Sharply dissect through the skin, subcutaneous tissues, and tendon sheath. Reflect the tendon sheath with the subcutaneous tissue to minimize subcutaneous dissection.

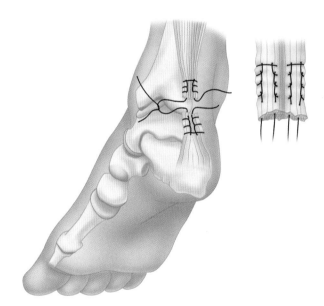

Figure 43-1

- Approximate the ruptured ends of the tendon with a 2-0 nonabsorbable suture (Figure 43-1).
- Check the repair for stability after the sutures are tied.
- Close the peritenon and subcutaneous tissues with 4-0 absorbable sutures.
- Close the skin, and apply a sterile dressing and a posterior splint or short-leg cast with the foot in gravity equinus.

OPEN REPAIR OF ACHILLES TENDON RUPTURE — LINDHOLM 〉

- With the patient prone, make a posterior curvilinear incision extending from the midcalf to the calcaneus.
- Incise the deep fascia in the midline and expose the tendon rupture.

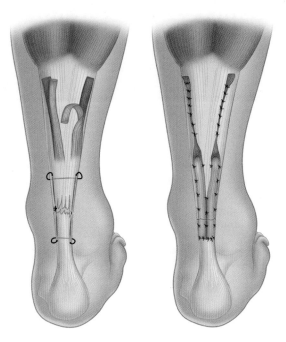

Figure 43-2

- Debride the ragged ends of the tendon and appose them with a box type of mattress suture of heavy non-absorbable suture material or wire; also use fine interrupted sutures (Figure 43-2).
- Fashion two flaps from the proximal tendon and gastrocnemius aponeurosis, each approximately 1 cm wide and 7 to 8 cm long. Leave these flaps attached at a point 3 cm proximal to the site of rupture.
- Twist each flap 180 degrees on itself so that its smooth external surface lies next to the subcutaneous tissue as it is turned distally over the rupture.
- Suture each flap to the distal stump of the tendon and to one another so that they cover the site of rupture completely.
- Close the wound, being careful to approximate the tendon sheath over the site of repair.

OPEN REPAIR OF ACHILLES TENDON RUPTURE — LYNN 〉

Lynn described a method of repairing ruptures of the Achilles tendon in which the plantaris tendon is fanned out to make a membrane 2.5 cm or more wide for reinforcing the repair. The method is useful for injuries less than about 10 days old. Later the plantaris tendon becomes incorporated in the scar tissue and cannot be identified easily.

- Make an incision 12.5 to 17.5 cm long parallel to the medial border of the Achilles tendon.
- Open the tendon sheath in the midline, and, with the foot held in 20 degrees of plantar flexion and without excising the irregular edges, sew the ends of the Achilles tendon together with 2-0 absorbable sutures.

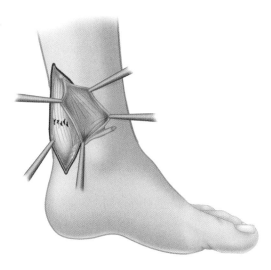

Figure 43-3

- If the plantaris tendon is intact divide its insertion on the calcaneus then, using forceps and beginning distally, fan out the tendon to form a membrane (Figure 43-3).

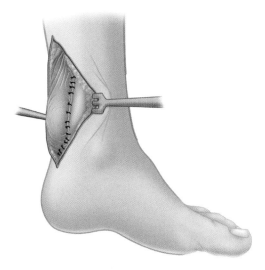

Figure 43-4

- Place this membrane over the repair of the Achilles tendon and suture it in place with interrupted sutures. When possible, cover the Achilles tendon for 2.5 cm both proximal and distal to the repair (Figure 43-4).
- If the plantaris tendon also is ruptured, dissect it free from the Achilles tendon for several centimeters and divide it proximally using a tendon stripper.
- Then pull the tendon distally into the incision, fan it out as a free graft, and cover the repair as already described.
- Close the sheath of the Achilles tendon as far distally as possible without tension and close the wound.

OPEN REPAIR OF ACHILLES TENDON RUPTURE — TEUFFER ❯

- Expose the Achilles tendon and the tuberosity of the calcaneus through a posterolateral longitudinal incision.
- Identify and retract the sural nerve in the proximal part of the wound.
- Detach the peroneus brevis tendon from its insertion through a small incision at the base of the fifth metatarsal.

- Excise the aponeurotic septum, separating the lateral and posterior compartments, and deliver the freed peroneus brevis into the first incision.
- Dissect the tuberosity of the calcaneus and drill a hole large enough for passage of the tendon through the transverse diameter of the bone.

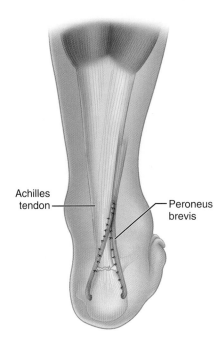

Achilles tendon — — Peroneus brevis

Figure 43-5

- Pass the peroneus brevis tendon through this hole and back proximally beside the Achilles tendon reinforcing the site of rupture and suture it to the peroneus brevis itself, producing a dynamic loop (Figure 43-5).

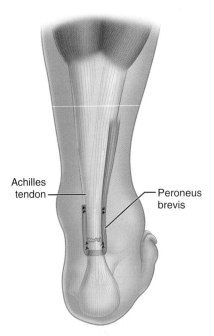

Achilles tendon — — Peroneus brevis

Figure 43-6

- Turco and Spinella described a modification in which the peroneus brevis is passed through a midcoronal slit in the distal stump of the Achilles tendon. The graft is sutured medially and laterally to the stump and proximally to the tendon with multiple interrupted sutures to prevent splitting of the distal tendon stump. This modification can be beneficial if a long distal stump is present (Figure 43-6).

POSTOPERATIVE CARE 〉

The cast is removed at 2 weeks, the wound inspected, and the staples or sutures removed unless subcuticular sutures were used for wound closure. Occasionally an additional week is required for proper wound healing before sutures are removed. A short-leg cast with the foot in gravity equinus is worn for an additional 2 weeks. At 4 weeks the cast is changed again and the foot is gradually brought to the plantigrade position over the following 2 weeks. Walking is gradually resumed with partial weight bearing on crutches during a 2-week period. At 6 to 8 weeks, a short-leg walking cast is applied with the foot in the plantigrade position and full weight bearing is allowed. Alternatively, a removable brace allowing only plantar flexion can be used as early as 4 to 6 weeks after surgery. Gentle active range-of-motion exercises for 20 minutes twice a day are begun. Isometric ankle exercises along with a knee-strengthening and hip-strengthening program can be instituted. Toe raises, progressive resistance exercises, and proprioceptive exercises, in combination with a general strengthening program constitute the third stage of rehabilitation. In reliable, well-supervised patients with good tissue repair this program can be accelerated with earlier use of dorsiflexion-stop orthoses and active range-of-motion exercises. Return to full unrestricted activity usually requires at least 6 months and often more.

A number of techniques have been developed to allow repair through smaller incisions to speed recovery and minimize complications, especially infection and sural nerve damage. Because of the risk of sural nerve injuries with "blind" suturing of the tendon, some of these techniques use multiple incisions (e.g., three-incision technique) endoscopy, or specially designed devices.

Comparisons of open repairs with minimally invasive or percutaneous techniques have shown functional results comparable to those obtained with open repair, with fewer complications, no apparent increased risk of rerupture, and better cosmetic results. Cited disadvantages of minimally invasive techniques include risk of sural nerve injury, failure to appose tendon ends or malalignment of tendon ends, and a lower strength of the repair. In a study of 211 patients with minimally invasive repairs, sural nerve injury occurred in 41 (19%) and reruptures in 17 (8%).

- In the operating room with the patient under local, regional, or general anesthesia, and with the extremity prepared as for open surgery, palpate the tendon defect and make small stab wounds on each side of the Achilles tendon 2.5 cm proximal to the rupture defect.

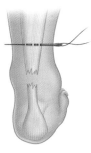

Figure 44-1

- Use a small hemostat to free the underlying tendon sheath from the subcutaneous tissue; pass a no. 0 or a no. 1 nonabsorbable suture threaded on a straight needle from the lateral stab wound through the body of the tendon and exit in the medial stab wound (Figure 44-1).

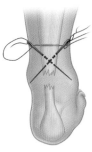

Figure 44-2

- With a straight needle on each end of the inserted suture, crisscross the needles within the body of the tendon and puncture the skin just distal to the site of tendon rupture. Enlarge the sites of needle puncture with a scalpel, and pull the suture completely through the stab wounds. Snug the suture within the proximal portion of the ruptured tendon (Figure 44-2).

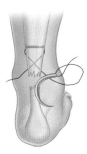

Figure 44-3

- With the lateral suture now threaded on a curved cutting needle, pass the suture back through the last stab wound to exit at about the midportion of the distal stump of the ruptured tendon on the lateral side. Enlarge the hole with a scalpel before pulling the suture through (Figure 44-3).

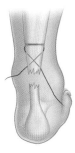

Figure 44-4

- Use a hemostat to free the subcutaneous tissue from the underlying tendon sheath (Figure 44-4).

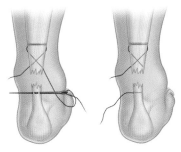

Figure 44-5

- Using a straight needle, pass the lateral suture through the body of the distal stump of the tendon. Enlarge the puncture wound in the skin as before (Figure 44-5).

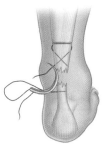

Figure 44-6

- Using a curved cutting needle, pass the suture from this distalmost stab wound on the medial side and exit at the middle stab wound on the medial side of the ruptured tendon (Figure 44-6).

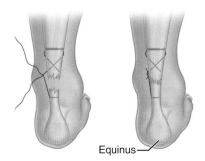

Figure 44-7   Equinus

- With the ankle maintained in equinus position apply tension to the suture in a crisscross manner and bring the tendon ends together. Tie the suture in this position and with a small hemostat bury the knot in the depths of the wound (Figure 44-7).
- Suturing the skin is unnecessary. Apply a sterile dressing to the stab wounds and apply a short-leg cast in gravity equinus position.

POSTOPERATIVE CARE ❯

The short-leg cast is worn with non–weight bearing for 4 weeks, at which time a weight-bearing, low-heeled, short-leg equinus cast is applied. At 8 weeks the cast is removed and a therapy program of toe-heel raising and gastrocnemius-soleus exercises is begun. The patient gradually restores the foot to a neutral position during a 4-week period. Then the patient begins heel cord stretching exercises for an additional 4 weeks.

The Bankart procedure is indicated when the labrum and capsule are separated from the glenoid rim or the capsule is thin; it is, however, technically difficult. Keys to the success of this procedure are (1) maximizing healing potential by abrading the scapular neck, (2) restoring glenoid concavity, (3) securing anatomical capsular fixation at the edge of the glenoid articular surface, and (4) re-creating physiological capsular tendon by superior and inferior capsular advancement and imbrication; supervised goal-oriented rehabilitation also is essential.

OPEN BANKART REPAIR ⟩

- Make an incision along the Langer lines beginning 2 cm distal and lateral to the coracoid process and going inferiorly to the anterior axillary crease.
- Develop the deltopectoral interval retracting the deltoid and cephalic vein laterally and the pectoralis major muscle medially. Leave the conjoined tendon intact and retract it medially.
- Split the subscapularis tendon transversely in line with its fibers at the junction of the upper two thirds and lower one third of the tendon and carefully dissect it from the underlying anterior capsule. Maintain the subscapularis tendon interval with a modified Gelpi retractor (Anspach, Inc, Lake Park, FL) and place a three-pronged retractor medially on the glenoid neck.

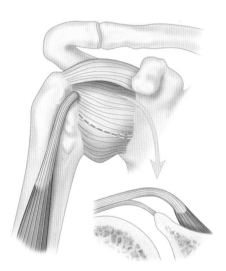

Figure 45-1

- Make a horizontal anterior capsulotomy in line with the split in the subscapularis tendon from the humeral insertion laterally to the anterior glenoid neck medially. Place stay sutures in the superior and inferior capsular flaps at the glenoid margin (Figure 45-1).
- Insert a narrow humeral head retractor and retract the head laterally. Elevate the capsule on the anterior neck subperiosteally. Leave the labrum intact if it is still attached. Decorticate the anterior neck to bleeding bone with a rongeur.

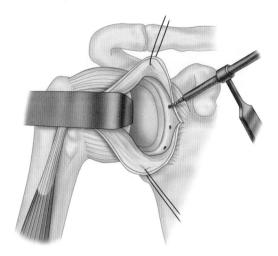

Figure 45-2

- Drill holes near the glenoid rim at approximately the 3-, 4-, and 5:30-o'clock positions, keeping the drill bit parallel to the glenoid surface (Figure 45-2).

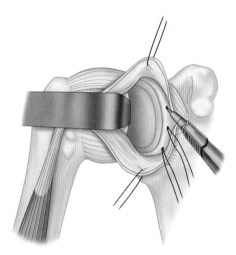

Figure 45-3

- Place suture anchors in each hole and check for security of the anchors. During this portion of the procedure maintain the shoulder in approximately 90 degrees of abduction and 60 degrees of external rotation for throwing athletes. Maintain the shoulder in 60 degrees abduction and 30 to 45 degrees external rotation in nonthrowing athletes and other patients (Figure 45-3).

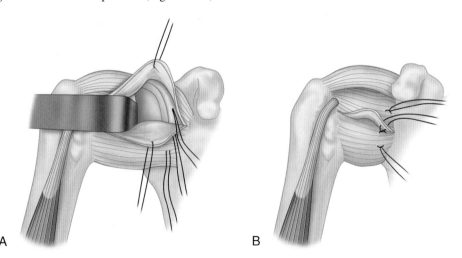

A   B

Figure 45-4

- Tie the inferior flap down in mattress fashion, shifting the capsule superiorly but not medially (Figure 45-4, **A**). The stay sutures help prevent medialization of the capsule. Shift the superior flap inferiorly, overlapping and reinforcing the inferior flap (**B**).

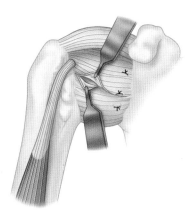

Figure 45-5

- Loosely close the remaining gap in the capsule. The reconstruction has two layers of reinforced capsule outside the joint (Figure 45-5).

POSTOPERATIVE CARE 〉

Postoperative rehabilitation is carried out as described in Box 45-1.

BOX　45-1　　Rehabilitation Program after Open Bankart Repair

Postoperative Period (0-3 Weeks)
- Abduction pillow
- Passive/active ROM: abduction (90 degrees), flexion (90 degrees), and external rotation (45 degrees); no extension
- Isometric abduction, horizontal adduction, and external rotation
- Elbow ROM
- Ball squeeze
- Ice

Phase I (3-6 Weeks)
- Discontinue brace/pillow
- Modalities as needed
- Progressive passive and active ROM, protecting anterior capsule
- Active internal rotation (full) and external rotation (neutral) using tubing and free weights
- Prone extension (not posterior to trunk)
- Shoulder shrugs and active abduction
- Supraspinatus strengthening
- Ice

Phase II (6 Weeks-3 Months)
- Continue ROM, gradually increasing external rotation (goal is full ROM by 2 months)
- Continue strengthening exercises with emphasis on rotator cuff and parascapular muscles
- Add shoulder flexion and horizontal adduction exercises
- Joint mobilization
- Begin upper body ergometer for endurance at low resistance
- Ice

Phase III (3-6 Months)
- Continue capsular stretching and strengthening and ergometer
- May include isokinetic strengthening and endurance exercises for internal and external rotation
- Add push-ups (begin with wall push-up with body always posterior to elbows)
- Start chin-ups at 4 to 5 months
- Total body conditioning
- Advance to throwing program or skill-specific training as tolerated
- Ice

ROM, Range of motion.

From Montgomery WH, Jobe FW: Functional outcomes in athletes after modified anterior capsulolabral reconstruction, *Am J Sports Med* 22:352, 1994.

ARTHROSCOPIC BANKART REPAIR

- Place the patient on the operating table in the lateral decubitus position with a beanbag and kidney rest. Carefully protect all bony prominences as well as the axillary area. Apply a heating blanket and serial compression devices around the lower extremities. Prepare and drape the patient so that there is wide exposure to the anterior, posterior, and superior aspects of the shoulder. Place the arm in 45 degrees abduction and 20 degrees forward flexion using 10 to 12 lb of traction.
- Outline the bony landmarks and mark the potential portals on the skin.
- Place the posterior portal 2 cm inferior to the posterolateral edge of the acromion.
- Before making additional portals, thoroughly examine the shoulder through the posterior portal to identify the most appropriate sites for placement of the anterior portals and for any additional posterior portals that may be necessary. Carefully visualize the entire labrum, 360 degrees of the shoulder joint, and the attachment of the glenohumeral ligament to the humerus from anterior to posterior. Thoroughly evaluate the glenohumeral joint for bony loss of the glenoid or humeral head. Defects of the humeral head larger than 6 mm in depth may need to be stabilized with a remplissage-type procedure. Glenoid bone loss greater than 6 mm should be restored with an open Laterjet procedure.

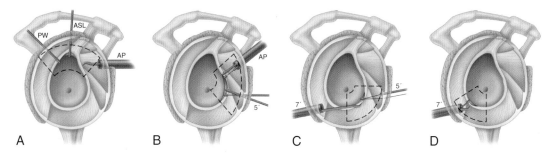

Figure 45-6

- After identifying the quadrant or quadrants of injury, create the planned portals using needle localization according to the quadrant approach (Seroyer et al.; Figure 45-6). **A,** In the superior quadrant, SLAP tears between 2 and 10 o'clock are accessible through anterior portal (AP), anterosuperior lateral (ASL), and the portal of Wilmington (PW). **B,** In the anterior quadrant, anteroinferior labral tears are accessible through the anterior portal (AP) and the 5-o'clock portal. **C,** In the anteroinferior quadrant, anteroinferior capsulolabral tears are accessible through the 5- and 7-o'clock portals. **D,** In the posteroinferior quadrant, posterior labral tears can be accessed through the 7-o'clock portal.

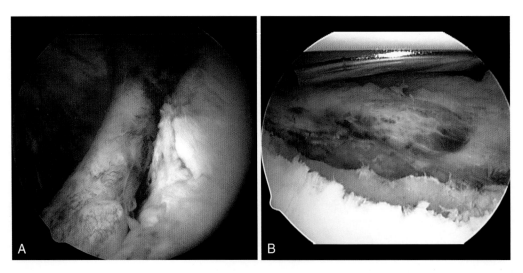

Figure 45-7

- Make an anterosuperior portal with the cannula entering the shoulder just posterior to the biceps tendon and anterior to the leading edge of the supraspinatus tendon (Figure 45-7). It is the best portal to visualize the full extent of the capsular ligamentous damage and to best identify the particular lesion as soft tissue (**A**) or bony (**B**).

- Make an anterior central portal to place an 8.25-mm clear cannula just above the superior edge of the subscapularis tendon at an angle of approximately 45 degrees to the glenoid articular surface. This is used for placement of anchors and for instrumentation using a spectrum suture passer.
- If the lesion extends posterior, make a 7-o'clock portal posteriorly using spinal needle localization. Enter the joint at an appropriate angle for placement of a suture anchor in the inferior part of the glenoid if necessary, or for placement of a spectrum for passing sutures along the capsular ligamentous complex.

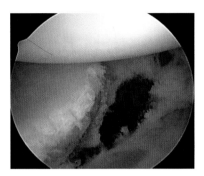

Figure 45-8

- While visualizing from the anterosuperior portal use an elevator to free up the capsule down to the subscapularis muscle, which should be visible. Abrade the glenoid neck to stimulate healing (Figure 45-8).
- While visualizing from the anterosuperior portal if necessary, perform a capsular plication procedure posteriorly extending along to the attachment of the posterior band of the inferior glenohumeral ligament. Using a rasp, freshen the soft tissue and the intended area of plication to incite some inflammation without damaging the tissue.
- Use a spectrum suture passer to pass PDS sutures starting at about the 6-o'clock position and taking approximately a 1 cm bite of capsule in a pinch-tuck technique. Make sure the needle comes out through the capsule and passes up under the labrum in its appropriate position. The sutures can be tied at the time they are passed but it may be easier to pass multiple sutures first, store them outside the cannula, and tie them later. Generally three sutures are passed with the upper extent being at the attachment of the posterior band of the inferior glenohumeral ligament.

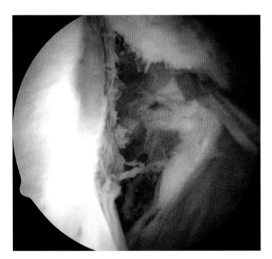

Figure 45-9

- Now perform the anterior part of the Bankart procedure. Abrade the anterior neck and free up the capsule and labral complex so it can be advanced superiorly. Plan the position of the suture anchors trying to get three or four anchors placed below the 3-o'clock position (Figure 45-9).

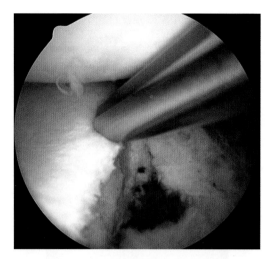

Figure 45-10

- The most inferior anchor often is best placed using a 5-o'clock percutaneous portal made with the help of a spinal needle for localization. Place the spinal needle at a 45-degree angle to the articular surface. The spear point guide can be placed at the 5:30 position on the neck, 1 to 2 mm on the articular surface for reaming and placement of the suture anchor. To obtain the best area of bone for drilling at a lower level, an angled reamer and anchor inserter, such as the JuggerKnot (Biomet), can be placed percutaneously. This provides excellent fixation in this position (Figure 45-10).

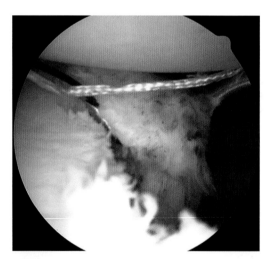

Figure 45-11

- The second and third anchors may be either single-loaded or double-loaded and usually are biocomposite double-loaded anchors. With this technique, take the most inferior suture out the posteroinferior cannula using a suture grasper. Obtain a good bite of the capsule and labrum just distal to the intended site of the anchor. Take this PDS out of the posterior inferior cannula and secure it around the inferior suture limb of the anchor and then retrieve it out the anterior cannula. Grasp the two sutures not involved in the first knot with a suture retrieval device from the posterior cannula, take them out the posterior cannula and store them for later tying. The arthroscopic knot is then tied (Figure 45-11).

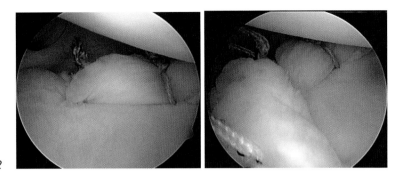

Figure 45-12

- Firmly secure the first suture that was passed through the labrum to the capsule and labrum up to the edge of the glenoid, creating an anterior bumper. Pass the superior of the two suture limbs that were passed out the posterior cannula back through the anterior cannula. Use the spectrum to pass a no. 1 PDS through the capsule and labrum. Carry this suture out the posterior cannula and shuttle the second suture through the capsule and out the anterior cannula, tying it down firmly to the capsule and labrum obtaining good secure fixation of the capsule (Figure 45-12).

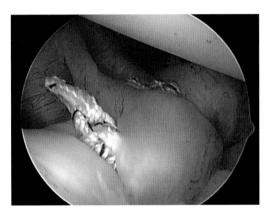

Figure 45-13

- Place a third anchor either single-loaded or double-loaded using the same technique. Sometimes some of the lower sutures can be used in either a single simple repair or as a mattress suture depending on the type of tear and tissue involved. This is determined at the time of surgery. Three or four anchors are placed each separated by 5 to 7 mm. Tie the knots securely, recreating a soft tissue. At this time, if the plication sutures have not been tied they should be tied posteriorly from the posterior cannula and secured. In our practice we generally tie these earlier in the procedure when they are placed but some authors prefer to tie them later (Figure 45-13).

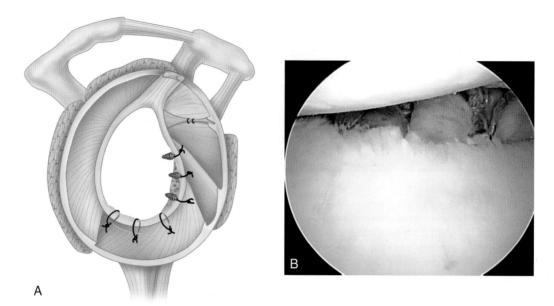

Figure 45-14

- If the patient had hyperlaxity and significant sulcus associated with the Bankart lesion, perform a rotator interval closure at this time by withdrawing the anterior central cannula to just outside the capsule. Pass a crescent spectrum needle through the inferior glenohumeral ligament several millimeters into the ligament and out into the joint. Maintain one limb outside the capsule while the limb in the joint is retrieved using a penetrator device through the anterior central cannula. Grasp the intraarticular limb of the suture at the level of the superior glenohumeral ligament and retrieve it out of the cannula for extracapsular tying using an SMC (Samsung Medical Center)-type knot. Generally, two sutures are passed in securing the rotator interval if it is thought that the slight loss of external rotation is offset by the added stability of these additional sutures (Figure 45-14).

- Upon completion close the portals with subcuticular poliglecaprone 25 (Monocryl). Apply a sterile dressing and an Ultrasling (DJD, Vista, CA).

POSTOPERATIVE CARE

A sling immobilizer is applied after surgery and worn for 4 to 6 weeks. Physical therapy is started 2 to 3 weeks after surgery. Active-assisted range of motion is performed from weeks 2 to 8 and isometric strengthening is performed from weeks 8 to 12. The athlete is allowed to return to preinjury conditioning programs and weight training at 12 weeks and at 6 months he or she is allowed to participate in contact sports based on range of motion and strength guidelines dictated by the contralateral shoulder (Table 45-1).

TABLE 45-1	Rehabilitation Protocol after Arthroscopic Bankart Repair*

PREOPERATIVE GOALS

1. Independent with postoperative exercise program
2. Independent with preoperative strengthening with isometrics and isotonics in pain-free stable range

PHASE I

Weeks 1-2 Postoperative

1. Pendulum exercises
2. Elbow, forearm, wrist AROM
3. Wrist isotonics and grip exercises
4. Sling at all times

No Formal PT If Patient Has Achieved Preoperative Goals

Weeks 3-4 Postoperative (PT QIW-TIW)

1. Initiate PT approximately 15 days postoperatively
2. PROM with the following restrictions
   FL < 160 degrees
   Scaption to < 150 degrees
   ER neutral to 30 degrees at 3 weeks and 40 degrees at 4 weeks
   IR in 45 degrees scaption < 60 degrees
3. Gentle AAROM with cane
   FL < 160 degrees
   ER neutral as above
4. Table slides in FL
5. Scapular mobility exercises
   Protraction/retraction
   Elevation/depression

Goals (by End of 4 wk)

1. Independent with HEP BID
2. PROM 150 degrees maximal FL
3. PROM 150 degrees maximal scaption
4. PROM 40 degrees maximal ER
5. PROM 60 degrees maximal IR in 45 degrees scaption
6. Full wrist, elbow AROM
Precautions
   1. Sling at all times except PT
   2. No true ABD PROM
   3. No ER with arm abducted from body

Weeks 5-6 Postoperative (PT QIW-TIW)

1. PROM with the following restrictions:
   FL < 170 degrees
   Scaption < 160 degrees
   ER 45 degrees, scaption < 60 degrees
   IR 45 degrees, scaption to 60 degrees
   Home ADD to WNL
2. AAROM—cane, pulley, wall walks
3. Submaximal (25%) isometrics at side for IR and ER, and ABD
4. Submaximal manual resistance scapular protraction/retraction and elevation/depression
5. AROM—prone EXT and rows, supine protraction and reverse Codman

Goals (by End of 6 wk)

1. Independent with HEP BID
2. PROM 170 degrees maximal FL
3. PROM 160 degrees maximal scaption
4. PROM 60 degrees maximal ER at 45 degrees scaption
5. PROM 60 degrees maximal IR at 45 degrees scaption
6. Home ADD to WNL
Precautions
   1. Use of sling during sleep and in crowds
   2. No true ABD PROM
   3. No ER with arm ABD from body > 45 degrees

Continued

TABLE	45-1	Bankart Repair Rehabilitation Protocol—cont'd

PHASE II—GRADED AROM AND STRENGTHENING

Weeks 7-8 Postoperative (PT BIW)

1. PROM with the following restrictions
   FL to WNL
   Scaption to WNL
   ER 70 degrees, scaption to 70 degrees by end of wk 7
   ER 90 degrees, scaption to 70 degrees by end of wk 8
   IR to WNL
2. Continued AAROM activities as needed
3. AROM FL and scaption to 90 degrees
4. Isotonics when able
   FL and scaption with 1-2 lb
   ER and IR with 1-2 lb (side lying) or Theraband (standing)
   Prone EXT, rows, and horizontal ABD < 90 degrees
   Biceps curls; triceps EXT
5. UBE for endurance
6. Proprioceptive training (ball wall dribble, weighted reverse Codman, submaximal manual resistance PNF)

Goals (by End of 8 wk)

1. Independent with HEP QID
2. Discontinue sling at all times without increased pain
3. PROM FL to WNL
4. PROM scaption to WNL
5. PROM 70 degrees maximal ER at 90 degrees scaption
6. PROM IR to WNL
7. AROM FL and scaption at least 90 degrees with proper scapular mechanics
8. Able to lift 2 lb to eye-level cabinet
9. Able to perform all grooming and dressing activities independently and with normal mechanics
10. Able to retrieve wallet from back pocket
11. Able to open/close car door
Precautions
1. Avoid terminal ER/ABD
2. Light-weight/high-repetition isotonics

Weeks 9-10 Postoperative (PT BIW)

1. PROM ER 90 degrees, scaption to WFL
2. Progress all AROM to WFL
3. Progress isotonic strengthening—Jobe rotator cuff program
4. Initiate isotonics—lateral pull-downs to chest, wall push-ups with elbows tight to side, step-ups, throwing lunges
5. Advance proprioceptive training to include progressive weight-bearing exercises on unstable surface
6. Advance endurance training for upper extremity and entire body

Goals (by End of 10 wk)

1. PROM WFL all directions
2. AROM WFL all directions
3. MMT 4/5 FL
4. MMT 4/5 scaption
5. MMT 4/5 ER
6. MMT 4+/5 IR
7. MMT 5/5 EXT
8. Able to place gallon milk in refrigerator
9. Able to lift 5 lb to eye-level cabinet
10. Able to lift 2 lb to overhead cabinet
Precaution
1. Evaluate for posterior capsular tightness; stretch if necessary

Weeks 11-14 Postoperative (PT BIM)

1. Progress isotonics—increase resistance
2. Progress ER and IR isotonics toward 90 degrees ABD (Theraband, weights)
3. Plyoball exercises if appropriate
   Chest pass
   Sideway throw
   Overhead throw
4. Isokinetic strengthening as needed

Goals (by End of 14 wk)

1. Independent with isotonic HEP
2. MMT 5/5 FL
3. MMT scaption 5/5
4. MMT ER 5/5
5. MMT IR 5/5
6. Able to lift 10 lb to eye-level cabinet
7. Able to lift 5 lb to overhead cabinet
8. Full return to strenuous work
Precaution
1. No bench press or flies until 6 mo postoperatively

AAROM, Active-assisted range of motion; *ABD*, abduction; *ADD*, adduction; *AROM*, active range of motion; *BID*, twice a day; *BIW*, twice a week; *BIM*, twice a month; *ER*, external rotation; *EXT*, extension; *FL*, flexion; *HEP*, home exercise program; *IR*, internal rotation; *MMT*, manual muscle testing; *PNF*, proprioceptive neuromuscular facilitation; *PT*, physical therapy; *QID*, four times a day; *QIW*, four times a week; *TIW*, three times a week; *UBE*, upper body exercise; *WFL*, within functional limits; *WNL*, within normal limits.

*The Bankart repair is intended to stabilize the anterior portion of the shoulder capsule that has lost integrity owing to repetitive or traumatic insult. It is paramount to protect healing tissue of anterior capsule during early stages of rehabilitation. Avoidance of terminal ABD/ER is crucial during this period. This protocol is a guideline and may be adjusted according to clinical presentation and physician's guidance.

TREATMENT OF SHOULDER INSTABILITY — CAPSULAR SHIFT, POSTERIOR CAPSULAR SHIFT, ARTHROSCOPIC CAPSULAR SHIFT

Barry B. Phillips

Capsular shift procedures are used for multidirectional shoulder instability. The principle of the procedure is to detach the capsule from the neck of the humerus and shift it to the opposite side of the calcar (inferior portion of the neck of the humerus), not only to obliterate the inferior pouch and capsular redundancy on the side of the surgical approach but also to reduce laxity on the opposite side. The approach can be anterior or posterior depending on the direction of greatest instability.

CAPSULAR SHIFT ⟩

- The patient is carefully examined and questioned preoperatively to determine the probable direction of greatest instability. After delivery of a general anesthetic, the instability of the shoulder is evaluated again. Anterior instability is tested with the arm in external rotation and extension at various levels of abduction. Inferior instability is tested with the arm in 0 degrees and 45 degrees of abduction. Posterior instability is tested with the arm in internal rotation at various levels of forward elevation. If this examination and the preoperative evaluation correlate with anteroinferior instability use an anterior approach.

- Place the patient in a tilted position with the front and the back of the shoulder exposed. Drape the arm free. Attach an arm board to the side of the table.

- Make a 9-cm incision in the skin creases from the anterior border of the axilla to the coracoid process.

- Develop the deltopectoral interval medial to the cephalic vein and retract the deltoid laterally. Divide the clavipectoral fascia and retract the muscles attached to the coracoid process medially.

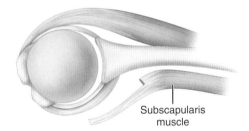

Subscapularis
muscle

Figure 46-1

- With the arm in external rotation, divide the superficial half of the thickness of the subscapularis tendon transversely 1 cm medial to the biceps groove. Leave the deep half of the subscapularis tendon attached to reinforce the anterior aspect of the capsule and tag the superficial half of the tendon with stay sutures and retract it medially. It is important that this superficial portion of the subscapularis tendon be free so that the action of the subscapularis muscle is not tethered (Figure 46-1).

- Close the cleft between the middle and superior glenohumeral ligaments with nonabsorbable sutures.

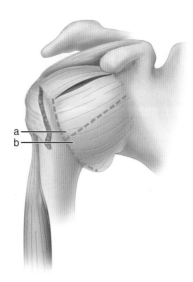

Figure 46-2

- Make a T-shaped opening by incising between the middle and inferior glenohumeral ligaments (Figure 46-2).

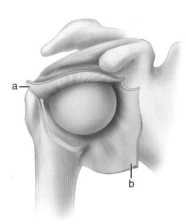

Figure 46-3

- With a flat elevator to protect the axillary nerve and with the arm in external rotation, develop a capsular flap by detaching the reinforced part of the capsule containing the inferior glenohumeral ligament from the inferior aspect of the neck of the humerus around to the posterior aspect of the neck of the humerus (Figure 46-3).
- Inspect the interior of the joint and remove any osteochondral bodies or tags of labrum.
- Test for posterior instability with and without forward traction on the inferior capsular flap to estimate the new location for the flap.
- Using curets and a small gouge, make a shallow slot in the bone at the anterior and inferior sulcus of the neck of the humerus, as shown in above. Suture the capsular flap to the stump of the subscapularis tendon and to the part of the capsule that remains on the humerus so that the capsular flap is held against the slot of raw bone. Suture anchors can be used to secure the capsule and generally are preferred.

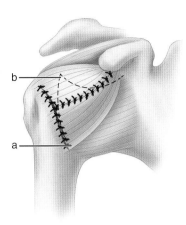

Figure 46-4

- The tension on the capsular flap that is selected must eliminate the inferior pouch and reduce the posterior capsular redundancy. Suture the inferior flap first and draw the superior flap down over it and suture it so as to cause the middle glenohumeral ligament to reinforce the capsule anteriorly and to act as a sling against inferior subluxation (Figure 46-4).

- Hold the arm in slight flexion and about 10 degrees of external rotation on the armboard while the anterior portion of the capsule is reattached with nonabsorbable sutures. Bigliani et al. recommended repairing the capsule with the arm held in approximately 25 degrees of external rotation and 20 degrees of abduction. For throwers, they recommended relatively more abduction and external rotation to ensure full range of motion.

- Bring the subscapularis tendon over the reattached anterior portion and reattach the tendon at its normal location.

- After closure of the deltopectoral interval with absorbable sutures and after closure of the skin with a skin stitch, maintain the arm at the side in neutral flexion-extension and in about 20 degrees of internal rotation by light plastic splints.

POSTOPERATIVE CARE 〉

Postoperatively the extremity is placed in a commercially available shoulder immobilizer with the shoulder in 30 to 40 degrees of abduction and slight external rotation. Range-of-motion exercises for the elbow, wrist, and hand are started immediately with Codman's exercises of the shoulder being added on the third postoperative day. External rotation to 10 degrees, forward elevation to 90 degrees, and isometric exercises are begun after 10 days. For 2 to 4 weeks isometric strengthening is continued and external rotation is increased to 30 degrees and forward elevation to 140 degrees. At 4 to 6 weeks resistive exercises are begun and external rotation is increased to 40 degrees and forward elevation to 160 degrees. At 6 weeks external rotation is increased to 50 degrees and forward elevation to 180 degrees. At 3 months external rotation can be progressed. In the dominant shoulder of throwers, external rotation should be progressed more quickly, however progression that is too quick can lead to recurrent instability, especially in patients in late adolescence.

The internal and external rotators curb anterior and posterior displacement and the supraspinatus and middle part of the deltoid curb inferior displacement. Complete recovery of the muscles probably is necessary to protect the repair because the capsule and ligaments normally function only as a checkrein. Lifting more than 9 kg and participating in sports are prohibited for 9 months and until muscle strength is normal on manual testing compared with the contralateral side. Ligament healing is more mature at 1 year and patients are advised against swimming with the backstroke or butterfly stroke, heavy overhead use of the involved arm, and participation in contact sports during the first year after surgery.

INFERIOR CAPSULAR SHIFT THROUGH A POSTERIOR APPROACH 〉

Neer and Foster described an inferior capsular shift procedure performed through a posterior approach. In this procedure, the posterior capsule is split longitudinally and the capsular attachment along the humeral neck is released as far inferiorly and anteriorly as possible. The superior capsule is advanced inferiorly and the inferior capsule is advanced superiorly. The infraspinatus is cut so that it is overlapped and shortened, adding further buttress to the posterior capsule. This procedure obliterates the axillary pouch and redundancy. It and other capsular shift procedures are indicated in posterior subluxation syndromes that are not true traumatic recurrent posterior dislocations.

▪ For the posterior approach, place the patient on the operating table in the lateral decubitus position with the involved shoulder up. The patient is held in position with a beanbag and kidney rest.

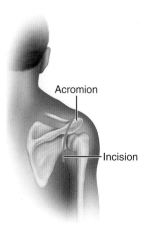

Figure 46-5

▪ Make a 10-cm incision vertically over the posterior aspect of the acromion and the spine of the scapula (Figure 46-5).

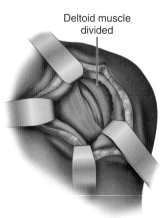

Figure 46-6

▪ Undermine the subcutaneous tissue to expose the deltoid muscle. Split the deltoid muscle from an area on the spine of the scapula beginning 2 to 3 cm medial to the posterolateral corner of the acromion and extending distally 5 to 6 cm. To protect the axillary nerve, the deltoid muscle should not be split distally beyond the teres minor. In a muscular individual the deltoid muscle can be reflected from the spine of the scapula or the acromion (Figure 46-6).

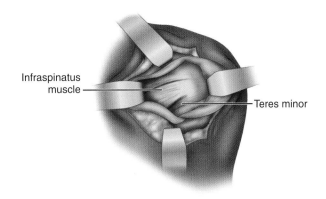

Infraspinatus muscle

Teres minor

Figure 46-7

- Expose the teres minor and infraspinatus muscles and develop the interval between these muscles (Figure 46-7).

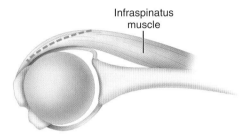

Infraspinatus muscle

Figure 46-8

- Detach the infraspinatus obliquely so that the superficial piece of tendon can be used later to reinforce the posterior part of the capsule (Figure 46-8).

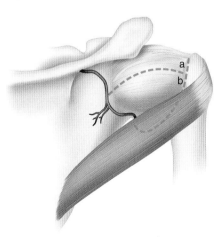

Figure 46-9

- Make a T-shaped opening in the posterior pouch in the posterior part of the capsule (Figure 46-9).
- Form a superior capsular flap by detaching 1.5 cm of capsule above the initial longitudinal capsular incision.
- Use a flat elevator to protect the axillary nerve and, with the arm in progressive internal rotation, form the inferior capsular flap by detaching the capsule from the neck of the humerus around to the anterior portion of the calcar.
- Elevate the teres minor from the capsule and leave it intact.

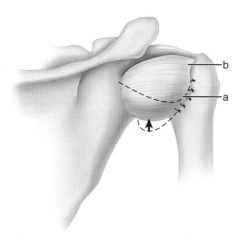

Figure 46-10

- Distract the joint (with the addition of muscle relaxants as necessary) so that the glenoid labrum can be inspected anteriorly. If the anterior portion of the glenoid labrum has been detached, make a second approach anteriorly through which the labrum is sutured to the bone of the glenoid (Bankart repair). If the anterior part of the labrum is intact, draw the posterior part of the capsule backward to eliminate the inferior pouch and to reduce anterior capsular laxity (Figure 46-10).

- With curets and a small gouge make a shallow slot in the sulcus of the humeral neck so that the capsular flap is approximated to raw bone. Hold the arm in slight extension and moderate external rotation as the capsule is reattached.

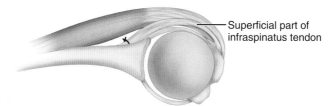

Superficial part of infraspinatus tendon

Figure 46-11

- During tensioning of the flaps, Bigliani suggested holding the extremity in 5 to 10 degrees of external rotation, 10 to 15 degrees of abduction, and neutral flexion and extension. Reattach the superior flap first while drawing it downward to eliminate the posterior pouch. Next, draw the longer inferior flap over it and turn back the excess part of the capsule for reinforcement posteriorly. Use the superficial portion of the infraspinatus to reinforce the posterior portion of the capsule further (Figure 46-11).

- Reattach the deep part of the infraspinatus superficially to preserve active external rotation and carefully reattach the deltoid if it has been detached.

- Close the wound, and immobilize the arm at the side in neutral flexion-extension and 10 degrees of external rotation by means of a light plaster splint extending from the wrist to the middle part of the arm and around the waist with the elbow bent 90 degrees. Rigid external immobilization is needed to ensure that 10 degrees of external rotation is maintained.

POSTOPERATIVE CARE 〉

The shoulder is immobilized with the arm at the side in slight abduction and neutral rotation for 6 weeks after surgery. A plastic brace maintains this position, supports the weight of the arm, and prevents inferior stress on the repair. Range-of-motion exercises with elevation in the scapular plane and external rotation and isometric exercises are begun 6 weeks after the surgery when the brace is removed. These exercises are progressed over the next 3 months to a full strengthening program. Elevation of more than 150 degrees and internal rotation exercises that might stress the repair are avoided for 3 months. Sports activities such as swimming and throwing are not allowed for 9 months to 1 year after surgery.

ARTHROSCOPIC CAPSULAR SHIFT ⟩

- Results of arthroscopic capsular volume reduction are comparable with that obtained with open techniques but with less morbidity.

- After examining the anesthetized patient and determining the amount of hyperlaxity present, place the patient in a lateral decubitus position and maintain the position with a beanbag and kidney rest. Carefully pad bony prominences. Apply a heating blanket and serial compression devices to the lower extremity. Place the arm in 45 degrees of abduction and 20 degrees of flexion with 10 lb of traction. During the procedure it is helpful to have an assistant to position the shoulder to obtain the most advantageous view and to place gentle pressure anteriorly or posteriorly when slight traction is necessary.

- Outline bony landmarks and potential portal sites on the skin. A posterior portal is made about 3 cm distal and slightly medial to the posterolateral acromial edge to evaluate the shoulder. The anterior portals are the anterosuperior lateral portal and the anterior central portal, which is usually about 1 cm lateral to the coracoid. Place working 8.25-mm cannulas later in the procedure in the posterior and anterior central portals. The anterosuperior portal is used for visualization.

- Use a small arthroscopic rasp to abrade the capsule and labrum around the area to be plicated. This generally extends from the length of the glenohumeral ligament attachment starting posteriorly at the 9-o'clock position and extending anteriorly through the 3-o'clock position. Freshen the soft tissue.

- Starting on the side of the shoulder where the most instability is present, plicate the capsule with 1-cm plication bites depending on the size of the patient and the extent of the capsular laxity. Plications are started inferiorly and with each plication the tuck is advanced superiorly and passed through the labrum with the suture shuttle device. A 45-degree spectrum can be used as a suture shuttle or a commercial shuttle device with a 45-degree angle can be used. Simple no. 1 PDS sutures are passed and tied with a sliding knot making sure the knots are tied off the edge of the articular surface.

- If nonabsorbable sutures are to be passed, a suture shuttle device is used with a pinch-tuck method. Grab about 1 cm of capsule bringing the needle up through the capsule and exiting lateral to the labrum. Pass the needle up and under the labrum while placing upward-directed tension on the capsule, advancing the capsule superiorly. Take the suture shuttle out the posterior cannula and carry a nonabsorbable suture out anteriorly through the working cannula.

- If a mattress suture is to be placed, use the same technique with the suture shuttle pinching the capsule up through the labrum and carry the suture out. Retrieve the second limb of the suture from the posterior cannula and carry it out to the anterior cannula. Tie the mattress suture. A figure-of-eight suture also can be used. Pass the same limb of the suture from anterior to posterior through the capsule and labrum twice and then retrieve it back out anteriorly for tying.

- Carry the capsular plication around inferiorly, taking care not to get too deep or too far from the labrum so as to catch the axillary nerve. Extend the plication up to about the 9-o'clock position.

- Close the rotator interval. For significant multidirectional instability this is done using a spectrum suture after having withdrawn the anterior cannula to just anterior to the capsule. Pass a PDS through the superior portion of the middle glenohumeral ligament and then retrieve it with a penetrator type grasper just superior to the superior glenohumeral ligament. Close the interval with two sutures anteriorly. On completion, close the posterior capsule similarly by passing a suture on each side of the rent and then closing it with the cannula just outside the capsule. These techniques can be done most easily by visualizing the anterior interval closure from the posterior portal and then moving the scope to the anterosuperior portal to visualize the posterior capsular closure.

- Close the arthroscopic portals with subcuticular Monocryl sutures and place sterile dressings.

POSTOPERATIVE CARE ⟩

An Ultrasling is applied with the arm in neutral rotation. The arm is kept in the sling postoperatively for 6 weeks.

The primary goal of rotator cuff repair is pain relief, and this can be accomplished with open or arthroscopic techniques. Functional improvement depends on the age of the patient, the size of the tear, and the postoperative rehabilitation program. Surgery is appropriate for acute rotator cuff injuries in patients with a defined injury who are suddenly unable to externally rotate the arm against resistance. Surgery is contraindicated in patients with rotator cuff tears and stiffness; the stiffness must be corrected before repair.

OPEN REPAIR OF ROTATOR CUFF TEARS

- Place the patient in a semi-upright position with the head elevated 30 to 35 degrees (beach chair position). Place a towel or an intravenous bag medial to the scapula to stabilize it. This degree of head elevation usually places the superior acromial surface perpendicular to the floor allowing the acromial osteotomy to be made perpendicular to the floor. Drape the arm free to permit shoulder rotation.
- Outline the bony contour of the shoulder including the lateral acromial border, coracoid, and acromioclavicular joint.
- Outline the proposed skin incision along the Langer line 4 to 6 cm long and infiltrate it with 10 mL of 1:500,000 epinephrine to minimize bleeding.

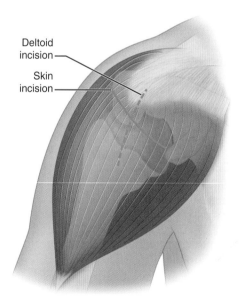

Deltoid incision

Skin incision

Figure 47-1

- Make the incision from lateral to the anterior acromion toward the coracoid and just lateral to it (Figure 47-1).

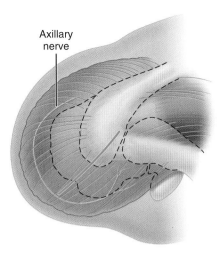

Figure 47-2

- After mobilization of the subcutaneous tissue, identify the raphe between the anterior and middle deltoid and split it from a point 5 cm or less distal to the acromial border (to avoid axillary nerve injury) toward the anterolateral acromion (Figure 47-2).
- The deltoid can be left attached or can be detached from the corner of the acromion depending on the surgeon's preference. We prefer to leave the deltoid attached initially, detaching it later if the procedure warrants.

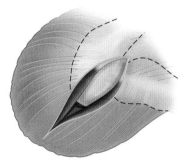

Figure 47-3

- To use this approach, elevate a flap of deltoid with its periosteal attachment and the periosteal attachment of the trapezius approximately 2 cm onto the superior acromial surface (Figure 47-3).
- Carry this medially as far as the acromioclavicular joint (the anterior capsule of which usually is included in the flap) and 1 cm along the lateral acromion. Occasionally these periosteal attachments are tenuous after elevation and the deltoid must be detached, to be secured later to the acromion through drill holes. We have found that using electrocautery with a Bovie needle for elevation usually ensures thicker flaps.
- The importance of correct deltoid detachment cannot be overemphasized. A secure cuff of tissue must be maintained for later defect closure or reattachment to the acromion. Without secure deltoid attachment, the results of the acromioplasty would be compromised by lack of deltoid function.
- After completing the anterior limb of the elevation, resect the coracoacromial ligament. We use the electrocautery for this as well because the acromial branch of the coracoacromial artery is contained within the ligament and electrocautery allows exposure of the entire subacromial space.
- With the subacromial space exposed, resect the bursa along with all adhesions and soft tissue coverage from the acromial undersurface. The bursa can be quite thick and easily mistaken for the rotator cuff tendon. The bursa can be identified by its continuity with the acromial undersurface and its unilaminar appearance as opposed to the multilaminar appearance of the rotator cuff.

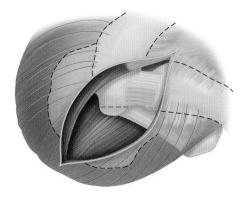

Figure 47-4

- After bursal resection use an oscillating saw or rongeur to remove the portion of the acromion that projects anterior to the anterior border of the clavicle. This removes a portion of the offending acromial hook and squares off the surface allowing easier completion of the acromioplasty with an oscillating saw or an osteotome. We prefer an oscillating saw for this portion of the procedure because it affords more control than an osteotome, which may propagate a fracture line into the posterior acromion (Figure 47-4).
- Begin the osteotomy at the anterosuperior aspect of the acromion and continue it through the junction of the anterior and middle thirds of the acromion, including the entire anterior acromion from medial to lateral.
- Use a curved, blunt Hohmann or malleable retractor to depress the humeral head and protect the cuff during this portion of the procedure.
- Smooth out any rough surfaces with a rasp.
- Palpate the acromioclavicular joint undersurface and remove any bony spurs.
- If severe degenerative changes are present, resect the distal 1.0 to 1.5 cm of the lateral clavicle. Preoperative radiographs and symptoms should indicate the necessity of this additional procedure, and it should not be done routinely.
- If the clavicle is resected, leave the superior acromioclavicular capsule intact to make deltoid repair in this area easier. Do not extend the clavicular cut beyond 1.5 cm to avoid violating the coracoclavicular ligaments and making the distal clavicle unstable.
- After standard acromioplasty, evaluate the rotator cuff tear carefully.
- Tears usually begin at the supraspinatus insertion, and the end retracts into its fossa under the acromioclavicular joint. Most tears not only are transverse but also have a longitudinal component making them oval or triangular. All but the smallest tears need to be advanced anteriorly and laterally, not just laterally, to restore anatomical position and correct muscle-tendon unit length. In tears of more than 2 to 3 cm the infraspinatus tendon is involved as well.
- When the defect has been identified and its size approximated, attention is turned to the repair itself. Usually some degree of mobilization is necessary.

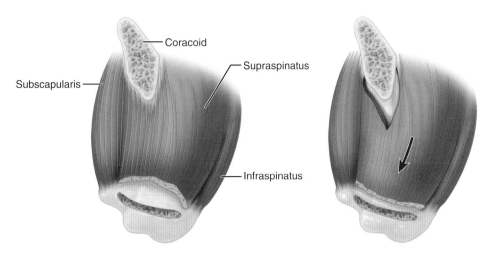

Figure 47-5

- Begin mobilization posteriorly with the infraspinatus, using a blunt probe or a finger to release adhesions inside and outside the joint. Do not dissect below the level of the teres minor to avoid injury to the axillary nerve in the quadrangular space or the suprascapular nerve in the area of the spinoglenoid notch near the inferior border of the supraspinatus fossa. Supraspinatus and subscapularis muscles have fascial attachments to the coracoid base via the coracohumeral ligament. Lateral mobilization of the retracted cuff is facilitated by release of these attachments (Figure 47-5).

- Continue mobilization anteriorly to the supraspinatus. If necessary more exposure can be gained by resecting the distal 1.0 to 1.5 cm of the clavicle at the acromioclavicular joint, but this should not be done unless concomitant acromioclavicular arthrosis exists. Release of the coracohumeral ligament in this area allows further mobilization of the supraspinatus laterally.

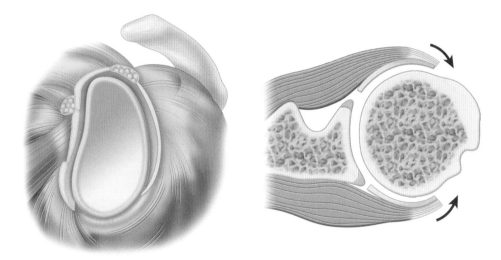

Figure 47-6

- If the supraspinatus and infraspinatus tendons are retracted so far that adequate length cannot be obtained with tendon mobilization, incise the capsule at its insertion into the glenoid labrum. If necessary carry this incision from the 8-o'clock position posterior to the 4-o'clock position posterior (Figure 47-6).

- The use of a second posterior incision over the scapular spine to increase mobilization has been described, but we have no experience with this technique.

- Debride the end of the mobilized tendon to obtain a raw edge, taking care not to confuse the tendon with the overlying bursa. The goals of mobilization are to obtain tissue of adequate strength, to position it anatomically for repair without damage to innervation and without compromise of deltoid function, and to decompress the subacromial space to prevent further mechanical impingement on repaired cuff tissue. When these goals are accomplished the actual repair can be performed. We believe that the best results are obtained with the double-row technique, suturing the tendon to bone in a cancellous trough in combination with suture anchor fixation. This reduces tension on the primary trough repair and increases the surface area of tendon-to-bone healing.

- With no. 2 nonabsorbable suture, use a double loop technique, superior to inferior and inferior to superior in a horizontal mattress manner. This helps push the tendon down into the trough.

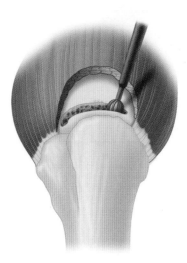

Figure 47-7

- Use a rongeur or burr to create a shallow trough running the length of the exposed bone of the greater tuberosity to accommodate the thickness of the supraspinatus and infraspinatus tendons. Bevel the proximal edge with a burr or rasp (Figure 47-7).

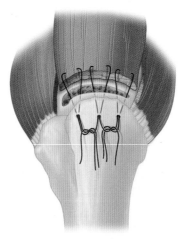

Figure 47-8

- Place two or three rotator cuff suture anchors immediately medial to the trough at a 45-degree angle and pass the suture through the rotator cuff tendon 3 to 5 mm medial to the sutures in the free end of the tendon (Figure 47-8).

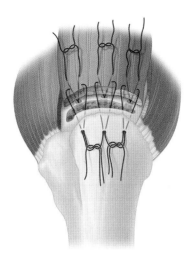

Figure 47-9

- Drill holes for sutures 2 to 3 cm distal to the trough and connect them to the trough using a no. 5 Mayo needle, a towel clip, or a specialized instrument (Concept, Largo, FL). Take care not to fracture the thin cortical bone in this area, which may be osteoporotic. Space the holes at least 5 mm (preferably 1 cm) apart on the cortical humeral surface to give an adequate surface over which to tie the knots (Figure 47-9).
- Tie the suture of the anchor down on top of the tendon with four or five knots to prevent impingement of the suture material. The use of strong sutures rather than Kocher clamps or hemostats to pull on the tendon while suturing avoids crush injury to the tendon. We occasionally make longitudinal incisions along the extremes of the free tendon edge to allow placement of the tendon in the trough. These can be sutured before closure.
- Next secure the sutures from the suture anchors over the tendon completing the double-row repair.
- If the lateral humeral cortex is fractured during tying down of the suture or construction of the suture tunnel, the anchors can be used as a salvage procedure. The anchors seem to have adequate holding power in cancellous bone and are reasonable alternatives in problematic situations. Use these sutures for additional leverage when tying down the trough sutures and tie them on top of the tendon with four knots to prevent impingement of the suture material.
- Suture the deltoid periosteum from side to side, or, if necessary, through drill holes into the acromion with nonabsorbable sutures, ensuring that the reattachment is secure. Close the wound in layers in routine fashion.

POSTOPERATIVE CARE

After standard repair, an abduction pillow, low-profile pillow sling, or shoulder immobilizer is worn for 6 weeks. It is removed for assisted exercises in flexion and external rotation to avoid adhesions, disuse atrophy, and disruption of the repairs. The repair is weakest at 3 weeks and tendon strength is less than at the time of surgery for the first 3 months after surgery. Empirically, we advance to isometric exercises of external rotation at 6 weeks, and at 12 weeks active motion is permitted. Patients are cautioned that overaggressive use of the extremity can lead to disruption of the repair for 6 to 12 months depending on the size of the repair and the quality of the tissue and repair.

See also Video 48-1.

ARTHROSCOPIC REPAIR OF ROTATOR CUFF TEARS 〉

- Before taking the patient to the operating room an interscalene block is administered. Place the patient in a lateral decubitus position maintained with a beanbag and kidney rest, making sure to relieve pressure from the axilla and all bony prominences. Maintain the extremity in 30 degrees of abduction and 10 degrees of forward flexion using sterile balanced suspension. Apply serial compression devices to the lower extremities to help avoid deep vein thrombosis. Control bleeding with the use of hypotensive anesthesia, with systolic pressure generally being around 100 mm Hg and the arthroscopic inflow pressure within 30 mm Hg of the systolic blood pressure.

- Wide draping is necessary to make sure that drapes do not interfere with the procedure. Also the distance from the patient's head to the shoulder is critical. Place the head in line with the body but take care that it does not interfere with the operating site. Anesthesia is placed at a 90 degree-angle to the chest also to free up the surgical site.

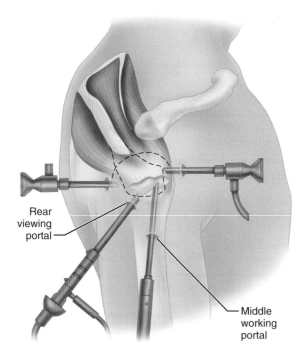

Rear viewing portal

Middle working portal

Figure 48-1

- Carefully outline the bony landmarks and potential portals on the skin. For large, muscular individuals and for large tears, an accessory posterolateral portal may be necessary. It is not routinely used for smaller tears or in smaller individuals. The anterior portal generally is a percutaneous portal used for retrieving and storing sutures. The suture anchors will be placed just off the lateral edge of the acromion using spinal needle localization and percutaneous insertion (Figure 48-1).

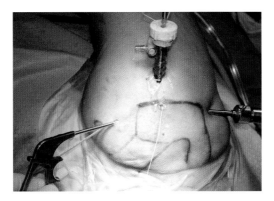

Figure 48-2

- A posterior portal 2 cm distal to the posterolateral acromion is used to fully evaluate intraarticular structures. Place the viewing cannula in the subacromial space. Identify the site and configuration of the tear. Create the lateral operating portal directly over the center of the tear, generally about 3 cm lateral to edge of the acromion and 2 to 3 cm posterior to the anterior edge of the acromion. Lateral distraction applied by an assistant can increase the space intermittently for visualization and for retrieving sutures (Figure 48-2).

- Perform a complete bursectomy to ensure good visualization and ease of retrieving sutures and perform subacromial decompression when indicated. Carefully define the depth of the tear and determine the type of tear (crescent, U-shaped, or L-shaped configuration). Determine the amount of retraction and mobility of the tendon and make sure the tendon can be placed back into the footprint, or if not, how it can be repaired to get the best fixation with minimal tension on the repair.

- Prepare the footprint by abrading the site without overly resecting bone. Abrasion can increase bleeding and marrow elements are released when the suture anchors are placed, both of which aid in healing.

- Define the potential location of the anchors, separating the insertion points by 1.2 to 1.5 cm to prevent tuberosity fracture. Determine where double-loaded or triple-loaded anchors should be used to get an appropriate number of sutures through the tendon and prepare either for a single-row repair, a double-row repair, or a transosseous equivalent repair. Double-row repairs with suture anchors can cause crowding of the anchors. A transosseous equivalent repair in which the lateral row is placed below the tuberosity does not produce as much crowding.

- For tears smaller than 1.5 cm, generally one double-loaded or triple-loaded anchor is used. For larger than 1.5 cm tears, two anchors should be planned, separating the starting points by 1.2 to 1.5 cm. If a tear is 3 cm or larger, generally a transosseous equivalent repair is performed with the medial anchors starting 5 mm off the articular suture and the lateral row about 5 mm lateral to the tuberosity thus separating the rows by 1.2 to 1.5 cm.

- After visualizing where the anchors will be placed in the lateral row, use electrocautery to resect the soft tissue to expose the site for insertion of a swivel lock device later in the procedure.

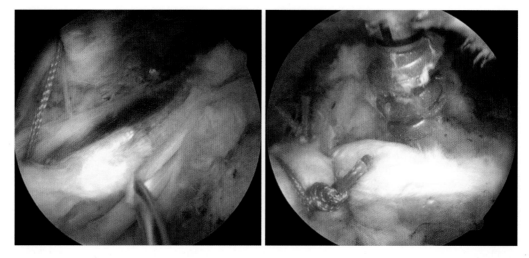

Figure 48-3

- Margin convergence and releases to reduce tension on the repairs should be contemplated. Particularly for U-shaped tears, margin convergence is always performed to reduce the size of the tear and more easily repair it back down to the tuberosity (Figure 48-3).
- For margin convergence of a U-shaped tear or medial extension of an L-shaped tear, use a large crescent-type suture shuttle device, passing it through both leaves, and then retrieve a no. 2 nonabsorbable suture back through the two leaves, storing them for later tying.

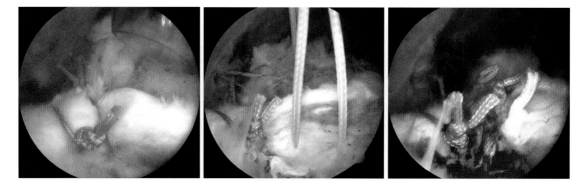

Figure 48-4

- Begin the convergence at the apex of the tear, working from medial to lateral. Make sure to visually line up the tear in its normal anatomy (Figure 48-4).

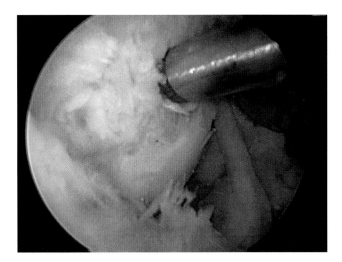

Figure 48-5

- For larger tears that can be repaired back into the anatomical footprint with no undue tension use a transosseous equivalent repair. Place suture anchors in a stepwise fashion placing the anterior anchor first, followed by the posterior anchor, through small percutaneous stab wounds just off the edge of the acromion so as to achieve a 45-degree angle to the shaft. Bury the anchors to make sure the edges are fully engaged in bone. The anterior anchor is placed at the insertion site of the rotator arch (Figure 48-5).

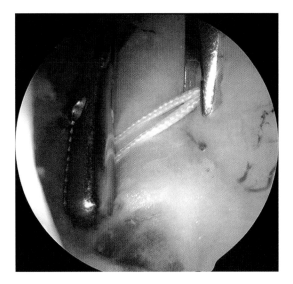

Figure 48-6

- Pass the mattress sutures through the tendon using a scorpion-type device about 4 mm lateral to the musculotendinous junction and separate by 7 mm (approximate width of the scorpion device). Capture the sutures and carry them through an anterior stab wound where they are paired and clamped. When passing sutures, pass the anterior sutures first and then work to posterior (Figure 48-6).
- Finally, after all sutures are passed and stored either through a separate stab wound anteriorly or through the previous stab wounds used for passing anchors, tie them starting posteriorly and then working to the anterior suture, which is generally tied last to secure the anterior edge of the cuff down to its anatomical position. As each suture is tied it is stored either outside the cannula or pulled back through one of the stab wounds.

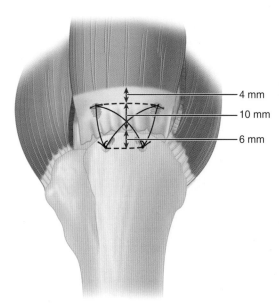
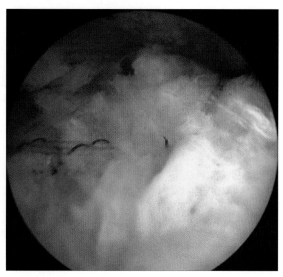

4 mm
10 mm
6 mm

Figure 48-7

- After all medial rows are tied, perform a transosseous equivalent repair. Place the lateral row fixation device about 1.5 cm lateral to the medial row about 6 mm lateral to the footprint. Use the swivel lock to secure the edge of the cuff down into the footprint but take care not to place this under excessive tension, which may cause the anchor to back out or place excessive compression on the cuff, interfering with the vascular supply (Figure 48-7).
- On completion put the arm through a range of motion to make sure there is no gapping of the anterior repair or impingement of the cuff on the acromion.

POSTOPERATIVE CARE

The postoperative course is critical in obtaining excellent results. Use of a sling is encouraged for 6 weeks in most all repairs. Strengthening exercises usually are not performed until 10 weeks after the repair to prevent overstrain on the cuff during the early healing phase.

ARTHROSCOPIC FIXATION OF TYPE II SLAP LESIONS

Barry B. Phillips

Type II SLAP (superior labrum anterior and posterior) lesions involve pathological detachments of the labrum and biceps anchor from the superior part of the glenoid. They should be repaired to avoid further destabilization of the shoulder. Patients older than 50 years have less potential for healing and greater potential for stiffness and pain and generally do better with a biceps tenodesis.

■ Place the patient in the lateral decubitus position and place the arm in 30 to 45 degrees of abduction and 20 degrees of forward flexion with 5 to 10 lb of balanced suspension. Administer general anesthesia and place a warming blanket to prevent hypothermia. Use an arthroscopic pump to maintain intraarticular pressure at 60 mm Hg. Use serial compression devices on the lower extremities.

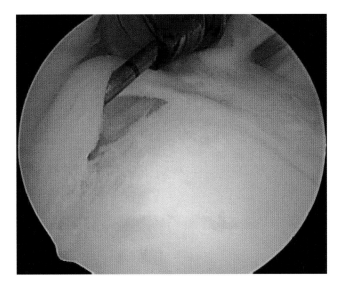

Figure 49-1

■ Establish a viewing portal 2 cm below the posterolateral acromion and an anterior central working portal for routine diagnostic arthroscopy. Findings such as a superior sulcus of more than 5 mm in depth, a displaceable biceps root, a positive drive-through sign, and a positive peel-back sign are indicative of a SLAP lesion (Figure 49-1).

■ Use an angled arthroscopic probe to test the stability of the biceps-superior labral attachments to the glenoid. A normal superior sublabral sulcus covered with articular cartilage can be seen 5 mm medially beneath the labrum. If the sublabral sulcus is deeper than 5 mm, or if the labral attachments at the medial limit of the sulcus are tenuous, a SLAP lesion may be present.

■ Assess whether the biceps root is easily displaceable with a probe. An unstable biceps root and superior labrum are easily displaced medially on the glenoid neck. Occasionally, the biceps root is unstable to probing yet tenuous superior labral attachments are present. Such cases represent interstitial disruption of medially located attachments and require completion of the lesions, bone bed preparation, and repair.

■ Sweep the arthroscope from superior to inferior between the glenoid and humeral head to see if the arthroscope can be easily "driven through" the joint. Although a positive drive-through sign is a sign of instability, "pseudolaxity" associated with SLAP lesions may also be the cause.

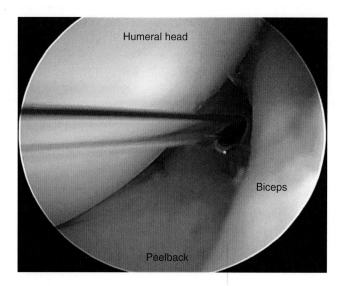

Figure 49-2

- The positive peel-back sign is diagnostic for a posterior SLAP lesion; however isolated anterior SLAP lesions often have a negative peel-back test but other arthroscopic signs, as described earlier, usually are positive. To perform the peel-back test, remove the arm from traction and observe the superior labrum arthroscopically as an assistant brings the arm to 90 degrees abduction and 90 degrees external rotation. Performing this dynamic peel-back maneuver in a shoulder with a posterior SLAP lesion causes the entire biceps-superior labrum complex to drop medially over the edge of the glenoid (Figure 49-2).

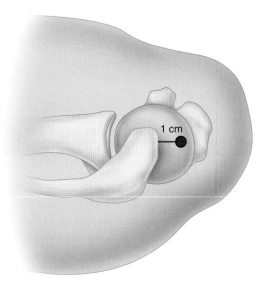

Figure 49-3

- When the diagnosis of a SLAP lesion is made, repair the lesion immediately because swelling may occur that obliterates the supralabral recess and obscures exposure. For the SLAP lesion repair, make three portals: a standard posterior viewing portal, an anterior portal located just above the lateral border of the subscapularis tendon, and an anterosuperior portal. The anterosuperior portal typically is located 1 cm off the anterolateral corner of the acromion (Figure 49-3). Use a spinal needle to locate this portal precisely so that it provides a 45-degree angle of approach to the anterosuperior corner of the glenoid for proper placement of the suture anchor.

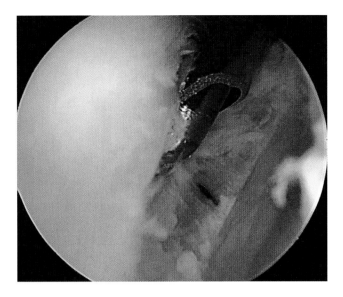

Figure 49-4

- Through the anterior portal, prepare the bone bed on the superior neck of the glenoid, beneath the detached labrum, using a motorized shaver. Débride the soft tissues carefully down to a bleeding base of bone but do not remove bone (Figure 49-4).

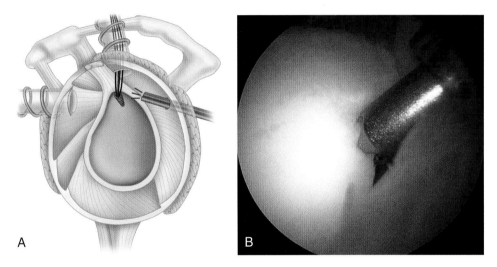

Figure 49-5

- For fixation of SLAP lesions use small size suture anchors and simple translabral loop sutures (Figure 49-5, A). The most critical element to resisting peel-back forces in a mechanically effective manner is to position a tight suture loop just posterior to the root of the biceps, with the loop attached to a suture anchor placed beneath the root of the biceps (B).

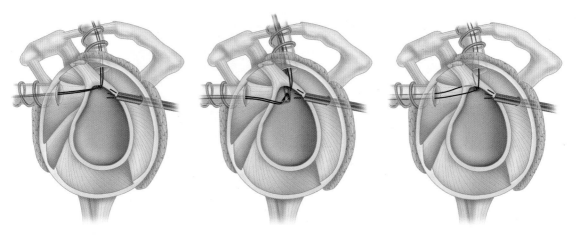

Figure 49-6

- To prevent suture or knot impingement, a vertical suture through the labrum or horizontal suture behind the biceps can be helpful in some cases. The strength of the different suture configuration is similar in laboratory studies. Knotless suture anchors also may be used to help prevent knot impingement (Figure 49-6).

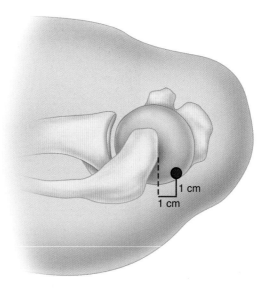

Figure 49-7

- For superior labral lesions that extend posteriorly to overlie the posterosuperior quadrant, place a second anchor through a posterolateral portal, which is located 1 cm lateral and 1 cm anterior to the posterior acromial angle (Figure 49-7).
- Pass the Spear Guide through the rotator cuff near the musculotendinous junction of the infraspinatus by this approach. Because the diameter of the Spear Guide is only 3.5 mm it is preferred over a standard 7-mm arthroscopy cannula for delivery of the suture anchor through the posterolateral portal. To minimize damage to the rotator cuff from portal placement place only the 3.5-mm Spear Guide through the posterolateral portal. This posterolateral portal is used for anchor placement only. Suture passage and knot-tying for the posterior anchor are accomplished through the anterosuperior portal.

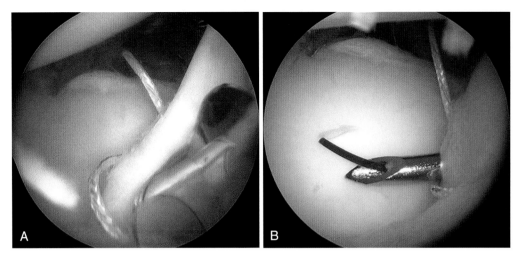

Figure 49-8

- Use the Birdbeak suture passers (Arthrex, Naples, FL) to pass the suture through the labrum. The 45-degree Birdbeak is ideal for passing sutures posterior to the biceps through the anterosuperior cannula and the 22-degree Birdbeak is best for passing sutures anterior to the biceps through the anterior cannula (Figure 49-8, **A**). Penetrate the labrum with the Birdbeak from superior to inferior and grasp the suture. Withdraw the Birdbeak to pull the suture out of the anterosuperior cannula. If the SLAP lesion extends anteriorly beyond the 1-o'clock position, place a separate suture anchor in that position for fixation of that portion of the labrum. A suture shuttle device also may be used and allows for more precise placement and less soft tissue damage (**B**).
- Securely tie the arthroscopic knots. The sutures create simple loops around the labrum that must be very tight to neutralize the peel-back forces. Use stacked reversing half-hitches tied with a knot pusher to create a secure knot. Alternatively use complex sliding knots backed up with three reversing half-hitches to provide adequate knot security.

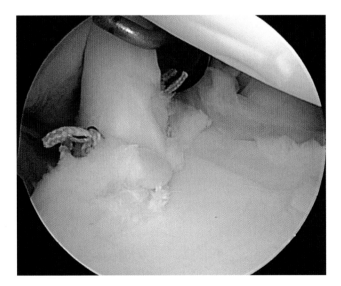

Figure 49-9

- Completed SLAP repair (Figure 49-9).
- After the repair perform the peel-back and drive-through test again to be sure that they are negative, indicating that the pathological process has been corrected. If the drive-through sign remains positive consider adjunctive measures for capsular tightening.

POSTOPERATIVE CARE ›

The operated arm is placed at the side in a sling with a small pillow. Passive external rotation of the shoulder with the arm at the side (not in abduction) and flexion and extension of the elbow are emphasized immediately. Patients who require posteroinferior capsulotomy are started on posteroinferior capsular stretches ("sleeper stretches") on the first postoperative day. The sling is discontinued after 3 weeks and passive elevation is initiated. From weeks 3 to 6 progressive passive motion as tolerated is permitted in all planes and sleeper stretches are begun in patients who did not have posteroinferior capsulotomy. From weeks 6 to 16 stretching and flexibility exercises are continued. Passive posteroinferior capsular stretching is continued, as is external rotation stretching in abduction. Strengthening exercises for the rotator cuff, scapular stabilizers, and deltoid are initiated at 6 weeks. Biceps strengthening can begin 8 weeks postoperatively.

At 4 months athletes begin an interval throwing program on a level surface. They continue a stretching and strengthening program with particular emphasis on posteroinferior capsular stretching. At 6 months pitchers may begin throwing full speed and at 7 months they are allowed full-velocity throwing from the mound. All throwing athletes are instructed to continue posteroinferior capsular stretching indefinitely. A tight posteroinferior capsule probably initiates the pathological cascade to a SLAP lesion and recurrence of the tightness can be expected to place the repair at risk in a throwing athlete (Table 49-1).

TABLE 49-1	Repair Protocol for Superior Labral Anterior-Posterior (SLAP) Lesion*

PHASE I—IMMEDIATE POSTSURGICAL

Weeks 0-2 Postoperative (Type II and IV)

1. P/AAROM with following restrictions
   - FL < 120 degrees
   - ER/IR < 30 degrees
2. Table slides in FL/pendulums
3. Scapular mobility exercises
4. Passive elbow FL
5. Active hand, wrist ROM and gripping exercises
6. Submaximal pain-free isometrics
   IR/ER
   ABD/ADD
   Scapular retraction/depression

Goals (By End of 2 Weeks)

1. Independent with HEP
2. PROM 120 degrees maximum FL/scaption
   - PROM 30 degrees maximal ER/IR
   - Full hand, wrist AROM
   - Active elbow EXT to 30 degrees, full passive elbow FL
Precautions
   - Sling compliance
   - No active biceps contraction
   - Full active elbow EXT

PHASE II—GRADED AROM/STRENGTHENING

Weeks 3-6 Postoperative

- Glenohumeral joint mobilizations (grades I and II)
- Progressing PROM to tolerance
- Progress AAROM/AROM
- Progress scapular mobility exercises (side lying)
- Elbow FL—no resistance
- UBE with low resistance
- Initiate Theraband ER/IR isometrics in neutral (sidestepping)
- Rhythmic stabilization progression
- PNF diagonals with light/moderate manual resistance

Goals (By End of 6 Weeks)

1. Independent with HEP
2. Gradually restore full PROM
3. Discontinue sling as pain decreases and proximal stability increases (week 3-4)
4. Restore correct shoulder girdle mechanics (scapulohumeral rhythm)
5. Full active elbow FL (pain-free)
6. Full EXT by 4-6 weeks depending on physician input
7. Able to comb hair (if dominant arm)
8. Sleep uninterrupted
Precautions
   1. No lifting
   2. ER with ABD > 90 degrees

TABLE 49-1	Repair Protocol for Superior Labral Anterior-Posterior (SLAP) Lesion—cont'd

Weeks 7-9 Postoperative

1. Continue progressing PROM—more aggressive mobilizations if needed (progress joint mobilizations grades III and IV as needed)
2. Elbow FL with light weights (1-5 lb)
3. UBE—increase intensity
4. Progress isotonics as able (Theraband/light weight)
5. Progress rhythmic stabilization/PNF diagonals
   - Progress closed-chain exercises (especially wall push-ups)

Goals (By End of 9 Weeks)

1. Independent with HEP
2. AROM WNL
3. Able to reach behind back for wallet
4. Able to lift plate into eye-level cabinet
Precaution
   No lifting > 5 lb

Weeks 10-11 Postoperative

1. Progress above exercises as tolerated
2. Theraband ER/IR 45 to 90 degrees increase speed/intensity (must be pain-free and demonstrate correct mechanics)
3. Closed-chain scapular stability exercises (quadruped, tripod, side lying)
4. Progress proprioceptive training to include progressive weight-bearing exercises on unstable surfaces

Goals (By End of 11 Weeks)

1. MMT elbow FL 4/5
2. MMT shoulder FL 4/5
3. MMT shoulder ABD 4/5
4. MMT shoulder ER 4/5
5. MMT shoulder IR 4/5
6. Able to lift 3 lb into overhead cabinet
7. Maintain scapulohumeral rhythm with strengthening and functional activities
8. Able to tuck shirt and fasten bra
Precaution
   No unilateral lifting over head > 5 lb

PHASE III—ADVANCED STRENGTHENING FOR RETURN TO SPORT

Weeks 12-15 Postoperative

1. Progress isotonics increasing resistance/repetitions (exercises, throwing, lunges)
2. Plyoball exercises if appropriate
   Chest pass
   Overhead throw
   Sideway throw
   One-handed ball on wall
3. Progress shoulder strengthening (lateral pull-downs, rows)
4. Isokinetic strengthening as needed

Goals (By End of 15 Weeks)

1. MMT shoulder musculature 5/5
   - Able to place ≥ 10 lb in overhead cabinet

Weeks 16-24 Postoperative

1. Initiate interval throwing (per physician input)
2. Initiate sport-specific/functional training
3. Isokinetic testing if requested

Goals (By End of 6 Months)

1. Return to sport/activity of choice
2. Independent with exercise progression

ABD, Abduction; *ADD,* adduction; *AROM,* active range of motion; *ER,* external rotation; *EXT,* extension; *HEP,* home exercise programs; *FL,* flexion; *IR,* internal rotation; *MMT,* manual muscle testing; *P/AAROM,* passive or active-assisted range of motion; *PNF,* proprioceptive neuromuscular facilitation; *PROM,* passive range of motion; *ROM,* range of motion; *UBE,* upper body exercises; *WNL,* within normal limits.

*Protocol was developed for patients after SLAP lesion repair. Surgery and rehabilitation differ depending on type of lesion. Types I and III usually are treated with débridement. The biceps tendon is stable, so postoperative rehabilitation usually progresses as tolerated. Types II and IV indicate an unstable biceps tendon requiring repair. This protocol addresses range-of-motion limitations and limited active biceps work necessary for type II/IV repairs. This is a guideline and may be adjusted to clinical presentation and physician's guidance.

Proximal biceps tendon ruptures are most common in individuals 40 to 60 years of age and often are due to impingement or chronic microtrauma on the tendon. These injuries also may occur in younger individuals during heavy weightlifting or other sports activities (e.g., football, rugby, soccer, snowboarding) or in a traumatic fall. Tenodesis techniques range from open to mini-open to all-arthroscopic. Fixation can be done with suture anchors, interference screws, or bone tunnels.

SUBPECTORAL BICEPS TENODESIS 〉

- With the patient in the beach chair position perform a standard diagnostic arthroscopic examination.
- Identify the rotator interval between the supraspinatus and subscapularis tendons and make a standard anterior portal from inside-out or outside-in.
- With a probe in the anterior portal, pull the biceps tendon into the glenohumeral joint to evaluate its mobility and any structural lesions. Because pathological processes of the biceps tendon are most often in the intertubercular groove portion it is critical that this part be drawn into the joint.
- Evaluate the coracohumeral ligament and supraspinatus and subscapular tendons for any pathological process.
- With an arthroscopic cutting instrument or thermal ablator through the anterior portal, tenotomize the biceps tendon at its base. A shaver can be used to débride the proximal portion for a stable base.

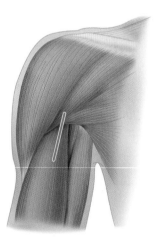

Figure 50-1

- With the arm abducted and internally rotated, palpate the inferior border of the pectoralis major tendon. On the medial aspect of the arm make an incision 1 cm superior to this inferior border and continue it to 3 cm below the inferior border (Figure 50-1).
- Inject the incision site with a local anesthetic plus epinephrine for subcutaneous hemostasis and perioperative analgesia.
- Dissect through the subcuticular tissue, using electrocautery to control bleeding, and clear the overlying fatty tissue until the fascia overlying the pectoralis major, coracobrachialis, and biceps is identified. If these anatomic landmarks are not seen the dissection may be too lateral. If the cephalic vein is seen in the deltopectoral groove the dissection is too proximal and too lateral.
- Once the inferior border of the pectoralis major has been identified, incise the fascia over the coracobrachialis and biceps in a proximal to distal direction. It is important to see the horizontal fibers of the pectoralis muscle and dissect below this level.
- Use blunt finger dissection under the inferior edge of the pectoralis muscle, palpating up the anteromedial humerus, to identify the longitudinal, fusiform structure of the biceps tendon.

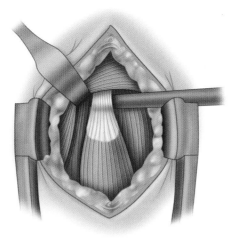

Figure 50-2

- Place a pointed Hohmann retractor into the pectoralis major tendon and on the proximal humerus to retract the muscle proximally and laterally (Figure 50-2).
- Position a blunt Chandler retractor on the medial aspect of the humerus and gently retract the coracobrachialis and short head of the biceps tendon. Avoid vigorous medial retraction to prevent injury to the musculocutaneous nerve.

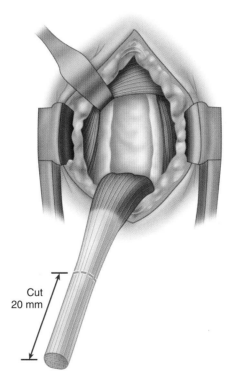

Cut
20 mm

Figure 50-3

- Once the biceps tendon is identified place a right-angle clamp deep to it and pull the tendon into the wound (Figure 50-3).
- One centimeter proximal to the pectoralis major tendon reflect the periosteum in a rectangle roughly 2 × 1 cm.
- To ensure appropriate tensioning of the biceps tendon resect the proximal portion to leave 20 to 25 mm of tendon proximal to the musculotendinous portion of the biceps.

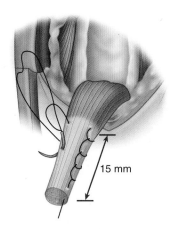

Figure 50-4

- Using a Krackow or whip stitch, weave a no. 2 nonabsorbable suture into the proximal 15 mm of the tendon. Secure enough of the tendon to ensure adequate interference fixation within bone and to position the musculotendinous portion of the biceps muscle beneath the inferior border of the pectoralis major tendon. This is critical for proper tensioning of the muscle-tendon unit as well as for cosmesis (Figure 50-4).

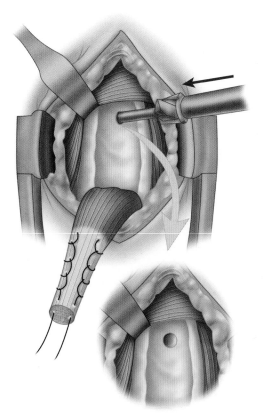

Figure 50-5

- Use a guidewire and an 8-mm reamer to make a 15-mm deep bone tunnel at the junction of the middle and distal thirds of the intertubercular groove between the lesser and greater tuberosities (Figure 50-5).
- Clear all debris from the field with irrigation.
- Thread one limb of the suture through a biotenodesis screwdriver and screw (8 × 12 mm) and wrap the end of the suture into the screw cleat.
- Place the tenodesis screwdriver into the bone tunnel and advance the screw over the tendon. When the screw is flush with the bone tunnel remove the screwdriver.

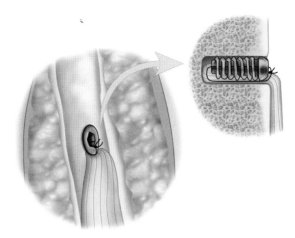

Figure 50-6

- Tie the limb of the suture next to the tendon and screw to the limb of the suture through the screw to provide both an interference fit and suture anchor stability (Figure 50-6).
- When the fixation is completed the musculotendinous junction should rest in its exact anatomic location underneath the inferior border of the pectoralis major tendon.
- Complete the procedure with standard wound closure.

POSTOPERATIVE CARE 〉

A sling is worn during sleep for the first 4 weeks and is used only while awake if the patient is having difficulty keeping the elbow flexed passively or if he or she is going into public areas. The sling is discontinued completely after 4 weeks. Activity typically is dictated by procedures done in conjunction with the biceps tenodesis. If biceps tenodesis alone is done strengthening activities should be restricted until 6 weeks after surgery. Many patients are able to resume activity as tolerated at 2 weeks but they should be informed of the risks.

Distal biceps tendon ruptures typically occur in middle-aged men during heavy lifting with the elbow flexed 90 degrees, or when the biceps muscle contracts against unexpected resistance. Distal biceps tendon ruptures can be repaired through a single-incision or two-incision (Boyd and Anderson) technique. The two-incision technique restores supination power and avoids the dangers of deep dissection in the antecubital fossa.

TWO-INCISION TECHNIQUE FOR REPAIR OF THE DISTAL BICEPS TENDON 〉

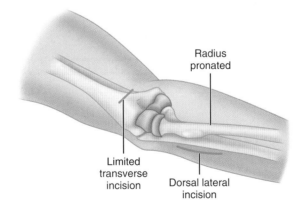

Radius
pronated

Limited
transverse
incision

Dorsal lateral
incision

Figure 50-7

- Make a 2-cm transverse anterior incision and a longer, 6- to 8-cm posterolateral incision over the radial aspect of the ulnar border (Figure 50-7).
- Open the deep fascia and identify the biceps tendon with palpation.
- Locate the original tunnel through the interosseous membrane.
- Place Krackow locking stitches in the tendon end. It is important to keep each locking throw in close proximity to the previous throw to avoid kinking the tendon and forming a bunched end to the tendon that would prohibit the tendon from seating into the groove or "trapdoor" created in the radial tuberosity.
- With a long curved hemostat deliver the tendon from the anterior incision to the posterolateral incision. Avoid making multiple passes through the membrane to minimize the risk of heterotopic ossification and subsequent synostosis.

- Deepen the posterolateral incision, identify the anconeus, and sharply dissect it off the bone. Pronate the arm to protect the posterior interosseous nerve.
- Use a small ¼-inch curved osteotome to make a trough or "trapdoor" in the tuberosity.

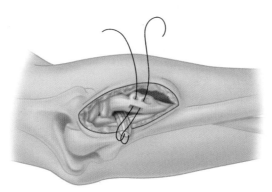

Figure 50-8

- Drill two holes in the dorsal aspect of the trough leaving a 10-mm bone bridge between them (Figure 50-8).
- Pass the sutures tied to the tendon, and with them the tendon, through the interosseous membrane.
- Use a suture passer to pass the first suture through the trough and out of the drill hole.
- Pass the second suture with the suture passer through the trough and out of the drill hole.
- Pulling carefully on the sutures in the tendon guide it into the trough in the bone.
- Tie the sutures securely over the bone and cut off the ends of the sutures.
- Close the anterior incision with the elbow flexed about 60 degrees.
- Release the tourniquet and close the posterolateral incision.

POSTOPERATIVE CARE

With the elbow flexed to 110 degrees and the forearm in moderate supination a posterior plaster splint is applied. At 2 weeks, the splint and the sutures are removed. A hinged brace is applied and worn for 4 weeks. Passive flexion is allowed, as is active extension, progressing 15 to 20 degrees per week. Supination/pronation range-of-motion exercises are added at 4 to 6 weeks. At 6 to 8 weeks full range of motion should be possible but return to full activities should be delayed for 12 to 16 weeks.

Reported advantages of the single-incision technique include limited exposure of the radial tuberosity, better cosmetic result, and decreased risk of heterotopic ossification. Disadvantages include increased costs (expensive hardware), possibility of less secure fixation, and no bony trough for tendon revascularization.

SINGLE-INCISION TECHNIQUE FOR REPAIR OF THE DISTAL BICEPS TENDON

- Make a 3- to 4-cm anterior longitudinal incision. Superficial antecubital veins may require ligation. Identify and preserve the lateral antebrachial cutaneous nerve.
- Identify the proximal torn biceps tendon and place it in a moist sponge.
- Ligate the radial recurrent vessels.
- Deep knee retractors allow excellent exposure of the radial tuberosity. Débride the remnant of the tuberosity free of remaining tendon and elevate the periosteum over the bone with a curet.
- Fix the tendon to the radial tuberosity with sutures through bone tunnels, suture anchors, button, or tenodesis or interference screws.
- Once the tendon is approximated move the forearm through a full range of pronation and supination to ensure that the tendon tracks smoothly.

POSTOPERATIVE CARE

The elbow is immobilized at 90 degrees for 2 weeks at which time the sutures are removed. A hinged elbow brace is applied with extension stopped at 80 degrees. Full passive flexion is allowed with passive pronation and supination to 90 degrees. At 6 weeks progressive extension in the brace is allowed at a rate of 20 degrees per week. At 8 weeks active flexion is begun and strengthening is started at 12 weeks. Full unrestricted use is allowed at 16 weeks.

ARTHROSCOPIC BICEPS TENODESIS WITH A PERCUTANEOUS INTRAARTICULAR TENDON ⟩

Sekiya et al. described a technique for repair of biceps rupture that should be used in middle-aged patients who are not doing high-level sports or heavy lifting. Indications are as for other biceps tendon problems with chronic bicipital tendinitis and an associated tear, medial subluxation, or bicipital pain with an associated SLAP tear.

- Place the patient in a "beach chair" or lateral decubitus position.
- Insert a spinal needle from the anterior aspect of the shoulder into the bicipital groove and through the transverse humeral ligament and the lateral aspect of the internal capsule.
- Under direct view pierce the biceps tendon with the spinal needle. Thread a no. 1 PDS (Ethicon, Cornelia, GA) through the spinal needle and pull it through the anterior portal with a grasper.
- Insert a second spinal needle through the transverse humeral ligament from the anterior shoulder and pierce the biceps tendon near the first suture. Thread a second no. 1 PDS through the spinal needle and pull it out of the anterior portal.
- These two sutures are used to pull a no. 2 braided nonabsorbable polyester suture (SURGIDAC; U.S. Surgical, Norwalk, CT) through the biceps tendon. Tie the no. 2 SURGIDAC suture to one strand of the PDS and pull it from the puncture wound in the anterior aspect of the shoulder through the biceps tendon and out of the anterior cannula. Tie the end of the SURGIDAC suture that was pulled through the anterior cannula to the other PDS and pull it back through the anterior cannula, through the biceps tendon, and out of the anterior shoulder puncture wound. This creates a mattress suture that secures the biceps tendon to the transverse humeral ligament in the bicipital groove.
- Repeat these steps to create a second mattress suture to secure the biceps tendon. Different color sutures may be used to simplify suture management.
- After the biceps tendon is adequately secured, use an arthroscopic scissors or biter to transect the biceps tendon proximal to the suture.
- Débride the stump of biceps anchor down to a smooth, stable rim on the superior labrum.
- At this point, direct the arthroscope into the subacromial space. Establish a lateral portal and perform any concomitant procedures such as a subacromial decompression or rotator cuff repair. Avoid transection of the previously passed sutures. We prefer to perform a subacromial bursectomy before passing tenodesis sutures.
- Locate the sutures securing the biceps tendon to the transverse humeral ligament in the bicipital groove in the subacromial space and pull through the lateral portal.
- Sequentially tie the sutures using standard arthroscopic knot-tying techniques.
- Remove all fluid and debris and close portals in the standard fashion. Dress the wound and place the shoulder in a sling.

POSTOPERATIVE CARE ⟩

If an isolated arthroscopic biceps tenodesis was done the patient is immediately started on passive pendulum exercises and active wrist and hand range-of-motion exercises. At 1 week after surgery gentle passive elbow and shoulder range of motion is begun in all planes under the guidance of a physical therapist. The sling is used for 4 weeks. Active motion and gentle strengthening of the shoulder and elbow can begin 8 weeks after surgery. By 12 to 16 weeks after surgery the patient is "weaned" from physical therapy to a home exercise program. Unrestricted use of the extremity is allowed 4 to 6 months after surgery.

BICEPS TENODESIS: ARTHROSCOPIC OR MINI-OPEN TECHNIQUE ⟩

Tenodesis can be done with a bioabsorbable biotenodesis screw or with two 5-mm screw-in suture anchors. The resistance to cyclic loading is comparable in both techniques whereas the ultimate pull-out strength of the biotenodesis screw is stronger than the suture anchors. Whether done arthroscopically or through a mini-open approach with a small anterior incision or a small subpectoral incision, long-term results are comparable and the technique should be chosen based on the skills and experience of the operating surgeon.

- Place the patient in the "beach chair" position with the arm in 30 to 60 degrees of forward flexion, 30 degrees of abduction, and 20 degrees of internal rotation resting on a padded Mayo stand.

- Pass an 18-gauge needle from the anterolateral corner of the acromion through the rotator cuff and into the biceps tendon.

- Pass a no. 1 monofilament suture through the 18-gauge needle, capture it with a grabber from the anterior portal, and then extract it.

- After the tendon is marked with a suture use an arthroscopic basket to release the tendon from its origin just lateral to the superior labrum. This completes the preparation for the biceps tenodesis during the glenohumeral joint arthroscopy.

- Make an anterolateral portal 2 to 3 cm below the palpable edge of the anterior acromion in the center of the anterior third of the acromion. Although visualization is maintained through the lateral portal the anterior portal is the working portal.

- Place an arthroscopic shaver in the anterior portal and remove all adventitial tissue. Anatomical landmarks and the monofilament suture are used for localizing the tendon in the groove. The falciform ligament of the pectoralis tendon is a reproducible landmark. The biceps tendon is directly under this structure.

- Using an arthroscopic basket identify the sheath and open it. Use electrocautery to clean surrounding tissues and use a probe to free the tendon. Extend the dissection proximally to the lateral aspect of the rotator interval. Avoid proceeding too far medially or the dissection to expose the biceps tendon from the biceps sheath may lead to a partial displacement of the superficial attachment of the subscapularis tendon.

- Retrieve the tendon by one of two methods. Capture the monofilament sutures with a crochet hook from the anterior portal and extract the tendon from that portal or localize the bicipital groove with a spinal needle in the anterolateral quadrant of the shoulder. After obtaining satisfactory angle and position, make a portal incision and retrieve the tendon with a hemostat. The amount of excursion of the biceps tendon is relatively small but can be improved by flexing the arm more than 90 degrees. Excessive distention of the soft tissues with fluid also may make the biceps tendon difficult to extract from the surgical wound. If this occurs, transfer the arthroscope to the anterior portal and use the modified lateral portal to extract the tendon.

- After the tendon is extracted from the anterolateral portal place a hemostat on the tendon at the level of the skin to prevent it from retracting underneath the skin.

- The placement and tension of the tenodesis are important for anatomical repair. To approximate the intraarticular distance remove 20 mm of tendon and place a "whip stitch" in 15 mm of tendon. This allows the tenodesis driver to "bury" the tendon with all of the suture and confirms correct placement in the bone tunnel.

- Place a braided suture on the end of the tendon using a tendon stitch technique as described by Krakow or a no. 2 Fiberwire (Arthrex, Naples, FL) that is 36 inches in overall length.

- Place a square knot at the end of the suture to maintain suture tension during insertion and to direct placement with the tenodesis driver.

- Allow the sutures to fall back into the subacromial space.

- Place cannulas into the anterior and anterolateral portals and shuttle the sutures into the anterior portal so that they are out of the way for the bone tunnel preparation.

- Use a lateral portal for exposure and identify the bicipital groove.

- Gently débride the soft tissue so that the bicipital groove can be easily seen. The lateral edge of the bicipital groove should be avoided because the ascending branch of the anterior circumflex vessel traverses along this edge. Débridement of the sheath and surrounding tissue avoids soft tissue interposition with the placement of the drill, tendon insertion into the bone tunnel, and placement of the interference screw. The groove should be easily seen before beginning the bone tunnel procedure.

- For instrumentation, use an 8.25-mm clear cannula in the anterior portal to enhance exposure and minimize soft tissue distention. Through the anterolateral portal, insert a cannulated reamer guidewire (2.4-mm) into the center of the bicipital groove 10 to 15 mm below the insertion of the supraspinatus lateral to the subscapularis insertion at the level of the transverse humeral ligament. The depth of insertion is 30 mm. Drilling beyond the posterior cortex of the humerus, which may increase the risk of complications during this operative procedure, is unnecessary. For most patients an 8-mm cannulated reamer is of adequate size to allow placement of the tendon into the bone tunnel and to secure fixation with an 8-mm bioabsorbable interference fit screw.

- Measure the tendon diameter with sizing holes found on the thumb pad of the biotenodesis driver. Advance the calibrated reamer over the guide pin to the 30-mm mark. The standard length of the proximal biceps biotenodesis screw is 23 mm.

- After the bone socket has been created the reamer and guide pin are removed.

- Assemble the biotenodesis driver and handle and place the bioabsorbable screw over the distal end of the driver. Typically an 8-mm screw is used for an 8-mm bone tunnel.

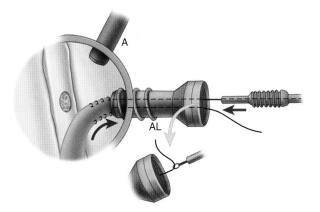

Figure 51-1

- Retrieve the sutures through the anterolateral portal. With a wire loop suture passer pull one limb of the suture through the driver and the screwdriver handle. Hold the other limb loosely. Pull the limb that is passed through the driver tightly until the end of the tendon is securely placed against the tip of the driver. Having the thumb pad against the driver handle so that it does not interfere with the insertion of the interference screw is important (Figure 51-1).

- Use the lateral portal for viewing and place the tenodesis driver through the anterolateral cannula. Observe the tip of the driver and the tendon as they exit the cannula.

- Place the tip of the driver at the superior aspect of the bone socket and manually insert it until the tendon reaches the base of the tunnel. Hold the free suture limb inside of the cannulated driver tight against the driver with a hemostat. After the driver and tendon have been seated at the bottom of the bone socket, use the thumb pad to hold the tendon and suture against the base of the bone tunnel. Appropriate insertion of the tendon is confirmed by seeing the suture disappear into the bone socket.

- Place the bioabsorbable interference screw directly over the top of the tendon until the head of the screw is below the level of the prominence of the medial and lateral intertubercular ridges. The head of the screw can be inserted until it is flush with the base of the bicipital groove.

- After the screw has been properly seated remove the driver from the anterolateral portal.

- Use a crochet hook to remove both limbs of the suture; one is through the center of the interference screw, and the other limb is captured between the interference fit screw and the bone tunnel.

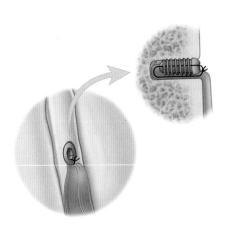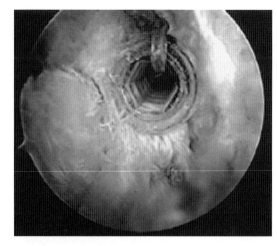

Figure 51-2

- Tie a knot composed of multiple half-hitches over the top of the interference screw, using arthroscopic knot-tying techniques (Figure 51-2).
- Irrigate the subacromial space, thoroughly removing any remaining soft tissue or debris.
- Rotate the arm from side to side to ensure that no prominence exists from the interference screw head and that no complications related to the procedure have occurred.

LATERAL DECUBITUS POSITION 〉

- The lateral decubitus position also can be used for subacromial surgery, including arthroscopic biceps tenodesis.
- Position the arm in 30 to 45 degrees of abduction with longitudinal traction. The advantage of this position is that the anatomy of the shoulder stays relatively fixed during the operative procedure. The disadvantage is that the traction is not easily removed. The elbow is not flexed during the operative procedure, which would provide a greater length of the biceps tendon available in the subacromial space. Thus, in the lateral decubitus position, the biceps tendon length is inadequate to extract routinely from the anterior portal.
- Romeo et al. recommended a modification of the technique from that used with the "beach chair" position previously described, which allows the biceps tendon to remain in the subacromial space at all times.
- After identifying the biceps tendon, by palpation or visualization below the transverse humeral ligament, remove the tendon from the groove. Place a single no. 2 Fiberwire into the tendon 2 cm cephalad to the intended tenodesis hole using a Viper punch (Arthrex, Naples, FL).
- Retrieve both suture limbs out of the anterior portal and tie a sliding locking knot over the tendon.
- Establish the bone socket and deliver the tendon using the same methods described with the "beach chair" position.
- Trim excess tendon at the conclusion of fixation.

POSTOPERATIVE CARE 〉

Postoperative management depends largely on the types of procedures that were performed in conjunction with the biceps tenodesis. If only a biceps tenodesis was done, the postoperative procedure is the same as for arthroscopic acromioplasty. Strengthening activities related to elbow flexion or forward elevation of the arm with the elbow extended should be restricted until 6 weeks after the biceps tenodesis.

Barry B. Phillips

ANTERIOR PORTAL

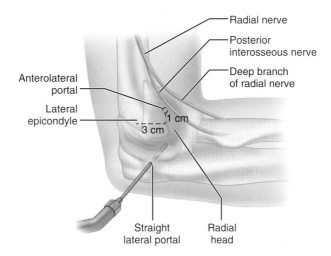

Figure 52-1

- Begin by distending the elbow joint. Insert an 18-gauge spinal needle at the direct lateral portal and aim it directly toward the center of the joint. The needle passes between the olecranon, radial head, and distal humerus. Avoid extending too far anteriorly and entering the soft tissues in the antecubital fossa. Extraarticular swelling from infiltration of irrigant into these anterior soft tissues can collapse the anterior joint space. Using a 61-mL syringe and connective tubing, distend the elbow with fluid. Free backflow of fluid confirms proper intraarticular location of the needle. Maximally distend the joint with 20 mL of fluid to displace the neurovascular structures anteriorly in the antecubital fossa and to increase the space available in the anterior aspect of the joint (Figure 52-1).

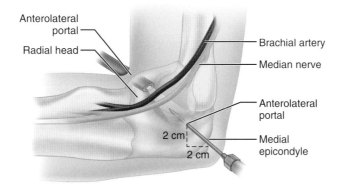

Figure 52-2

- Leaving the first needle in place and maintaining distention, insert a second 18-gauge spinal needle through the midanterolateral portal. Aim this needle toward the center of the joint. Free backflow of the solution confirms an intraarticular location (Figure 52-2).

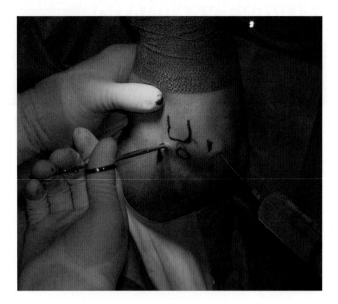

Figure 52-3

- Remove the needle and incise the skin with the tip of a no. 11 blade by pulling the skin against the cutting edge. Use a mosquito hemostat to dissect bluntly down to the fascia to minimize the chance of injury to cutaneous or radial nerves (Figure 52-3).
- Pass the arthroscopy cannula with a blunt trocar along the same course as the needle, just proximal and anterior to the radiocapitellar articulation. Use the trocar to capture the joint capsule laterally. Increase the angle of insertion to approximately 70 degrees to horizontal, moving toward the center of the joint. It is important to prevent the trocar from skiving more medially before penetrating the joint capsule. If this occurs viewing and instrumentation from the anterolateral portal are compromised.

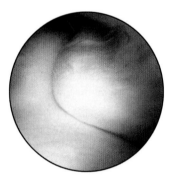

Figure 52-4

- Insert the arthroscope through this cannula with inflow through the arthroscope. This portal allows examination of the coronoid process of the ulna and the trochlear ridge (Figure 52-4).
- Examine the capsule medial to the articulation. Synovitis or capsular damage in this area may indicate medial instability. Confirm instability by releasing traction, supinating the forearm, and applying valgus stress to the elbow at varying degrees of flexion from 30 to 90 degrees. Opening of the joint medially of more than 1 mm indicates medial laxity. Flexing and extending the elbow also allows viewing of the trochlea. Retracting the arthroscope brings the radial head into view, and the radioulnar articulation is viewed as the forearm is pronated and supinated.
- Turn the scope to observe the capsule and its insertion on the distal humerus. Observe the adequacy of the coronoid fossa. Embedded loose bodies, osteophytes, and adhesions may impinge the coronoid as the elbow is fully flexed.

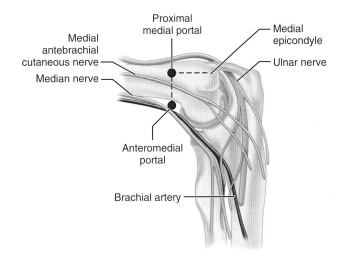

Figure 52-5

- The anteromedial portal can be established with the Wissinger rod technique or under direct arthroscopic vision through the anterolateral portal. Some authors believe the anteromedial or the proximal medial portal should be established first in the manner described for the anterolateral portal (Figure 52-5).

- With the Wissinger rod technique, push the arthroscope up to the medial capsule at the desired location for the medial portal, remove the arthroscope, and hold the cannula flush against the capsule. Insert the Wissinger rod and advance it until it tents the skin medially, incise the skin, and push the rod through the skin. Place a cannula sheath over the rod and advance it into the joint. Remove the rod and the portal is established.

- Alternatively an 18-gauge spinal needle can be inserted through the anticipated anteromedial portal site into the joint while confirming a satisfactory position arthroscopically. After the skin is incised, and the fascia is reached with a hemostat, insert a blunt trocar following the same course as the needle heading toward the center of the joint. Push the blunt trocar against the capsule where the exactness of the entry point can be confirmed proximal and anterior to the articulation, allowing maneuverability. Withdraw the arthroscope from harm's way before pushing the cannula while twisting back and forth to penetrate the joint capsule. This method prevents the cannula from sliding anteriorly over the joint capsule and damaging neurovascular structures.

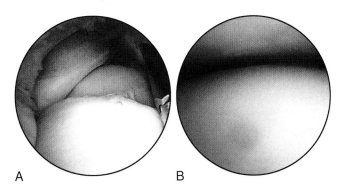

Figure 52-6   A   B

- Leaving the cannula in the anterolateral portal, the arthroscope can be switched to the anteromedial portal to view the radioulnar and radiocapitellar articulations and the annular ligament (Figure 52-6, **A**). Extending the elbow reveals more of the capitellum, and pronating and supinating the forearm exposes more of the radial head. Chondromalacia of the radiocapitellar joint may develop as a result of repetitive trauma from throwing or racquet sports. Osteophytes and loose bodies likewise may form. By placing varus stress to the joint the articular surface of the capitellum can be seen better as the elbow is extended (**B**). The annular ligament can be examined using the shaver tip or blunt cannula to lift the capsule anteriorly and distally over the radial head. The anterolateral capsule and gutter should be examined for synovitis. A synovial plica in the lateral gutter may be a normal finding. With repetitive trauma this band may become thickened and fibrotic and may need to be excised. Slowly retracting the arthroscope and turning the lens toward the ulna reveals the coronoid process.

DIRECT LATERAL PORTAL 〉

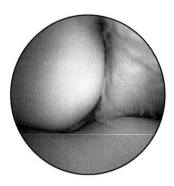

Figure 52-7

- This portal is made proximal and posterior to the radiocapitellar articulation, just posterior to the previously established anterolateral portal. Use a blunt trocar to enter the joint carefully to avoid scuffing the articular cartilage. Become anatomically oriented by finding the two articulations and the posterior aspect of the radiocapitellar and the radioulnar articulations (Figure 52-7).

- Examine the concavity of the radial head articulating on the convex capitellum. Turn the lens to look anteriorly and gently move the elbow through flexion and extension to examine the surface of the capitellum. Examine for chondromalacia and any chondral defects producing instability and incongruence. Probe osteochondritis dissecans lesions through an accessory portal and evaluate the stability of the articular cartilage. Sweep the scope back posteriorly to the area of the two articulations.

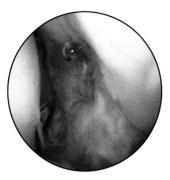

Figure 52-8

- Examine the articulation between the olecranon and the trochlea. Small loose bodies may hide in this area. A normal bare area exists in the olecranon articulation at the site of the physeal scar. Follow the articulation proximally to view the posteromedial olecranon tip. Chondromalacia of the olecranon tip may progress to osteophyte formation, which is indicative of posteromedial elbow impingement. This spectrum of lesions is a continuum of a pathological response related to medial elbow laxity from repetitive throwing (Figure 52-8).

- Sweep the arthroscope more proximally and turn the lens to observe the anticipated site of establishment of the posterolateral portal.

POSTEROLATERAL PORTAL 〉

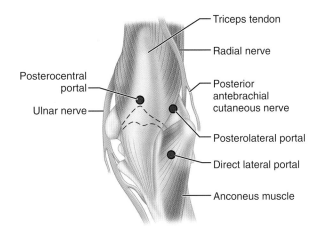

Triceps tendon

Radial nerve

Posterocentral portal

Ulnar nerve

Posterior antebrachial cutaneous nerve

Posterolateral portal

Direct lateral portal

Anconeus muscle

Figure 52-9

- The posterolateral portal can be established under arthroscopic guidance with the arthroscope in the direct lateral portal and the lens directed posteriorly. First insert an 18-gauge needle, aiming toward the olecranon fossa, and confirm satisfactory position. If the direct lateral portal is to be a working portal as for treating an osteochondritis dissecans lesion, the posterolateral portal should be made at or just proximal to the olecranon tip in line with the radial gutter. A 70-degree arthroscope is inserted and directed toward the radiocapitellar joint for visualization. This allows for separation of the scope and the working portal for easier triangulation (Figure 52-9).

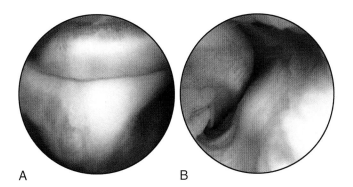

Figure 52-10   A   B

- Incise the skin and use a small hemostat to spread down to the capsule. Use a blunt trocar to enter the joint. The arthroscopic view includes the olecranon fossa, olecranon tip, and posterior trochlea (Figure 52-10, **A**) and a portion of the posterior band on the ulnar collateral ligament (**B**). With the patient prone, arthroscopic procedures in the posterior compartment are technically easier and orientation is improved. Loose bodies frequently gravitate to the posterior compartment and osteophytes form on the posteromedial tip of the olecranon. Palpation along the ulnar nerve locates it immediately superficial to this posteromedial osteophyte, separated only by the joint capsule, and the proximity of this nerve should be considered when using motorized instruments or osteotomes posteriorly.

- If a second operative portal is needed, establish the straight posterior portal under arthroscopic guidance as described.

POSTOPERATIVE CARE 〉

Rehabilitation begins immediately. The patient is encouraged to move the elbow within the postoperative dressing as soon as pain and swelling permit. Flexibility and strengthening exercises are begun when pain and swelling are sufficiently diminished.

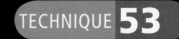
LATERAL EPICONDYLITIS 〉

Lateral epicondylitis (tennis elbow) occurs more frequently in nonathletes than athletes, with a peak incidence in the early fifth decade. Most patients with tennis elbow can be treated nonoperatively; for those who do not improve with nonoperative treatment, resection of diseased tendon and repair of normal tendon to bone can provide pain relief and improve function. We currently prefer to expose the diseased extensor carpi radialis brevis orgin, resect degenerative tissue, and repair the tendon to bone.

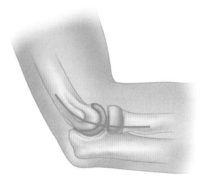

Figure 53-1

- Make a gently curved incision 5 cm long centered over the lateral epicondyle (Figure 53-1).

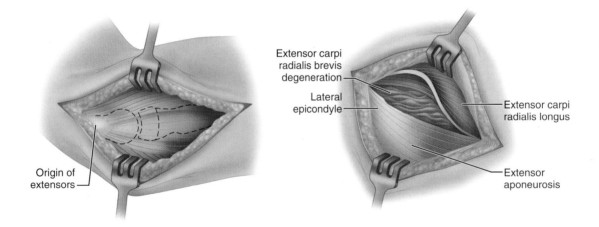

Figure 53-2

- Incise the deep fascia in line with the incision and retract it. Identify the extensor carpi radialis longus and the origin of the extensor digitorum communis, which partially obscure the origin of the deeper extensor carpi radialis brevis (Figure 53-2).
- Elevate the brevis portion of the conjoined tendon at the midportion of the lateral epicondyle toward the elbow joint.
- Because normal-appearing Sharpey fibers are elevated, excise abnormal-appearing tendon. The diseased tissue may appear fibrillated and discolored and may contain calcium deposits.
- Occasionally, the disease process will have spread to the origin of the extensor digitorum communis and a portion of this can be excised. We see no reason to enter the joint itself unless preoperative evaluation indicates intraarticular processes, such as a loose body, degenerative joint disease, effusion, or synovial thickening.

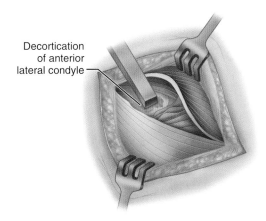

Figure 53-3

- Decorticate a small area of the lateral epicondyle with a rongeur or osteotome, taking care not to enter the joint and damage the articular cartilage (Figure 53-3).
- Suture the remaining normal tendon to the fascia or periosteum, or attach it with nonabsorbable sutures through drill holes in the epicondyle. The use of suture anchors has been reported to be successful in attaching the tendon but we do not believe it is necessary.
- Close the extensor carpi radialis longus and extensor digitorum communis interval with absorbable sutures (which cover the knots made for the extensor carpi radialis brevis repair to bone if anchors are used).
- Close the skin incision with absorbable 4-0 sutures and adhesive strips.

POSTOPERATIVE CARE 〉

The splint is removed within the first week of surgery and range-of-motion (ROM) exercises are begun. After the wound has healed (10 to 14 days) therapy is continued, including edema control and ROM exercises followed by strengthening exercises. Strenuous activity can be resumed within the limits of pain in 8 to 10 weeks and full power should return in approximately 3 months. The rehabilitation protocol is not time dependent but rather goal dependent, with patients passing from one phase to the next after certain goals have been met.

MEDIAL EPICONDYLITIS 〉

Medial epicondylitis is similar to lateral epicondylitis but is much less common and more difficult to treat. If nonoperative treatment fails, excision of the diseased tendon origin and reattachment usually are successful. If ulnar nerve symptoms are present, the ulnar nerve should be decompressed and transposed.

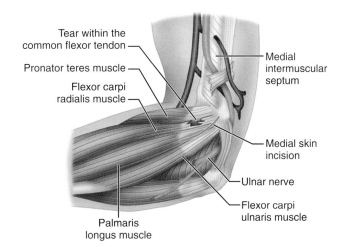

Figure 53-4

- Make a slightly curved 5-cm incision starting approximately 1 cm proximal and just posterior to the medial epicondyle. Placement of the incision posteriorly avoids sensory branches of the medial antebrachial cutaneous nerve anterior and distal to the epicondyle (Figure 53-4).
- Retract the subcutaneous tissue and skin over the medial epicondyle to expose the common flexor origin.

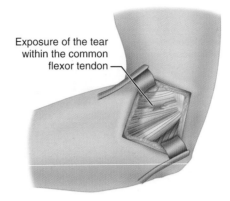

Figure 53-5

- Make a longitudinal incision in the tendon origins beginning at the tip of the medial epicondyle and distally for 3 to 4 cm to expose the pathological tissue (Figure 53-5).

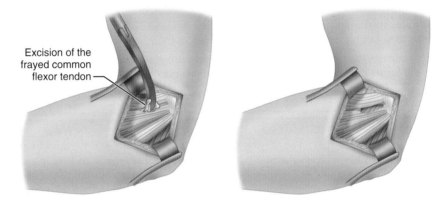

Figure 53-6

- Excise the pathological tissue elliptically, including the joint capsule if necessary, while leaving the normal tissue of the attachment to the medial epicondyle intact (Figure 53-6).

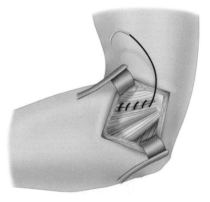

Figure 53-7

- Close the elliptical defect with absorbable sutures (Figure 53-7).
- Transpose the ulnar nerve in patients with symptoms or pathological anatomy found at the time of surgery.
- Close the subcutaneous tissue with absorbable suture and the skin with a running subcuticular suture.
- Apply a dressing and a posterior splint with the elbow in 90 degrees of flexion.

POSTOPERATIVE CARE ❯

The splint is removed 1 week after surgery and elbow ROM exercises are initiated. Strengthening exercises are started when full range of motion is achieved, typically 3 weeks after surgery. Strenuous activity can resume when the patient achieves normal strength without pain, typically 3 months after surgery. A longer period of immobilization and slower progression of rehabilitation are indicated in patients who had ulnar nerve transposition.

ARTHROSCOPIC TENNIS ELBOW RELEASE ⟩

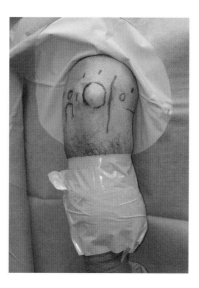

Figure 53-8

- After intubation, place the patient prone on the operating table. Place two rolled towels longitudinally under the patient's thorax. Pad all bony prominences well. Position the affected extremity with the ipsilateral shoulder abducted to 90 degrees, and support the arm with a precut foam holder (Figure 53-8).

- After marking anatomical landmarks and portal sites, distend the joint with 20 to 30 mL of saline through an 18-gauge needle introduced through the direct lateral portal.

- Establish the proximal medial or superomedial portal, which is located approximately 2 cm proximal to the medial epicondyle and 1 cm anterior to the intermuscular septum. Introduce the trocar and sheath anterior to the intermuscular septum, maintaining contact with the anterior aspect of the humerus at all times as the trocar is directed toward the radial head. Insert a 2.7-mm, 30-degree arthroscope into the joint and perform the diagnostic portion of the procedure.

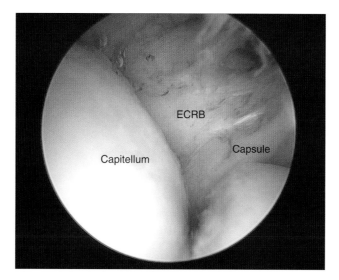

Figure 53-9

- After the pathological tissue is identified, establish the superolateral portal with an 18-gauge needle through the lesion. Using a full-radius resector, excise the capsule to identify the undersurface of the extensor carpi radialis brevis tendon. View the origin of the extensor carpi radialis brevis (Figure 53-9).

- Using a curet and motorized shaver, débride the capsule and the pathological tendinous attachment of the extensor carpi radialis brevis and decorticate the lateral epicondyle. Decortication of the lateral epicondyle and lateral epicondylar ridge can be done with an arthroscopic burr, hand-held instruments, or electrocautery. Although a 30-degree arthroscope is adequate to view around the corner for most of the procedure, a 70-degree arthroscope may be required in rare instances.

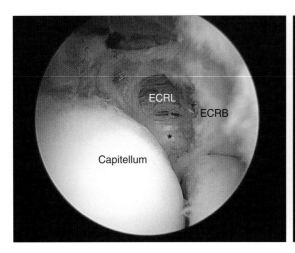 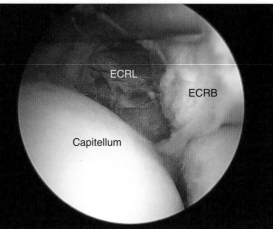

Figure 53-10

- After release of the extensor carpi radialis brevis tendon and decortication of the lateral epicondyle, view the overlying muscle belly of the extensor musculature. Protect the lateral ulnar collateral ligament by limiting the amount of posterior resection (Figure 53-10).

POSTOPERATIVE CARE ⟩

Postoperatively the arm is placed in a sling with the elbow in 90 degrees of flexion. Gentle active and passive ROM exercises are encouraged. The patient progresses to wrist extension-strengthening exercises and overall upper extremity rehabilitation exercises.

CREDITS

Figures 53-4 through 53-7 redrawn from Dlabach JA, Baker CL. Lateral and medial epicondylitis in the overhead athlete, Oper Tech Orthop 11:46, 2001.

Figures 53-9, 53-10 from Morrey BF, Sanchez-Sotelo J. Advanced Techniques. Arthroscopic Management of Lateral Epicondylitis. In Morrey BF, Sanchez-Sotelo J, eds. Elbow and Its Disorders, 4th ed, Philadelphia, Elsevier, 2009, Fig. 41-9.

ULNAR COLLATERAL LIGAMENT RECONSTRUCTION

Barry B. Phillips

ANDREWS ET AL. TECHNIQUE

The goal of this procedure is to reconstruct the anterior bundle of the ulnar collateral ligament. Preoperatively, the presence or absence of the palmaris longus tendon should be documented. Alternative sources of tendon graft include the contralateral palmaris longus tendon, a trimmed gracilis tendon, the plantaris tendon, or the extensor tendon from the fourth toe.

- Drape the arm so that the entire volar forearm to the palm is exposed. Place a tourniquet on the upper arm for hemostasis. If an acute medial rupture of the elbow is not present, perform a limited arthroscopic examination through the anterolateral portal to evaluate intraarticular structures and valgus stability.
- After arthroscopic evaluation make an incision centered over the medial epicondyle and extend it approximately 3 cm proximally and distally.
- Identify the medial antebrachial cutaneous nerve, which is a single large branch with a variable course and possibly other branches. Protect the nerve throughout the procedure.
- Elevate the skin flaps to expose the deep fascia covering the flexor pronator muscles and identify the ulnar nerve.
- Incise the cubital tunnel to mobilize the nerve. Continue the mobilization proximally to include the arcade of Struthers and excise a portion of the intermuscular septum to prevent impingement of the nerve when it is anteriorly transposed. Incise the flexor carpi ulnaris distally along the course of the nerve. Sacrifice the small branches of the nerve that supply the elbow joint if necessary but protect the branches to the flexor pronator muscles.
- Transpose the ulnar nerve anteriorly and follow the split in the flexor carpi ulnaris down to the insertion of the anterior band of the ulnar collateral ligament on the sublime tubercle of the ulna.
- Develop the interval between the ulnar collateral ligament and the flexor muscle mass, starting at the insertion on the ulna where a good tissue plane exists, and working proximally to the medial epicondyle.
- Use small Hohmann retractors to retract the flexor muscles anteriorly to provide full exposure of the ligament. This exposure uses the split in the flexor carpi ulnaris that is required to mobilize the ulnar nerve and avoids detachment of the flexor-pronator insertion on the medial epicondyle.
- After exposure is complete evaluate the ligament. If it appears normal, make a longitudinal incision in line with the fibers of the anterior bundle to evaluate for internal degeneration or detachment of the undersurface of the ligament consistent with a partial rupture. Preserve the remnants of the ligament and augment them with the tendon graft.
- Make a 2-cm transverse incision on the distal wrist flexor crease to harvest the palmaris tendon (or alternate tendon source).
- Identify the median nerve and isolate the tendon with a hemostat.
- Make serial transverse incisions proximally at 7- to 9-cm intervals to the level of the musculotendinous junction. Usually three incisions are required.
- Release the tendon distally. Deliver it through each incision proximally and divide just proximal to the musculotendinous junction to give a length of 15 to 20 cm.
- Strip off the muscle and trim the tendon graft.
- Place a 1-0 nonabsorbable suture in both ends of the graft with a locking stitch to assist in graft passage.
- If posterior olecranon osteophytes are present remove them before placing the graft.
- Make a vertical arthrotomy posteriorly to expose the olecranon tip. Use a small osteotome and rongeur to remove the tip of the olecranon, taking approximately 5 mm to 1 cm of bone and cartilage.
- Close the arthrotomy.

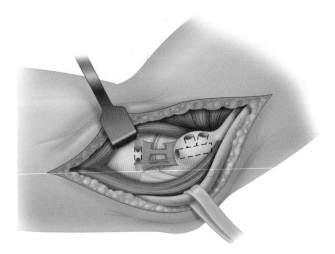

Figure 54-1

- Using a ⁵⁄₆₄-inch bit (3.2 mm for palmaris graft or 3.5 mm for hamstring graft) drill two holes distally at the level of the insertion of the anterior bundle on the sublime tubercle of the ulna. Place the drill holes just anterior and posterior to the sublime tubercle at right angles to each other, staying approximately 5 mm distal to the articular surface. Connect the drill holes with curets and a towel clip. Proximally, drill two convergent ⁵⁄₆₄-inch (3.2 mm or 3.5 mm) tunnels to meet at the insertion of the ligament on the medial epicondyle (Figure 54-1).

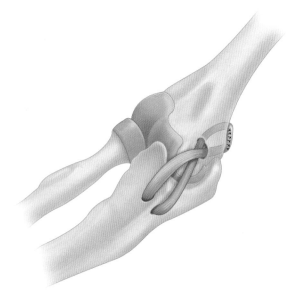

Figure 54-2

- Using a Hewson suture passer, pass the graft through the ulna in a figure-of-eight pattern across the joint. Bring each end out through the two tunnels in the humerus and, if the graft is long enough, pass one end through a second time (Figure 54-2).
- Place the arm in 30 degrees of flexion with a varus stress applied at the elbow to allow optimal tensioning of the graft.
- Secure the graft with nonabsorbable 2-0 suture over the medial epicondyle and suture the remaining ligament to the graft for added stability. Do not place more sutures than necessary because they may become symptomatic over the medial epicondyle.
- Loosely close the split in the flexor carpi ulnaris avoiding constriction of the ulnar nerve.
- Transpose the ulnar nerve anterior to the epicondyle by making a flap in the flexor pronator fascia, leaving attachments proximally at the medial epicondyle. The flap is approximately 3 cm long × 1 cm wide. Dissect muscle tissue away to leave a thin fascial flap.

- Close the defect in the fascia to prevent herniation and transfer the nerve subcutaneously and anteriorly to lie under the fascial flap.
- Loosely reattach the flap distally over the ulnar nerve with nonabsorbable 3-0 sutures to provide a sling to keep the nerve in position without compressing it.
- Place a drain subcutaneously and close the skin with absorbable 3-0 subcuticular sutures.
- Apply a posterior splint with the elbow in 90 degrees of flexion.

POSTOPERATIVE CARE 〉

The splint is worn for 1 week. When it is removed a functional brace set at 30 to 100 degrees is applied. Wrist gripping exercises are begun during the first week and elbow isometric flexion and extension exercises are started during the second week. The brace is advanced from 15 to 110 degrees by week 3. Light isotonic exercises are started the fourth week and full motion should be regained by 6 to 8 weeks. From 9 to 13 weeks, advanced strengthening exercises are begun with eccentric elbow exercises and isometric and isotonic exercises. An interval throwing program is started during week 14 and return to competitive throwing is allowed in 22 to 26 weeks.

ALTCHEK ET AL. TECHNIQUE 〉

The technique described by Altchek et al. uses a muscle-splitting approach and a single closed-end humeral tunnel.

- Place the patient supine on the table, and prepare and drape the arm in a sterile fashion. To assist in the arthroscopic examination use a McConnell arm holder to hold the forearm against the chest.
- Examine the elbow arthroscopically for ulnar collateral ligament laxity by applying valgus stress with the elbow in 90 degrees of flexion. Remove loose bodies and posteromedial osteophytes as necessary.
- After arthroscopy has been completed release the arm from the arm holder and place on the hand table below.
- If a reconstruction is planned, harvest the graft at this time. Usually the ipsilateral palmaris longus is harvested through a 5-mm to 1-cm incision placed in the distal wrist crease. Rather than make multiple incisions, use a tendon stripper specially made for this purpose.
- Place a no. 1 braided nonabsorbable suture using a no. 1 Ethibond Excel OS-2 needle (Ethicon, Inc, Johnson & Johnson, Westwood, MA) in a Krackow fashion in one end of the tendon. After harvest, place the tendon on a moist sponge on the back table.
- To expose the medial collateral ligament, use a tourniquet to exsanguinate the arm.
- Make an incision from the distal third of the intermuscular septum across the medial epicondyle to a point 2 cm beyond the sublime tubercle of the ulna. While exposing the fascia of the flexor pronator, identify and preserve the antebrachial cutaneous branch of the median nerve, which frequently crosses the operative field.

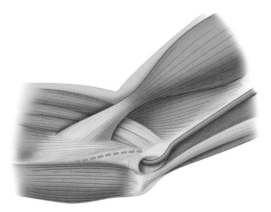

Figure 54-3

- Incise the fascia of the flexor carpi ulnaris longitudinally and split the underlying ligament (Figure 54-3).

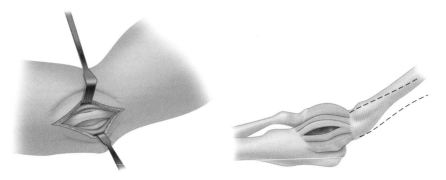

Figure 54-4

- Place a deep, blunt, self-retaining retractor to maintain the exposure. Incise the anterior bundle of the medial collateral ligament longitudinally, exposing the joint. At this point medial collateral ligament laxity can be confirmed by observing 2 mm or more separation of the joint surfaces with valgus stress (Figure 54-4).
- Expose the tunnel positions for the ulna. For the posterior tunnel, subperiosteally expose the posterior ulna at all times and meticulously protect the nerve. If the nerve subluxes anteriorly so that it cannot be protected, transpose it.
- Using a no. 3 burr create tunnels anterior and posterior to the sublime tubercle so that a 2-cm bridge exists between them. Connect the tunnels using a small curved curet. Do not violate the bony bridge. Pass a looped 2-0 suture with a no. 1 Ethibond Excel OS-2 needle.

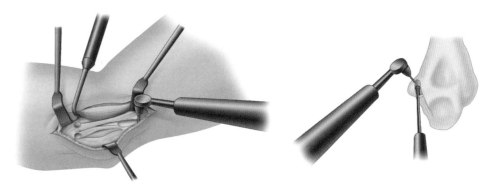

Figure 54-5

- The humeral tunnel position is located in the anterior half of the medial epicondyle in the anterior position of the existing medial collateral ligament. Using a no. 4 burr create a longitudinal tunnel up the axis of the epicondyle to a depth of 15 mm. Expose the upper border of the epicondyle just anterior to the intermuscular septum. Create two small tunnels separated by 5 mm to 1 cm with a dental drill with a small bit. This allows suture passage from the primary humeral tunnel. Use a suture passer from each of the two upper humeral tunnels to pass a looped suture for later graft passage (Figure 54-5).
- With the elbow reduced, repair the longitudinal incision in the medial collateral ligament with a 2-0 absorbable suture.

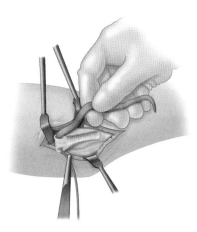

Figure 54-6

- Pass the graft through the ulnar tunnel from anterior to posterior. Pass the limb of the graft that has sutures already in place into the humeral tunnel exiting into one of the small superior humeral tunnels (Figure 54-6).
- With the first limb of the graft securely docked in the humerus, reduce the elbow with forearm supination and gentle varus stress. Maintain tension on the graft while flexing and extending the elbow to avoid potential creep within the graft.

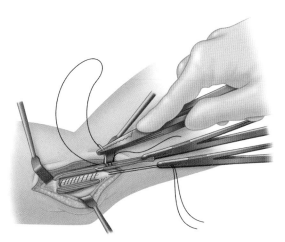

Figure 54-7

- Measure the final length of the graft by placing the free limb of the graft adjacent to the humeral tunnel and visually estimating the length of the graft that can be tensioned within the humeral tunnel. Mark this point with dye and place a no. 1 braided nonabsorbable suture in a Krackow fashion. Dock this end of the graft securely in the humeral tunnel with the sutures exiting the small superior humeral tunnel. The graft may be quadrupled and secured with one braided nonabsorbable suture in a Krackow fashion in the looped end as well as in both tails. These are then folded over and secured on the docking position as described by Paletta et al (Figure 54-7).
- Perform final graft tensioning by moving the elbow through a full range of motion with varus stress placed on the elbow.
- When satisfied with graft tension, tie two sets of graft sutures over the bony bridge on the humeral condyle.
- Deflate the tourniquet and copiously irrigate the wound.
- Approximate the flexor carpi ulnaris fascia and perform subcutaneous and subcuticular closure.
- Place the elbow in a plaster splint at 60 degrees of flexion.

POSTOPERATIVE CARE ❯

After the first week of surgery the sutures are removed and the elbow is placed in a hinged brace. Motion is allowed between 45 degrees of extension and 90 degrees of flexion. Over the next 3 weeks motion is gradually advanced to full. A formal physical therapy program is begun at 6 weeks and gradual strengthening of the forearm and shoulder is started. Care is taken to prevent a valgus load across the elbow during this phase of rehabilitation. At 12 weeks the strengthening program is more vigorous and bench-pressing with light-to-moderate weights is allowed. At 4 months a throwing program is begun for throwing athletes.

LATERAL ULNAR COLLATERAL LIGAMENT RECONSTRUCTION FOR POSTEROLATERAL ROTATORY INSTABILITY 〉

For posterolateral rotatory instability that persists because of disruption of the lateral ulnar collateral ligament and incompetence of the lateral capsular structures, Nestor, O'Driscoll, and Morrey described the use of a Kocher lateral incision for repair or reconstruction of the lateral side.

- Approach the elbow through a modified Kocher incision.
- By sharp dissection carefully elevate the common extensor origin, including a portion of the extensor carpi radialis, to reveal the origin of the radial collateral ligament complex at the lateral epicondyle.
- Distally, reflect the anconeus muscle posteriorly and the extensor carpi ulnaris anteriorly. Reflect the extension of the origin of the anconeus to the lateral aspect of the triceps fascia sufficiently to expose the ligament adequately. Identify the supinator crest of the ulna.
- Typically a lax ulnar band of the radial collateral ligament is observed and the abnormal portion of the ligament is proximal to the annular ligament. The pivot-shift maneuver reveals laxity of the anterior part of the capsule over the radial head and of the posterior part of the capsule at the posterior aspect of the radiohumeral joint. The subluxation of the joint clearly shows the stretched ulnar part of the collateral ligament.
- Enter the joint and inspect for loose bodies and abrasion of the articular surfaces.

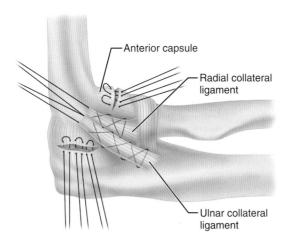
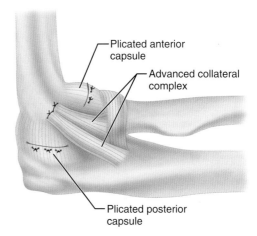

Figure 54-8

- Tighten the anterior and posterior aspects of the capsule with plication sutures but do not tie these sutures (Figure 54-8, left). If the radial collateral ligament complex appears intact but stretched or detached from its origin, imbricate and advance it with a Bunnell suture technique. Suture and plicate the ulnar and the radial parts of the radial collateral ligament complex. Advance the suture through holes placed in the bone at the humeral anatomical origin of the ligament (Figure 54-8, right).
- If the tissue of the collateral ligament is of poor quality, as is usually the case, reconstruct the ulnar part of the radial collateral ligament with an autogenous graft from the palmaris longus tendon.

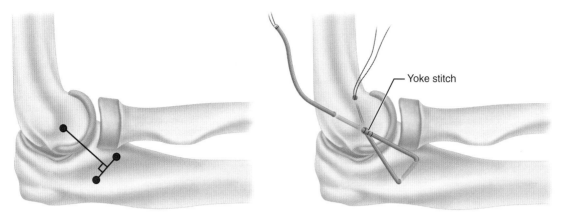

Figure 54-9

- Pass the tendon through an osseous tunnel created by a small burr just posterior to the tubercle of the crest of the supinator. Make the entry holes about 7 mm apart to lessen the likelihood of rupture of the osseous tunnel roof. Thread the tendon through a humeral tunnel that emerges at the origin of the ligaments. Determine the location of the tunnel in the humerus by placing a temporary suture in the ulnar tunnel and holding the ends of the suture against the humerus with a hemostat while the elbow is moved. Reflect the tendon graft back onto itself, crossing the joint again, and attach it into its origin with 1-0 nonabsorbable sutures (Figure 54-9).
- If the tendon graft seems to be inadequate for the size of the arm or for the anticipated activity or stress, use an autogenous or allograft hamstring tendon to reinforce the reconstruction with the same sites of attachment to bone and crossing the joint twice.
- Tie all the sutures with the elbow flexed 30 degrees and with the forearm fully pronated.
- After completing the reconstruction test the elbow for anterolateral rotatory instability. Allow the anconeus and triceps muscles to assume their normal positions and close the interval between the anconeus and the extensor carpi ulnaris with absorbable sutures.
- Apply a splint with the forearm flexed 90 degrees and pronated.

We prefer to use a closed-end tunnel and docking technique in the humerus comparable to that used with the ulnar collateral ligament. When the palmaris is deficient we use a 3.2-mm thick portion of the gracilis tendon. One hamstring may be split for medial and lateral reconstructions in the case of global instability after dislocation. The humeral tunnel is drilled at the point on the epicondyle where the line drawn along the anterior humeral cortex intersects a line through the center of the radiocapitellar axis between the 3:00 and 4:30 position on the epicondyle (Fig. 54-10). Stability and isometry are less affected by the location of the ulnar tunnels. Placement of drill holes 4 mm posterior to the radial head at the crista supinatoris and at the proximal aspect of the lesser sigmoid notch provides reproducible landmarks.

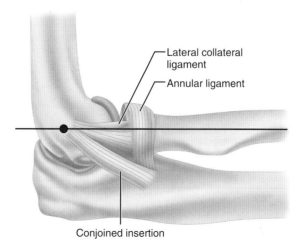

Lateral collateral
ligament

Annular ligament

Conjoined insertion

Figure 54-10

POSTOPERATIVE CARE 〉

With the forearm in full pronation the elbow is placed in 70 to 80 degrees of flexion and held in this position for 10 to 14 days. Protected movement is allowed in a hinged brace 2 to 6 weeks after surgery. After 6 weeks the hinged brace can be removed for light activity. The brace is discontinued completely at the end of an additional 6 weeks but patients are encouraged to protect the elbow from heavy activity. Full activity is allowed at 6 months and participation in contact sports is allowed at 1 year. The patient is advised to protect the elbow from stresses during activities of daily living such as lifting weights. We recommend that patients lift weights only in the plane of elbow flexion and extension, keeping the shoulder adducted and the elbow close to the body.

FIXATION OF THE LATERAL AND MEDIAL MALLEOLI

Matthew I. Rudloff

Bimalleolar ankle fractures disrupt the medial and lateral stabilizing structures of the ankle joint; operative treatment has been shown to obtain better outcomes than nonoperative treatment of these fractures. For most displaced bimalleolar fractures, we recommend ORIF of both malleoli.

FIXATION OF THE LATERAL MALLEOLUS 〉

- If the fractured fibula is part of a bimalleolar fracture pattern, we usually reduce and internally fix the lateral malleolar or fibular fracture before fixing the medial malleolar component. The exception to this is a comminuted lateral malleolus as part of a bimalleolar or trimalleolar pattern. Occasionally, if comminution is severe, the lateral malleolus can be overreduced in the coronal plane, which inhibits anatomical reduction of the medial malleolar component of the injury. In this circumstance it may be advisable to proceed with medial malleolar fixation initially.

- Expose the lateral malleolus and the distal fibular shaft through a lateral longitudinal incision. Protect the superficial peroneal nerve. Alternatively, a posterolateral incision can be used, and the plate can be inserted with a posterior antiglide technique.

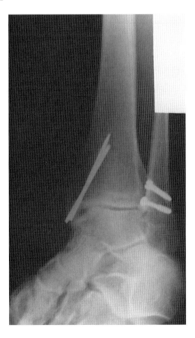

Figure 55-1

- If the fracture is sufficiently oblique, the bone stock is good, and there is no comminution, fix the fracture with two lag screws inserted from anterior to posterior to establish interfragmentary compression. Place the screws approximately 1 cm apart. The length of the screws is important as they must engage the posterior cortex for secure fixation but must not protrude far enough posteriorly to encroach on the peroneal tendon sheaths (Figure 55-1).

- If the fracture is transverse an intramedullary device may be used. Expose the tip of the lateral malleolus by splitting the fibers of the calcaneofibular ligament longitudinally.

- Insert a Rush rod, interlocking fibular rod, or other intramedullary device across the fracture line into the medullary canal of the proximal fragment. If using an intramedullary device do not tilt the lateral malleolus toward the talus. The insertion point for intramedullary fixation tends to be the lateral surface of the malleolar tip. Because the intramedullary appliance is straight, the lateral malleolus may be inadvertently tilted toward the talus resulting in narrowing of the ankle mortise and reduced motion. This mistake can be avoided by contouring the intramedullary pin.

- If the fracture is below the level of the plafond, if the distal fragment is small, and if the patient has good bone stock, use an intramedullary 3.5-mm malleolar screw for fixation. A 4.5-mm lag screw can be used in large patients. Alternatively, orient the malleolar screw slightly obliquely to engage the medial cortex of the fibula proximal to the fracture.
- In patients with poor bone quality place Kirschner wires obliquely from lateral to medial through the distal and proximal fibular fragments and secure them further with a tension band wire.
- Anatomical reduction and maintenance of fibular length are necessary.
- If the fracture is above the level of the syndesmosis, use a small fragment, one-third tubular plate for fixation after anatomical reduction has been obtained; a 3.5-mm dynamic compression plate can be used in larger individuals or for more proximal fractures. The plates can be used to supplement lag screw fixation or to span a comminuted segment. In general place three cortical screws in the shaft of the fibula above the fracture and two or three screws distal to the fracture. Unicortical cancellous screws are placed below the level of the plafond. If the plate is placed posterolaterally it acts as an antiglide plate. Several commercially available precontoured fixed angle distal fibular locking plates provide alternative fixation options distally, often however at the expense of increased hardware prominence.
- For fractures in osteoporotic patients or patients with poor soft tissue coverage, reduce and stabilize the fracture with Kirschner wires placed obliquely through the distal fibular fragment and into the tibia.

FIXATION OF THE MEDIAL MALLEOLUS 〉

- Make an anteromedial incision that begins approximately 2 cm proximal to the fracture line, extends distally and slightly posteriorly, and ends approximately 2 cm distal to the tip of the medial malleolus. We prefer this incision for two reasons: (1) the posterior tibial tendon and its sheath are less likely to be damaged, and (2) the surgeon is able to see the articular surfaces, especially the anteromedial aspect of the joint, which permits accurate alignment of the fracture. However, this incision cannot be made extensile distally if associated foot injuries must be treated.
- Handle the skin with care, reflecting the flap intact with its underlying subcutaneous tissue. The blood supply to the skin of this area is poor and careful handling is necessary to prevent skin sloughing. Protect the greater saphenous vein and its accompanying nerve.
- Usually the distal fragment of the medial malleolus is displaced distally and anteriorly and a small fold of periosteum is commonly interposed between the fracture surfaces. Remove this fold from the fracture site with a curet or periosteal elevator, exposing the small serrations of the fracture.
- Débride small, loose osseous or chondral fragments; large osteochondral fragments should be preserved and supported with a bone graft.

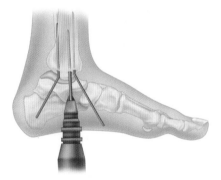

Figure 55-2

- With a bone-holding clamp or towel clip, bring the detached malleolus into the normal position and, while holding it there, internally fix it with two 2-mm smooth Kirschner wires drilled across the fracture site as temporary fixation devices (Figure 55-2).

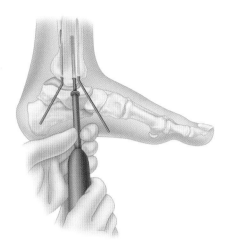

Figure 55-3

- Check the fracture reduction with anteroposterior and lateral radiographs. If the reduction is satisfactory, remove one of the Kirschner wires and insert a 4-mm lag screw; remove and replace the other Kirschner wire. Alternatively, a drill with a 2.5- and a 3.5-mm bit can be used to create a path for the screws; a long pelvic drill bit will be necessary if bicortical lag screw fixation is chosen (Figure 55-3).
- Carefully inspect the interior of the joint, particularly at the superomedial corner, to ensure the screw has not crossed the articular surface.
- Use radiographs to verify the position of the screw and the fracture.
- If the medial malleolar fragment is very small or comminuted, fixation with a screw may be impossible; in these cases use several Kirschner wires or tension band wiring for fixation. Large vertical fractures of the medial malleolus that involve proximal comminution often require a buttress plate to prevent loss of reduction; a small, one-third tubular plate usually is sufficient. To avoid wound complications extreme care must be taken when applying bulky hardware to this area of poor skin coverage.

POSTOPERATIVE CARE ⟩

The ankle is immobilized in a posterior plaster splint in a neutral position and elevated. If the bone quality is good, and the fixation is secure, the splint can be removed on the first postoperative visit and replaced with a removable splint or fracture boot. Range-of-motion exercises are begun. Weight bearing is restricted for 6 weeks, after which partial weight bearing can be started if the fracture is healing well and progressed accordingly.

If skin conditions, bone quality, or other factors have prevented secure fixation, the fracture must be protected longer. The patient is placed in either a short-leg or a long-leg non–weight-bearing cast, depending on the stability of the fixation. If a long-leg cast is used it can be converted to a short-leg cast in 4 to 6 weeks. The patient is not allowed to bear weight on the ankle until fracture healing is progressing well (8 to 12 weeks). A short-leg walking cast is worn and weight bearing is progressed. The cast is removed when the fracture has united.

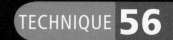
Locked intramedullary nailing currently is considered the treatment of choice for most tibial shaft fractures and is especially useful for segmental and bilateral tibial fractures.

Fracture Table

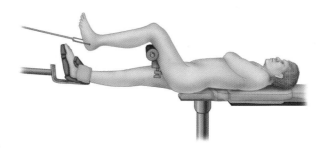

Figure 56-1

- If a fracture table is used, place a calcaneal traction pin before positioning. Place the patient supine with the hip flexed 45 degrees and the knee flexed 90 degrees (Figure 56-1).
- Place a well-padded crossbar proximal to the popliteal fossa to support the thigh in the flexed position. Adequate padding should reduce the risk of compression neuropathy.
- Attach the calcaneal pin to the traction apparatus on the fracture table, apply traction, and reduce the fracture under fluoroscopic guidance.
- To decrease the risk of traction injury to neurological structures release the traction after the ability to reduce the fracture has been confirmed.
- Prepare and drape the limb allowing full exposure of the knee to above the patella and enough access to the distal tibia for locking screw placement. Reapply traction after the entry portal is made.

Standard Operating Table

- If a standard operating table is used place the patient supine with the thigh supported in a flexed position over a padded bolster.
- A skilled assistant is needed to assist with fracture reduction and help support the limb during the procedure.
- A femoral distractor or two-pin external fixator can be used to help maintain reduction. Place a Schanz pin 1 cm distal to the knee joint, and place a second pin 1 cm proximal to the ankle joint. The proximal pin must be placed in the posterior portion of the tibial condyle to avoid the path of the nail.

Measurement of Rotation

- Before nailing measure rotation by the method described by Clementz. Measure the amount of tibial torsion in the uninjured extremity with the knee fully extended and a C-arm image intensifier placed in the lateral position with the beam parallel to the floor.
- Rotate the leg until a perfect lateral view of the distal femur is obtained with the condyles superimposed exactly. Hold the knee and foot in this position while the C-arm is brought into the anteroposterior position with the beam perpendicular to the floor to image the ankle.
- Rotate the C-arm until a tangential image of the inner surface of the medial malleolus is seen. This is the reference line at the ankle.
- Tilt the beam cranially 5 degrees to obtain a better image of the ankle. Center the structures to be imaged in the radiographic field.
- The amount of tibial torsion is equal to the difference between the reference line at the ankle and a line perpendicular to the floor. If the tangential view of the medial malleolus is obtained with the C-arm rotated laterally 10 degrees from perpendicular, tibial torsion is 10 degrees.

- Alternatively, obtain rotational alignment by aligning the iliac crest, patella, and second ray of the foot.
- Close attention to operative technique can greatly decrease the risk of complications after tibial nailing.

Nail Placement

- Begin the entry portal by making a 3-cm incision along the medial border of the patellar tendon extending from the tibial tubercle in a proximal direction. It may be necessary to extend the incision farther proximally through skin and subcutaneous tissue only to protect the soft tissues around the knee during reaming and nail insertion.

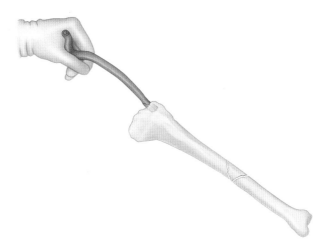

Figure 56-2

- Insert a threaded tip guidewire through the metaphysis anteriorly to gain access to the medullary canal. With the appropriate soft tissue sleeve advance the guidewire into the correct starting portal as noted on multiplanar imaging. This typically is located along the medial slope of the lateral tibial eminence on the anteroposterior view and just anterior to the articular margin on lateral imaging (Figure 56-2).
- Confirm the proper position on anteroposterior and lateral fluoroscopic views before guidewire insertion. Obtain a true anteroposterior view of the tibia when assessing the placement of the guidewire. If the limb is externally rotated, the portal may be placed too medially and violate the tibial plateau and injure the intermeniscal ligament. A portal placed too distally may damage the insertion of the patellar tendon or cause the nail to enter the tibia at too steep of an angle, which may cause the tibia to split or cause the nail to penetrate the posterior cortex. Check the process of insertion on lateral fluoroscopic views. The safe zone for tibial nail placement is just medial to the lateral tibial spine on the anteroposterior view and immediately adjacent and anterior to the articular surface on the lateral view.
- Direct the guidewire nearly perpendicular to the shaft when it first penetrates the cortex but gradually bring it down to a position more parallel to the shaft as it is inserted more deeply to prevent violation of the posterior cortex. Once appropriate provisional guidewire trajectory is achieved, the entry portal is created by using the cannulated entry reamer with matching soft tissue protection sleeve. Alternatively, the starting portal can be initiated by use of a cannulated curved awl.

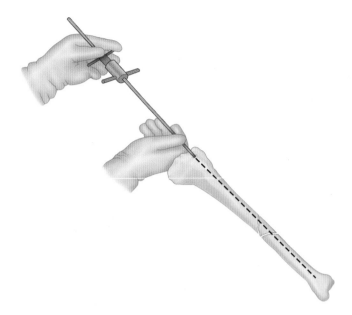

Figure 56-3

- Insert a ball-tipped guidewire through the entry portal into the tibial canal and pass it across the fracture site into the tibia under fluoroscopic guidance. The guide rod should be centered within the distal fragment on anteroposterior and lateral views and advanced to within 1.0 cm to 0.5 cm of the ankle joint (Figure 56-3).

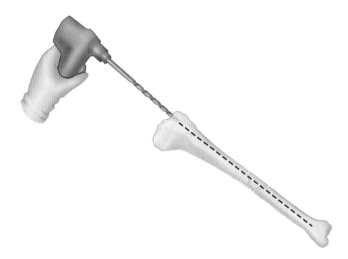

Figure 56-4

- If a reamed technique is chosen, ream the canal in 0.5-mm increments starting with a reamer smaller than the measured diameter of the tibial canal. Ream with the knee in flexion to avoid excessive reaming of the anterior cortex. Hold the fracture reduced during reaming to decrease the risk of iatrogenic comminution. Prevent the guide rod from being partially withdrawn during reaming. We prefer "minimal" reaming with no more than 2 mm of reaming after cortical contact ("chatter") is first initiated (Figure 56-4).
- Choose a nail diameter that is 1.0 to 1.5 mm smaller than the last reamer used. Ream the entry site large enough to accept the proximal diameter of the chosen nail. It is important never to ream with the tourniquet inflated because this may lead to thermal necrosis of bone and soft tissue especially in individuals with small-diameter medullary canals.
- If an unreamed technique is chosen, ream only the cancellous bone of the entry portal to accommodate the proximal portion of the nail. The canal diameter can be determined in open fractures after débridement by passing sounds of different sizes through the fracture site and across the isthmus.
- Alternatively, flexible reamers or flexible sounds can be manually pushed without power through the entry portal and across the isthmus. The largest sound or reamer that can be inserted without excessive force corresponds to the correct nail diameter.

- Canal diameter also can be measured radiographically but this is less accurate. Never insert a nail with a diameter larger than the canal. It also is important not to undersize the nail because a loose-fitting nail would be less stable and the smaller implants are not as strong and may be more prone to hardware failure. In general the largest implant suitable for a given patient should be used.

- When reaming is completed, determine the length of the nail by using the system-specific depth gauge to accurately determine the necessary implant length. Alternatively, place the tip of a guidewire of the same length at the most distal edge of the entry portal. Subtract the length of the overlapped portions of the guide rods from the full length of the guide rod to determine the length of the nail, making sure the fracture is held out to length during this measurement. Comminuted fractures may require preoperative radiographic measurement of the contralateral tibia to assess length properly.

- Attach the insertion device and proximal locking screw guide to the nail. Direct the apex of the proximal bend in the nail posteriorly. Some nail systems use oblique proximal locking screws that are directed anteromedial to posterolateral and anterolateral to posteromedial. Insert the nail with the knee in flexion (except in some proximal third fractures) to avoid impingement on the patella. Evaluate rotational alignment by aligning the iliac crest, patella, and second ray of the foot. Tremendous force should not be necessary to insert the nail. Moderate manual pressure with a gentle back-and-forth twisting motion usually is sufficient for nail insertion. If a mallet is used, the nail should advance with each blow. If the nail does not advance, withdraw the nail and perform further reaming or insert a smaller diameter nail. It is important to keep the fracture well aligned during nail insertion to prevent iatrogenic comminution and malalignment.

- When the nail has passed well into the distal fragment, remove the guidewire to avoid incarceration, and during final seating of the nail, release traction to allow impaction of the fracture. Do not shorten fractures excessively with segmental comminution. When the nail is fully inserted the proximal end should lie 0.5 to 1.0 cm below the cortical opening of the entry portal. This position is best seen on a lateral fluoroscopic view. If the nail protrudes too far proximally knee pain and difficulty with kneeling may result. Excessive countersinking also should be avoided because it makes nail removal more difficult. The distal tip of the nail should lie 0.5 to 2.0 cm from the subchondral bone of the ankle joint. Distal fractures require nail insertion near the more distal end of this range.

- Insert proximal locking screws using the jig attached to the nail insertion device. Place the drill sleeve through a small incision down to bone. Measure the length of the screw from calibrations on the drill bit. The number of interlocking screws is dependent on fracture characteristics. Tighten all connections between the insertion device, drill guide, and nail before screw insertion.

- Perform distal locking by using a freehand technique after "perfect circles" are obtained by fluoroscopy. In the lateral position adjust the fluoroscopic beam until it is directed straight through the distal screw holes and the holes appear perfectly round.

- Place a drill bit through a small incision overlying the hole and center the tip in the hole. Taking care not to move the location of the tip, bring the drill bit in line with the fluoroscopic beam and drill through the near (medial) cortex. Detach the drill from the bit and check the position of the drill bit with fluoroscopy to ensure that it is passing through the screw hole. When proper position is confirmed, drive the drill bit through the far (lateral) cortex.

- Measure the screw length using drill sleeves and calibrated bits or check the anteroposterior view on the fluoroscopy screen using the known diameter of the nail as a reference for length.

- After screw insertion, obtain a lateral image to ensure the screws have been inserted through the screw holes. Two distal locking screws are used in most fractures.

- Some nail systems have the option of placing an anteroposterior distal locking screw. "Perfect circles" are obtained in the anteroposterior fluoroscopic view. Do not injure the anterior tibial tendon or extensor hallucis longus or nearby neurovascular structures. Meticulous attention to technique can minimize complications from anteroposterior distal interlocking. Careful soft tissue protection and retraction both during drilling and screw insertion are critical to prevent soft tissue injury or tethering as the screw head engages anterior tibial cortex. A drill sleeve can be valuable for protection of the associated soft tissues during this portion of the procedure.

- Before interlocking, inspect the fracture site for possible distraction. If the fracture is distracted place the distal locking screws first. Some intramedullary implants now have the capability to provide axial compression, for properly selected fracture patterns, during the process of interlocking.

- After distal locking is complete impact the fracture by carefully driving the nail backward while watching the fracture site under fluoroscopy. Keep the knee flexed until the nail insertion instruments are removed to avoid damage to the soft tissues around the patella.

- Most nails are statically locked. Minimally comminuted transverse diaphyseal fractures can be dynamically locked however comminuted or metaphyseal fractures should be statically locked. If there is any question about stability perform static locking. Because the nail may not prevent malalignment of unstable fractures before it is locked it is crucial to maintain accurate reduction until proximal and distal locking is complete.

- Modifications in technique have decreased the incidence of malalignment in proximal-third fractures. The reduction can be manipulated more freely if nailing is not done on a fracture table.

- To prevent valgus start the entry portal in line with the lateral intercondylar eminence and center it on the medullary canal on the anteroposterior fluoroscopic image. An incision lateral to the patellar tendon can be used.

- To prevent anterior angulation and displacement move the portal more proximally and posteriorly and direct it more vertically in a line more parallel with the anterior tibial cortex. Interlocking the nail proximally with the knee extended relaxes the pull of the patellar tendon and prevents anterior angulation. Many nail systems require removal of the insertion jig however, to extend the knee to avoid impingement on soft tissues.

- Tornetta et al. recommended nailing proximal-third tibial fractures in a semiextended position (15 degrees of flexion) using two thirds of a medial parapatellar arthrotomy to retract the patella laterally. This technique prevents the patella from causing the portal to be angled from medial to lateral and allows proximal interlocking to be performed with the knee extended. Using a nail with a more proximally located bend decreases the risk of anterior displacement of the proximal fragment. A nail with proximal locking screws oriented obliquely at 90 degrees to each other provides more resistance to varus-valgus angulation than one-plane, medial-to-lateral screws.

- In contrast to diaphyseal fractures the nail does not "automatically" reduce the fracture because it is inserted through the wide tibial metaphysis. Accurate fracture reduction before nail insertion helps to decrease the risk of malalignment. Reduction can be accomplished by using an AO distractor medially or by limited open reduction and application of a unicortical plate as described by Benirschke et al. This technique can be particularly useful in open fractures.

- Evaluate the stability of the fracture after surgery. If the fracture is so proximal that only one proximal locking screw can be placed, consider alternative methods of fixation.

- If instability is present, use a two-pin medial external fixator to enhance stability during the early phases of healing.

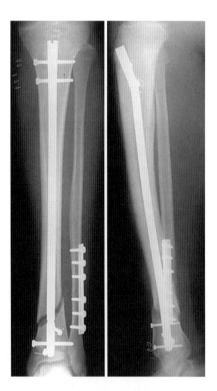

Figure 56-5

- Malalignment also can be prevented by using blocking screws. Overcorrect the deformity and insert blocking screws anteriorly to posteriorly on the concave side of the deformity. The screws effectively reduce the diameter of the metaphysis and physically block the nail, preventing angulation. Use blocking screws to prevent malalignment in distal metaphyseal fractures (Figure 56-5).

POSTOPERATIVE CARE ⟩

The patient initially is placed in a removable splint and early range-of-motion exercises are begun. Noncompliant patients or patients with unstable fracture fixation are placed in a patellar tendon-bearing brace or orthosis until enough healing occurs to ensure stability. Axial stable patterns (i.e., transverse diaphyseal) can be permitted unrestricted weight bearing. Weight bearing is restricted until early callus occurs (4 to 6 weeks) and then is progressed as tolerated in fractures without axial stability and those at the proximal or distal metadiaphyseal junction. Nail removal is not routinely necessary but may be needed to relieve pain in patients with prominent hardware. Nail removal usually is delayed until at least 12 to 18 months after injury when all fracture lines are obliterated and there is full cortical remodeling.

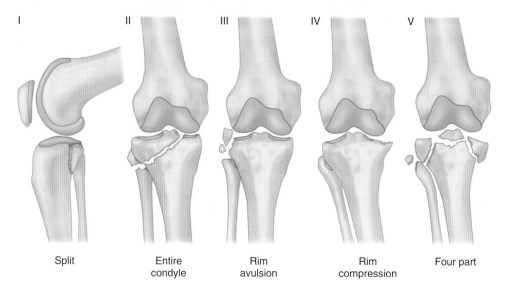

I	II	III	IV	V
Split	Entire condyle	Rim avulsion	Rim compression	Four part

Figure 57-1

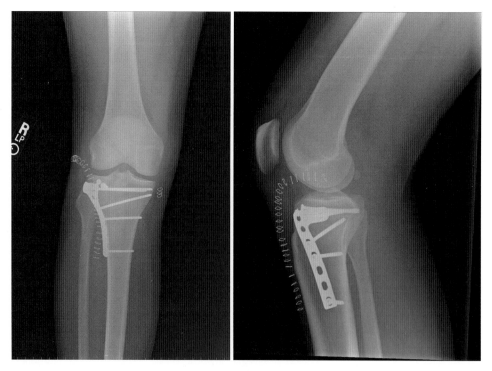

Figure 57-2

The fracture-dislocation patterns classified by Hohl and Moore (Figure 57-1) occur with frequent associated ligamentous, meniscal, and neurovascular injuries. Goals of treatment include restoration of articular congruity, axial alignment, joint stability, and functional motion. Unstable fractures of the entire condyle are best treated with closed or open reduction and internal fixation. Depressed articular segments require elevation through a cortical window, bone grafting, and fixation with either large cancellous screws or a buttress plate (Figure 57-2).

- Apply a tourniquet except in patients with severe soft tissue injury.

- For fractures of the lateral condyle make a straight or slightly curvilinear anterolateral incision starting 3 to 5 cm above the joint line proximally and extending distally below the inferior margin of the fracture site from just anterior to the lateral femoral epicondyle to Gerdy's tubercle. This incision provides good exposure while avoiding skin complications. Alternatively, an L-shaped incision may be used.

- Make the fascial incision in line with the skin incision. Do not undermine soft tissue flaps more than necessary. If necessary for exposure, reflect a portion or all of the iliotibial band from its insertion on Gerdy's tubercle. Gain intraarticular exposure by incising the coronary or inframeniscotibial ligament and retract the meniscus superiorly after placement of nonabsorbable meniscocapsular tagging sutures.

- Inspect and débride or repair any meniscal tears to preserve as much of the menisci as possible.

- To expose the longitudinal fracture of the lateral condyle, elevate the origin of the extensor muscles from the anterolateral aspect of the condyle in an extraperiosteal fashion. Reflect the muscle origin laterally until the fracture line is exposed.

- Retract the lateral fragment to gain access to the central part of the tibial condyle. This lateral fragment often hinges open like a book, exposing the depressed articular surface and cancellous bone of the central depression.

- Alternatively, make a cortical window below the area of depression to allow reduction of this fragment. This approach generally requires less soft tissue dissection than hinging open the lateral condylar fragment.

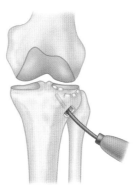

Figure 57-3

- Insert a periosteal elevator well beneath the depressed articular fragments and by slow and meticulous pressure elevate the articular fragments and compressed cancellous bone in one large mass. This produces a large cavity in the metaphysis that must be filled with bone graft or substitute. Unless this is done redisplacement and settling can occur. Various types of grafts have been proposed, from transverse cortical supports to full-thickness iliac grafts. We prefer injectable bone substitutes such as calcium sulfate or phosphate bone cements for metaphyseal subchondral defect management after elevation of depressed articular segments (Figure 57-3).

- The standard lateral approach gives only a limited view of the posterolateral plateau and provides no access to the posterior wall of the lateral tibial plateau. Certain fractures located in the posterolateral plateau require a more extensile approach. In this situation, the fascial incision follows the insertion of the extensor muscles and continues over the subcapital fibula. The entire layer is stripped distally as required. Expose the peroneal nerve and cut the fibular neck with an oscillating saw. This allows retraction of the upper segment to the back or rotation of the fibular head upward exposing the posterolateral plateau and the lateral and posterior flare of the proximal tibia.

- If displacement of the peripheral rim is slight, and central depression of the condyle is the main deformity, remove an anterior cortical window with its proximal edge distal to the articular surface.

- Insert a small thin osteotome, periosteal elevator, or curved bone tamp through the cortical window or fracture line into the cancellous subchondral bone and elevate to the normal level the depressed fragments of the articular surface. As the fragments are elevated and reduced, temporarily fix them with multiple small Kirschner wires. Stabilize with subchondral raft screw fixation.

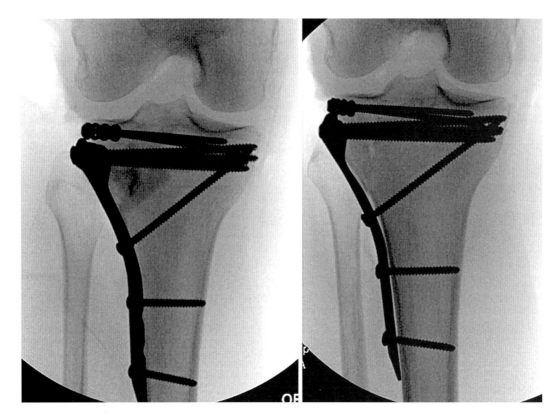

Figure 57-4

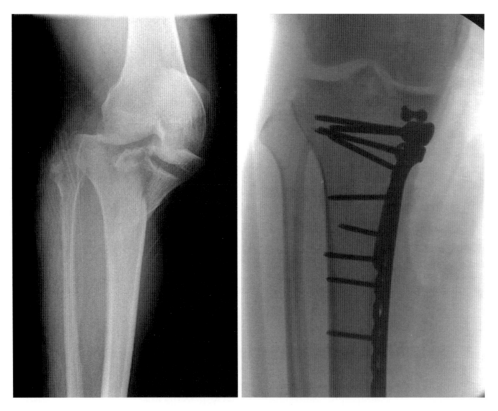

Figure 57-5

- Apply a buttress plate to the anterolateral proximal tibia (Figure 57-4). Precontoured periarticular plates designed for tibial plateau fractures are readily available typically in either a 3.5- or 4.5-mm dimension. Depending on the fit of the implant, one may choose to place separate raft screws before affixing the plate to ensure subchondral support of newly elevated articular segments (Figure 57-5). Typically, for simple lateral condylar fractures alone (Shatzker I & II), nonlocking 3.5-mm implants are sufficient.

- Augment the defect with cancellous bone or bone graft substitute.
- If the meniscus has been detached peripherally, carefully suture it back to its coronary ligament attachment. If the iliotibial band has been reflected from its insertion at Gerdy's tubercle, reattach it.

POSTOPERATIVE CARE 〉

The knee is placed into a removable knee immobilizer. At 1 to 2 days postoperatively physical therapy is initiated with quadriceps exercises; gentle active-assisted exercises are begun, or a passive motion machine can be used. Crutch walking is begun but no weight bearing is permitted for 12 weeks. If extensive suturing of the periphery of the meniscus was necessary, immobilization for approximately 3 weeks is required before motion exercises are permitted.

Matthew I. Rudloff

Wiring techniques are used most often for transverse fractures. They also can be used in comminuted fractures if the fragments are large enough to lag together with screws, converting it to a transverse fracture. Many wiring techniques have been described, including cerclage wiring, alone or in combination; tension-band wiring, alone or modified with longitudinal Kirschner wires or screws; Magnusson wiring; and Lotke longitudinal anterior band wiring (Figure 58-1). By proper placement of the wires the distracting or shear forces tending to separate the fragments are converted into compressive forces across the fracture site, resulting in earlier union and allowing immediate motion and exercise of the knee. Generally, two sets of wire are used. One is passed transversely through the insertion of the quadriceps tendon immediately adjacent to the bone of the superior pole and then passed anteriorly over the superficial surface of the patella and in a similar way through the insertion of the patellar tendon. This wire is tightened until the fracture is slightly overcorrected or opened on the articular surface. The second wire is passed through transverse holes drilled in the superior and inferior poles of the anterior patellar surface and tightened.

The capsular tears are repaired in the usual manner. The knee is immobilized in flexion and early active flexion produces compressive forces to keep the edges of the articular surface of the patella compressed together. Early active flexion exercises are essential for the tension band principle to work. Schauwecker described a similar technique in which the wire is crossed in a figure-of-eight over the anterior surface of the patella (Figure 58-2). Supplemental lag screws or Kirschner wires can be used to increase fixation in comminuted fractures.

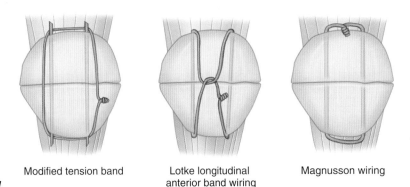

Modified tension band   Lotke longitudinal anterior band wiring   Magnusson wiring

Figure 58-1

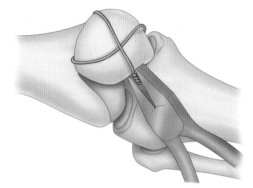

Figure 58-2

- Approach the patellar fracture through a longitudinal midline or lateral parapatellar incision.
- Carefully clean the fracture surfaces of blood clot and small fragments.
- Explore the extent of the retinacular tears and inspect the trochlear groove of the femur for damage.
- Thoroughly lavage the joint.

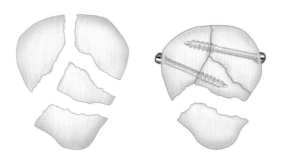

Figure 58-3

- If the major proximal and distal fragments are large reduce them accurately, with special attention to restoring a smooth articular surface (Figure 58-3).
- With the fracture reduced and held firmly with clamps, drill two 2-mm Kirschner wires from inferior to superior through each fragment. Place these wires about 5 mm deep to the anterior surface of the patella along lines dividing the patella into medial, central, and lateral thirds. Insert the wires as parallel as possible. In some cases it is easier to insert the wires through the fracture site into the proximal fragment in a retrograde manner before reduction. This is made easier by tilting the fracture anteriorly about 90 degrees.
- Withdraw the wires until they are flush with the fracture site, accurately reduce the fracture and holding it with clamps drive the wires through the distal fragment. Leave the ends of the wires long, protruding beyond the patella and quadriceps tendon attachments to the inferior and superior fragments.
- Pass a strand of 18-gauge wire transversely through the quadriceps tendon attachment as close to the bone as possible, deep to the protruding Kirschner wires over the anterior surface of the reduced patella, transversely through the patellar tendon attachment on the inferior fragment and deep to the protruding Kirschner wires, and back over the anterior patellar surface; tighten it at the upper end. Alternatively, place the wire in a figure-of-eight fashion.
- Check the reduction by palpating the undersurface of the patella with the knee extended. If necessary make a small longitudinal incision in the retinaculum to allow insertion of the finger.
- Bend the upper ends of the two Kirschner wires acutely anteriorly and cut them short.

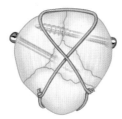

Figure 58-4

- When they are cut, rotate the Kirschner wires 180 degrees; with an impactor embed the bent ends into the superior margin of the patella posterior to the wire loops. Cut the protruding ends of the Kirschner wires short inferiorly (Figure 58-4).
- Repair the retinacular tears with multiple interrupted sutures.

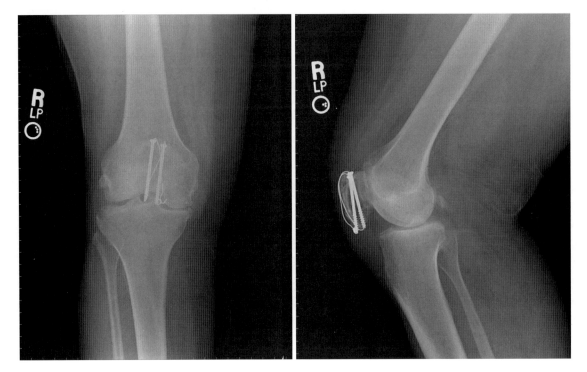

Figure 58-5

- Alternatively, 4.0-mm partially threaded cannulated screws can be used instead of Kirschner wires. Mini-fragment lag screws also can be placed horizontally to join comminuted fracture fragments, converting a comminuted fracture to a transverse fracture pattern. A modified anterior tension band technique can be used. If the anterior cortex is split from the articular surface in the coronal plane, the fragment usually can be secured with the anterior tension band wire. If this is unsuccessful the fragment can be excised (Figure 58-5).

POSTOPERATIVE CARE 〉

The limb is placed in extension in a posterior plaster splint or removable knee brace. The patient is allowed to ambulate while bearing weight as tolerated on the first postoperative day. Isometric and stiff-leg exercises are encouraged beginning on the first postoperative day. The extent of active motion permitted in the immediate postoperative period is determined intraoperatively based on the fracture repair stability. Active range-of-motion exercises can be performed when the wound has healed at 2 to 3 weeks. Progressive resistance exercises can be begun and the brace discontinued at 6 to 8 weeks if healing is evident on radiograph. Unrestricted activity can be resumed when full quadriceps strength has returned, at 18 to 24 weeks. In patients with less stable fixation or extensive retinacular tears active motion should be delayed until fracture healing has occurred. Initiating range-of-motion exercises by the sixth postoperative week is desirable but not always possible. A controlled motion knee brace can be used allowing full extension and flexion to the degree permitted by the fixation as determined intraoperatively.

Closed nailing is an exacting technique. A full set of nails, reamers, extractors, and related equipment and an image intensifier must be available. Also, a radiolucent flat-topped or suitable radiolucent fracture table that permits unencumbered rotation of the image intensifier for fracture visualization is a prerequisite. Preoperative radiographs of the uninjured femur can be used to estimate proper nail diameter, expected amount of reaming, and final nail length for severely comminuted fractures. Radiographic templates are available for preoperative planning. Proper length must be attained with traction before closed antegrade intramedullary nailing. The nail length should permit the proximal end to lie flush with the tip of the greater trochanter and the distal end to lie between the proximal pole of the patella and the distal femoral epiphyseal scar.

ANTEGRADE FEMORAL NAILING 〉

Patient Positioning and Preparation

- Based on preoperative templating and surgical plan, decide on a radiolucent flat-topped or fracture table and patient position. We prefer the use of a fracture table.

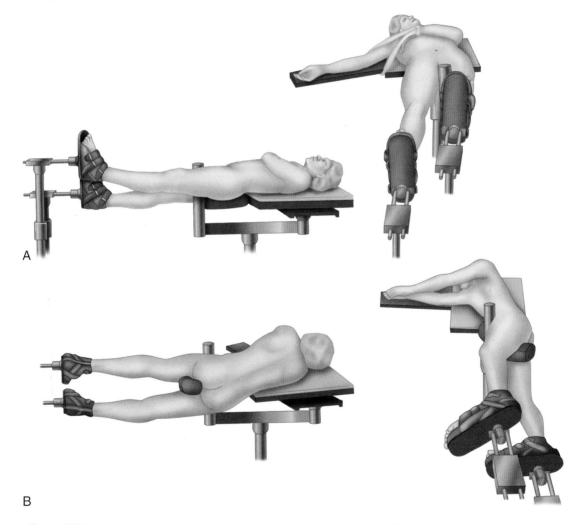

A

B

Figure 59-1

- We have used the lateral and supine positions extensively and each has its relative indications (Figure 59-1). The supine position is more universal. It provides easier access for the anesthesiologist, especially in severely injured patients. The circulating and scrub nurses and the radiographic technicians are also more comfortable with the patient in this position. It is most useful for bilateral femoral fractures, fractures of the distal third of the femur, and femoral fractures with contralateral acetabular fractures. Gaining the correct entry portal to the proximal femur usually is only somewhat more difficult with the patient supine, primarily in obese patients.

- If the patient is supine adduct the trunk and affected extremity. Flex the affected hip 15 to 30 degrees.
- Apply traction through a skeletal pin or to the foot with a well-padded traction boot. A well-padded perineal post is positioned and the uninjured extremity is placed in a well-padded traction boot. The legs are positioned in a scissor configuration.
- Estimate correct rotational alignment with respect to the normal anteversion of the hip as determined with the image intensifier. This can be accomplished by taking fluoroscopic views of the uninjured knee and hip at the same rotation of the image intensifier and saving these for later reference. Comparable anteroposterior fluoroscopic views of the injured limb, both knee and hip, can then allow for rotational correction based on the profile of the lesser trochanter. Similarly the angle difference between a radiographic true lateral of the knee and hip will represent hip anteversion.
- Rotate the foot and distal fragment of the femur to match the proximal fragment by observing the image C-arm. By taking successive views with the C-arm it is possible to obtain a lateral view of the proximal femur in which the femoral neck and shaft are parallel but offset about 1 cm. The angle of the C-arm necessary to obtain this "true lateral" usually can be read directly off the C-arm. Taking into account the normal femoral anteversion of 15 to 20 degrees, it is possible to determine exactly the angle at which to place the foot. For example, if the femoral neck and shaft were superimposed when the C-arm was angled 40 degrees from the horizontal, assuming a femoral anteversion of 20 degrees, it would be necessary to externally rotate the foot 20 degrees to match proximal and distal fragments.
- If the patient is in the lateral decubitus position with the perineal post, ensure that most of the trunk weight is on the trochanteric rest of the unaffected hip.
- Place the fractured side in 15 to 30 degrees of hip flexion. The normal side is in neutral to slight hip extension. Use the image intensifier to view the entire femur in the anteroposterior and lateral projections from the knee to the hip.
- Prepare the patient in the standard manner. Drape the buttocks and lateral thigh to the popliteal crease. Cover the image intensifier arm with a sterile isolation drape.

Preparation of Femur

- Make a short oblique skin incision starting 2 to 3 cm from the proximal tip of the greater trochanter and continue it proximally and medially. A longer incision may be necessary in obese patients.
- Incise the fascia of the gluteus maximus in line with its fibers.
- Identify the subfascial plane of the gluteus maximus and palpate the piriformis fossa or trochanteric portal.

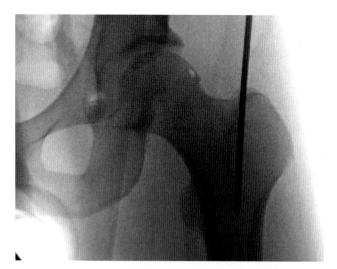

Figure 59-2

- Advance the threaded tip guidewire to the approximate level of the piriformis fossa. If a trochanteric antegrade technique is used the entry point is along the medial slope of the greater trochanter (Figure 59-2).
- Image the trochanteric region to adjust the position of the guidewire such that the trajectory will permit placement into the center of the medullary canal distally.

- Check the pin position with anteroposterior and lateral imaging. If the pin is not central in the femoral canal, but appropriate on one image plane, then the soft tissue guide with multiple-pin "honeycomb" insert may be used. This device permits fine tuning of the starting guidewire to the proper position by the addition of a second pin.
- When the pin is properly placed advance it to below the lesser trochanter.

Proximal Entry Portal Preparation

- Remove the honeycomb insert, leaving the guidewire and the entry portal tool in the wound. If the insert was not needed, place the soft tissue sleeve before creating the entry portal to protect the abductor muscular insertion.

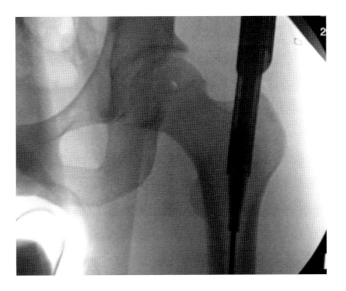

Figure 59-3

- Place the entry reamer assembly consisting of a 14-mm channel reamer, entry reamer connector, and entry reamer, into the entry portal tool and over the guidewire (Figure 59-3).
- Ream the assembly into the femur until it bottoms out on the entry portal tool.
- Check the position of the reamer during the insertion with anteroposterior and lateral imaging.
- Remove the entry reamer and guidewire leaving the entry portal tube and the channel reamer in place.
- Alternatively, the cannulated entry reamer can be positioned over the starting guidewire. For simple diaphyseal fractures the channel reamer generally is not necessary. The device's advantages become clearly evident with more proximal fractures as a means of externally controlling the characteristic deformity often seen in subtrochanteric fracture patterns.

Reduction and Guidewire Insertion

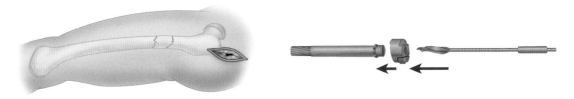

Figure 59-4

- Place the reduction tool consisting of the reducer and a T-handle into the channel reamer and connector in the femur (Figure 59-4).

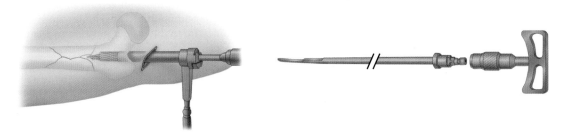

Figure 59-5

- Advance the reduction tool to the fracture site. Use the tool to manipulate the proximal fragment and engage the distal fragment with the tool's tip. Alternatively, if the intramedullary reduction tool is not used, percutaneous unicortical reduction "joysticks" can be used to facilitate reduction or external reduction devices also are available (Figure 59-5).

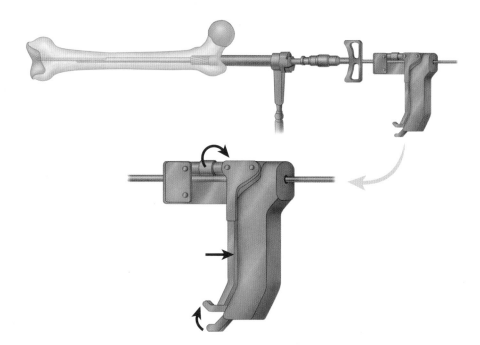

Figure 59-6

- When the distal fragment is reached and engaged, advance the 3.0-mm ball-tipped guidewire across the fracture. Use the vice grip device to advance the guidewire (Figure 59-6).

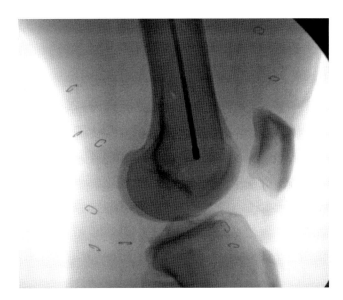

Figure 59-7

- Confirm the reduction and position of the guidewire with anteroposterior and lateral images at multiple levels. The goal should be concentric central placement of the wire distally to the level of the epiphyseal scar (Figure 59-7).
- Remove the reduction tool with the T-handle if used.

Canal Preparation

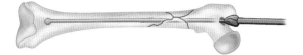

Figure 59-8

- Remove the reducer, and ream the canal sequentially at 0.5-mm intervals until there is moderate "chatter" or until the reaming exceeds the selected nail diameter by 1.0 to 1.5 mm. The channel reamer must be removed for reamers larger than 12.5 mm. An obturator is used to prevent inadvertent removal of the ball-tipped wire from the proper position within the distal segment of the femur. This must be done during withdrawal of the reamer with each pass. If the wire is withdrawn, reposition and confirm the location on fluoroscopy before further reaming (Figure 59-8).
- Confirm the proper nail length by positioning the guidewire at the point of desired distal position, usually between the superior pole of the patella and the level of the distal epiphyseal scar on the anteroposterior image.
- The proper nail length can be determined by either of two methods.
- Using the guidewire method, with the distal end of the rod between the proximal pole of the patella and the distal femoral epiphyseal scar, overlap a second guide rod on the portion of the reduction guide rod extending proximally from the femoral entry portal. The difference in length of the two guidewires is the desired length of the nail.
- Alternatively, most nail systems now supply cannulated depth gauges designed to be placed over the 3.0-mm wire permitting length determination. This is the preferred method. Insert the ruler over the guidewire and place it at the level of the femoral insertion. Check this with the anteroposterior image. Read the measurement off the measurement device.

Nail Insertion

- Attach the drill guide assembly to the selected nail.
- Remove the entry portal tube and channel reamer leaving the guidewire in place.
- Place the nail into the femur and advance it manually. The nail may require gentle impaction to fully seat.

- If there is significant resistance, remove the nail and ream the canal 0.5 mm larger.
- Seat the nail completely as confirmed on multiplanar image intensification.

Interlocking of Nail

- For proximal and distal interlocking use the 5-mm locking screws. Depending on the chosen implant's configuration, proximal and distal locking options may vary. Standard static locking with this implant is from the greater trochanter directed obliquely to the lesser trochanter.
- Place the gold drill sleeve into the proximal guide and dimple the skin.
- Make a stab wound at that point and spread the tissue to the bone.
- Insert the gold drill sleeve with the silver inner liner and use the long pilot drill to go to the inner cortex but not through it.
- Measure the length on the calibrated drill bit at the silver guide top and then penetrate the far cortex. Remove the drill and silver sleeve.
- Insert the screw of the proper length and advance it manually until seated.
- Check the position with an anteroposterior image.
- Evaluate that satisfactory length and rotational alignment has been restored before proceeding with distal interlocking.

Freehand Technique for Distal Targeting

- Place the image intensifier in the lateral position and scan the distal femoral metaphysis. A true lateral image should be sought. This is confirmed with visualization of the distal interlocking screw holes appearing as perfect, clear circles. If the holes appear oblong or to have double density then the proper image has not been obtained. Note that this represents a true lateral image of the nail and not necessarily the distal femur.
- When the holes are completely circular, center a ring forceps or the tip of a scalpel over the chosen interlocking hole on the lateral side of the leg. Make a longitudinal stab incision through the skin, subcutaneous tissue, and iliotibial band centered over the interlocking hole in the nail.

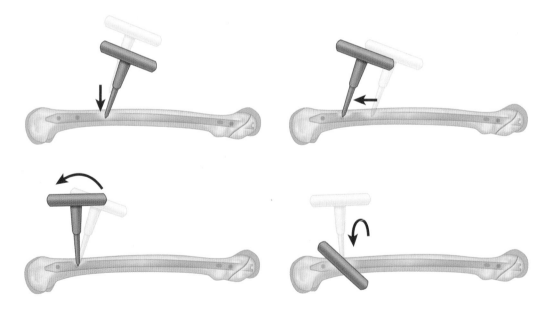

Figure 59-9

- Place a trocar-tip drill bit over the screw hole angled approximately 45 degrees to permit viewing under fluoroscopy. Make appropriate adjustments until the tip is centered over the desired hole; each adjustment should be accompanied by a fluoroscopic image until the proper position is obtained (Figure 59-9).
- Bring the drill parallel and in line with the fluoroscopic beam. Take care to maintain constant pressure to avoid movement of the drill tip.

- Penetrate the lateral cortex. Remove the drill bit from the driver and confirm on the lateral image the drill bit placed within the interlocking hole. If it is not, make appropriate adjustments in alignment. Then reattach the driver and penetrate the medial cortex.
- Calibrated drill bits are used for this portion of the procedure and it greatly increases the ease of determining screw length. Alternatively, a standard depth gauge can be used. Place the appropriate length interlocking bolt by hand confirming satisfactory purchase.
- Repeat if additional distal interlocking screws are desired.
- Anteroposterior and lateral imaging should confirm appropriate screw position and length.
- Irrigate and close the wounds in a standard layered fashion.

Final Evaluation

- Before leaving the operative suite several key elements must be evaluated.
- First, if the nail has been locked in standard fashion, evaluate the femoral neck with multiplanar fluoroscopic imaging to ensure that no occult femoral neck fracture is identified.
- Next, confirm the length and rotational reductions and compare with the uninjured limb to ensure symmetry.
- Evaluate the thigh compartments and if clinical concern exists obtain objective compartment measurements.
- Examine the ligaments of the ipsilateral knee.
- A postoperative anteroposterior pelvis radiograph with both hips internally rotated provides the optimal profile view of the femoral neck as a further check for occult femoral neck fractures and should be obtained and reviewed before anesthesia is discontinued.

POSTOPERATIVE CARE 〉

Weight bearing depends on the stability of the fracture fixation. Weight bearing to tolerance is allowed immediately regardless of the nail size if satisfactory cortical contact is achieved. In the rare circumstance that an adolescent nail is used in an adult, protected weight bearing should be initiated until early radiographic healing is noted. Touch-down or partial weight bearing is allowed in comminuted injuries. Hip and knee range of motion are encouraged. Quadriceps-setting and straight-leg raising exercises are begun before hospital discharge. Hip abduction exercises are begun after wound healing. Weight bearing is progressed as callus formation occurs. Ambulatory aids such as crutches or a walker are used for the first 6 weeks. Hip and knee range of motion and strengthening exercises are recommended during this time. Unassisted ambulation is permitted as strength recovery and radiographic healing progress.

Retrograde femoral nailing may be beneficial in the following clinical situations: (1) obese patients in whom it is difficult to obtain an antegrade entry portal; (2) patients with ipsilateral femoral neck and shaft fractures to allow the use of separate fixation devices for the shaft and neck fractures; (3) patients with floating knee injuries to allow fixation of the femoral and tibial fractures through the same anterior longitudinal incision; (4) multiply injured trauma patients to decrease operative time by not using a fracture table, which allows multiple injuries to be treated by preparing and draping simultaneously; and (5) pregnant patients, so that intraoperative fluoroscopy is minimized around the pelvis. Retrograde nailing is more reliable in controlling distal shaft fractures, whereas antegrade nailing provides better control of proximal shaft fractures.

RETROGRADE FEMORAL NAILING 〉

- Place the patient on a radiolucent flattop operating room table. A small bolster can be positioned under the ipsilateral hip to prevent external rotation of the proximal femur. Surgical preparation and draping must include the hip girdle and lower flank.
- Position the leg over a sterile bump or triangle. Tibial traction may be used and affixed to the traction bow holder. Alternatively, a tibial traction pin and traction bow can be used as a "handle" for more exacting control of the distal segment when manual traction is used.

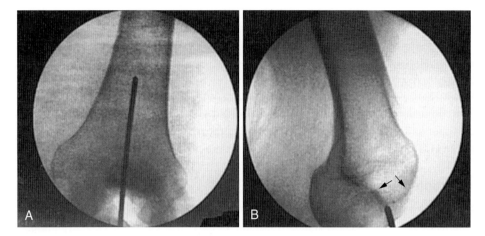

Figure 59-10

- Make an incision through the lateral parapatellar, medial parapatellar, or transpatellar tendon based on surgeon preference. The retropatellar fat pad must be incised and an arthrotomy performed. Insert a 3.2-mm guidewire into the intercondylar notch (Figure 59-10, **A**). Position the pin directed centrally into the medullary canal on anteroposterior imaging. Confirm its position and trajectory on lateral imaging; the pin placement should be in line with the medullary canal at the anterior extent of Blumensaat's line (**B**).
- Advance the guidewire into the distal femoral metaphysis. Place the soft tissue protection sleeve over the guidewire for protection of the articular surfaces and patellar tendon.
- Similar to the antegrade technique, a multiple-pin "honeycomb" insert can aid in perfecting the guidepin placement. If this is used remove the honeycomb insert and place the cannulated entry reamer over the initial guidewire.
- Advance into the femur until the reamer is within the distal femur taking special care to maintain the soft tissue protection sleeve in place to avoid iatrogenic intraarticular injury. (Do not use the channel reamer and entry reamer connector for this procedure.)
- Take care to ensure appropriate trajectory of the pin in the distal segment particularly with fractures involving the distal femoral metaphysis. Otherwise coronal and sagittal plane malalignments can result secondary to nail-canal mismatch. Blocking screws may be indicated to maintain alignment.
- Remove the reamer and guidewire and insert a 3-mm bead-tipped guidewire into the distal fragment.
- Reduce the fracture and advance the guidewire into the proximal segment to the level of the lesser trochanter. A cannulated reduction tool or external devices, such as a large distractor, can be used for reduction maneuvers in combination with axial traction. Small bumps or bolsters can be placed along the posterior surface of the thigh as determined by fluoroscopy to aid in sagittal plane reduction.
- Prepare the medullary canal by introducing cannulated reamers over the guidewire to a diameter 1.0 to 1.5 mm larger than the nail to be used.
- Recheck the position of the guidewire to confirm its position at the lesser trochanter.
- Apply traction to the leg to ensure proper length. Measure for the appropriate length of the nail with a ruler placed over the guidewire. Check to ensure the ruler is countersunk. This is most easily performed on the lateral image plane.

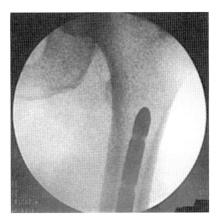

Figure 59-11

- Remove the entry portal tool and insert the nail attached to the targeting guide, seating it to the level of the lesser trochanter (Figure 59-11).
- Maintain traction on the leg to avoid shortening.
- Check the lateral image to ensure the nail is properly inset.
- When the nail is at the proper level, remove the guidewire.
- Proceed with distal locking of the nail using the guide.
- Insert the drill sleeve and trocar through the targeting guide and dimple the skin.
- Make a stab wound at the site and enlarge the hole with blunt dissection to bone.
- Reinsert the drill guide to bone. Advance the drill until the far cortex is encountered and read the measurement off the drill bit calibrations for length approximation. Complete the penetration of the cortex.
- Insert the screw by hand until fully seated.
- Check the length and position of the screws with anteroposterior and lateral imaging.
- Repeat this procedure until the desired number of interlocking screws have been positioned.
- Recheck the alignment and length of the femur using a Bovie cord from the anterior superior iliac crest, middle of the femoral head, middle of the knee, and middle of the tibial plafond. Check the lateral reduction.
- When the final reduction and length are acceptable, move to the proximal locking hole, which should be placed in the anteroposterior plane at the level of the lesser trochanter to avoid nerve and vessel injury. Identify the hole by the perfect circle technique.
- Using the image intensifier, localize the interlocking holes proximally because this will assist in placement of the incision. Make a longitudinal skin incision, sharply dividing the subcutaneous tissue and deep fascia, and bluntly dissect to bone. Avoid damage to the branches of the femoral nerve.
- Drill into the femur when the position is acceptable by the perfect circle technique.
- Use the same technique to determine the screw length as described previously.
- Place the interlocking screw using the captured screwdriver.
- Recheck the alignment and reduction with multiple anteroposterior and lateral views.
- Image the hip in full fluoroscopic mode with internal and external rotation and push-pull to check for an occult femoral neck fracture.
- Close the wounds in a standard layered fashion and apply a dressing.
- Perform the same series of checks as described for antegrade nailing.

POSTOPERATIVE CARE 〉

Postoperative rehabilitation depends on the stability of fixation, and the fracture pattern and must be individualized for each patient. All patients are initially placed in a knee immobilizer. Patients with stable fixation can be started on a continuous passive motion program in the first 24 to 48 hours after surgery. Fractures with less secure fixation may require hinged bracing. Initial weight bearing depends on fracture stability after fixation. Patients with intercondylar fractures or supracondylar fractures require protected weight bearing until radiographic progression permits advancement of weight bearing (usually between 10 and 12 weeks).

COMPRESSION HIP SCREW FIXATION OF INTERTROCHANTERIC FEMORAL FRACTURES

John C. Weinlein

Internal fixation is appropriate for most intertrochanteric femoral fractures. Optimal fixation is based on the stability of the fracture. The mainstay of treatment of intertrochanteric fractures is fixation with a screw-side plate device or intramedullary device.

Patient Positioning

- Place the patient on a fracture table with a perineal post.

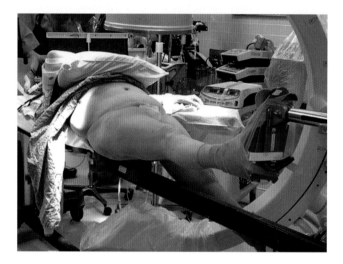

Figure 60-1

- Either place the foot of the contralateral lower extremity in a boot and scissor the leg (unaffected hip extended relative to the injured side) or use a well-leg holder (Figure 60-1).
- Place the affected extremity into a boot after the reduction maneuver has been carried out (further details later). We typically place the affected extremity in 20 to 30 degrees of hip flexion.
- Position the fluoroscopy unit on the contralateral side or between the patient's legs depending on the position of the uninjured leg. Adequate fluoroscopy must be attainable before proceeding.

Reduction

- Reduction of the affected extremity typically is done with traction and internal rotation. The typical sagittal plane deformity, posterior sag, may require correction with an anterior applied force to the posterior distal fragment before completing the reduction with traction and internal rotation.
- Once the fracture has been provisionally reduced, place the affected leg in the boot and obtain fluoroscopy views in the sagittal and coronal planes. Make any necessary adjustments by increasing or decreasing traction or altering abduction/adduction and internal/external rotation. Carefully scrutinize the fluoroscopic images to avoid the most common malalignments: varus deformity, posterior sag, and excessive internal rotation.

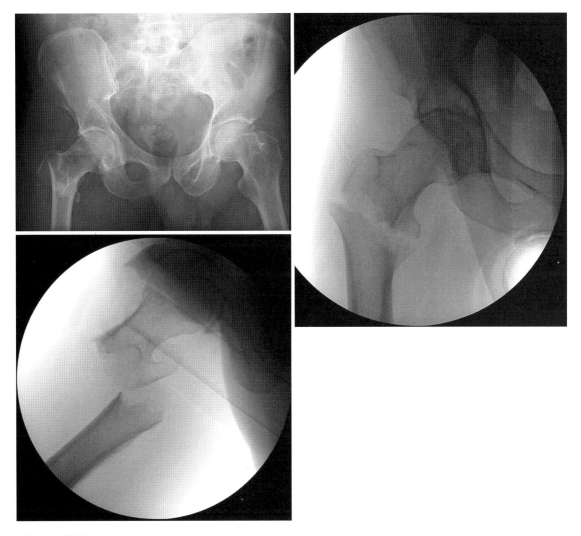

Figure 60-2

- The fracture mechanism (low-energy and high-energy) should have already been noted because standard reduction maneuvers are not likely to be successful with high-energy intertrochanteric femoral fractures and open reduction through a Watson-Jones approach probably will be required (Figure 60-2).

Exposure

- Begin the incision at the vastus ridge and carry it distally. Continue dissection through the iliotibial band and split the fascia of the vastus lateralis longitudinally.
- Elevate the vastus lateralis anteriorly off the lateral intermuscular septum while coagulating branches of the profunda femoris artery as they are encountered.
- Complete the exposure by sharply incising the origin of the vastus lateralis to allow retraction and subsequent plate placement.

Stabilization

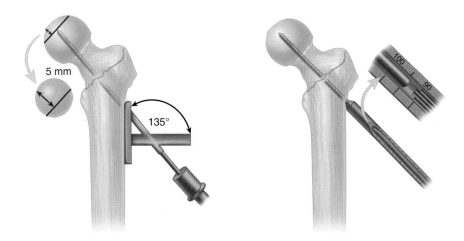

Figure 60-3

- Insert a guide pin through the angled guide into the center-center position within the femoral head. A guide pin can be placed anteriorly along the femoral neck to approximate the anteversion. Insert the guide pin to approximately 5 mm from the articular surface and measure (Figure 60-3).

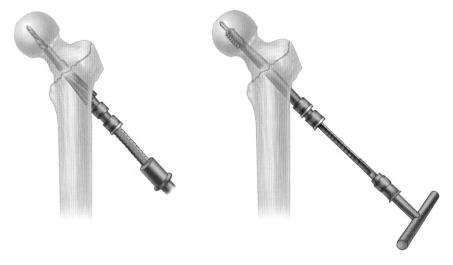

Figure 60-4

- Set a triple reamer 5 mm less than the above measurement and ream. Be sure not to advance the guide pin into the pelvis when reaming. A tap may need to be used in patients with good bone quality (Figure 60-4).
- Select a lag screw that is the same length as the measurement from the triple reamer. If significant shortening is expected or desired, choose a lag screw that is 5 mm shorter than the measurement from the triple reamer. Ensure that the lag screw is sufficiently covered by not placing a lag screw any shorter than 5 mm less than the measurement from the triple reamer.

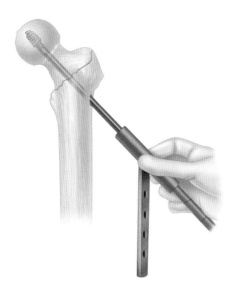

Figure 60-5

- Using the insertion wrench insert the lag screw with the plate to the appropriate depth. 90 degrees of rotation of the lag screw results in 0.75 mm of lag screw advancement. When advancement is completed the handle of the insertion wrench must be perpendicular to the axis of the femur and not the axis of the floor (Figure 60-5).

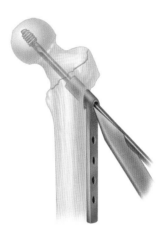

Figure 60-6

- Advance the side plate onto the lateral aspect of the femur. Use a tamp to fully seat the plate onto the lag screw. Unscrew the lag screw retaining rod and remove the insertion wrench and then the guide pin (Figure 60-6).

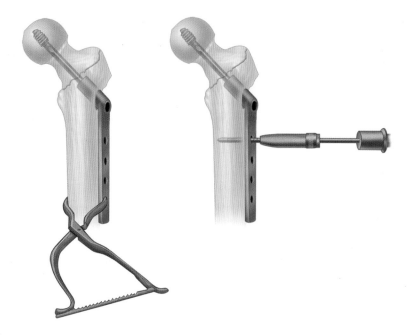

Figure 60-7

- Secure the plate to bone with a screw or a plate clamp. Place two to three bicortical screws in total in the shaft, typically through a two- to four-hole plate. If a screw is used to reduce the plate to the bone the initial screw usually must be changed because it is too long (Figure 60-7).

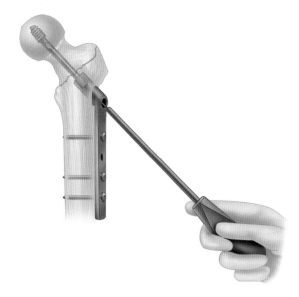

Figure 60-8

- Release traction and insert a compression screw if desired. Alternatively, apply manual compression. Obtain fluoroscopic images to evaluate reduction and hardware placement (Figure 60-8).

POSTOPERATIVE CARE 〉

Patients with intertrochanteric femoral fractures treated with a compression hip screw are allowed to bear weight as tolerated in most circumstances because this device is used in more stable fracture patterns.

See also Video 61-1.

The mainstay of treatment of subtrochanteric femoral fractures is intramedullary nailing. Evidence exists that intramedullary implants are superior to extramedullary implants in the treatment of most fractures in this difficult region. Certainly, there are circumstances in which blade plates and proximal femoral locking plates are useful, and we use both of these devices.

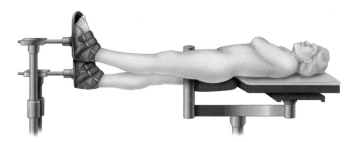

Figure 61-1

- Place the patient supine (or lateral) on a fracture table with the injured extremity in traction through a skeletal traction pin or boot and the hip flexed 30 to 40 degrees (Figure 61-1).
- Use anteroposterior and lateral fluoroscopy to calculate the amount of rotation of the proximal fragment. This calculation is based on a true lateral image of the femoral neck on which the degree of the C-arm from the horizontal is noted and 15 degrees (average anteversion) is subtracted. Alternatively and more accurately, determine the anteversion of the contralateral side by obtaining a true lateral image of the hip and knee from the uninjured side. This more accurate value of anteversion is then subtracted from the degree the C-arm is from the horizontal on the true lateral view of the injured side.
- Externally rotate the distal fragment through the traction pin or boot to match the calculated rotation of the proximal fragment, typically 5 to 15 degrees.

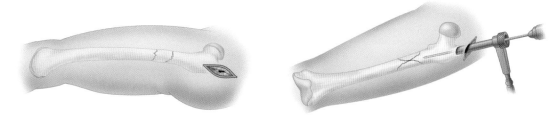

Figure 61-2

- After making an incision, place a guide pin on the proximal femur in a position to proceed with a modified medial trochanteric portal (or piriformis fossa portal) and insert the guide pin. If localization of the guide pin is difficult because of abduction, flexion, and external rotation of the proximal fragment, enlarge the proposed lateral incision for placement of reconstruction screws and introduce a large bone-holding forceps to correct the proximal segment deformity and simplify guide pin placement (Figure 61-2).
- If a piriformis nail is used, the guide pin must be "cheated" approximately 5 mm anteriorly on the lateral view to allow placement of the two cephalomedullary screws.

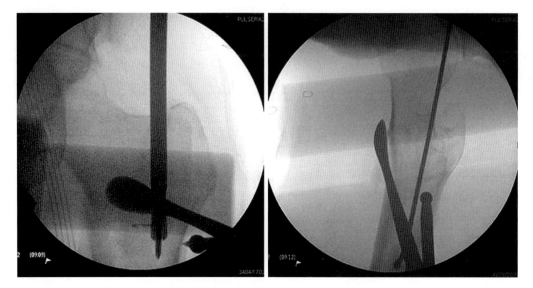

Figure 61-3

- Correct the typical deformities of the proximal segment and hold them corrected before reaming the proximal segment. Correct any residual abduction and flexion with a combination of ball spike pusher and elevator (Figure 61-3).

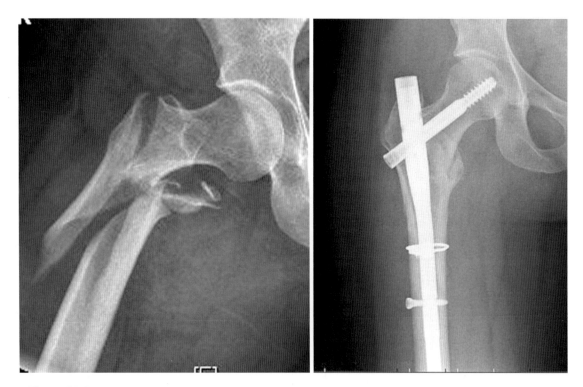

Figure 61-4

- Alternatively, place a clamp through the same incision that will be used for insertion of the cephalomedullary screws. If instability persists after clamp removal, a cerclage wire can be used to hold the deformities corrected (Figure 61-4).

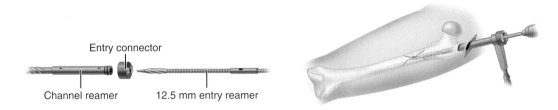

Figure 61-5

- Use the combination entry reamer/channel reamer to ream the proximal femur, avoiding eccentric reaming (Figure 61-5).

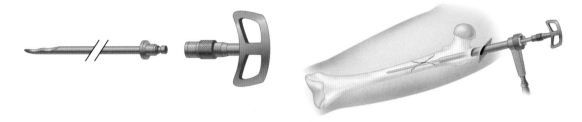

Figure 61-6

- Use the reduction tool to aid with fracture reduction (Figure 61-6).

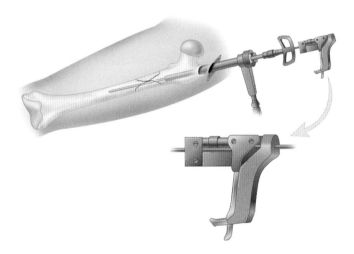

Figure 61-7

- Insert the ball-tipped guide rod across fracture (Figure 61-7).

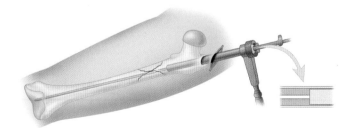

Figure 61-8

- Measure for length of the intramedullary nail (Figure 61-8).

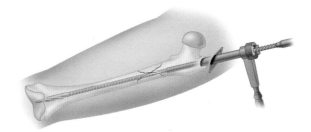

Figure 61-9

- Ream the femoral shaft sequentially through the channel reamer (Figure 61-9).

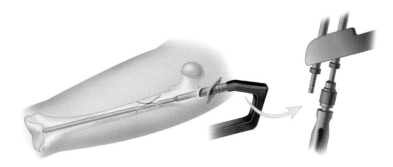

Figure 61-10

- Place the appropriate-size intramedullary nail and lock it proximally in reconstruction mode (Figure 61-10).
- Drill a hole for the most distal of the cephalomedullary screws first, just above the calcar. Leave the drill bit in place while drilling for the second screw and also leave this drill bit in place. Place the distal screw first and then the more proximal screw, placing both screws in the center of the femoral head on the lateral view.
- Lock the nail distally with a free-hand technique.
- Check rotation for any external or internal rotational malalignments. Move the hip through a range of motion at 90 degrees of flexion and compare this range of motion to the contralateral side. A significant side-to-side difference can be corrected by removing the distal interlocking screws, correcting the rotation, and then relocking the nail.

POSTOPERATIVE CARE 〉

Patients with subtrochanteric femoral fractures treated with an intramedullary device typically are allowed touch-down weight bearing for the first 6 weeks and advanced based on healing as shown on follow-up radiographs.

INTRAMEDULLARY FIXATION OF CLAVICULAR FRACTURES

Edward A. Perez

Suggested advantages of intramedullary fixation of clavicular fractures include small skin incision, less periosteal stripping, and relative stability to allow callus formation. Disadvantages include frequent complications such as intrathoracic migration, pin breakage, and damage to underlying structures.

- Place the patient in a semi-sitting position on a radiolucent table with an image intensifier on the ipsilateral side. By rotating the image 45 degrees caudal and cephalad, orthogonal views of the clavicle can be obtained.

- Make a 2- to 3-cm incision over the posterolateral corner of the clavicle 2 to 3 cm medial to the acromioclavicular joint. Little subcutaneous fat is in this region, so take care to prevent injury to the underlying platysma muscle.

- Use scissors to free the platysma muscle from the overlying skin and split its fibers in line with the muscle. Take care to prevent injury to the middle branch of the supraclavicular nerve, which is usually found directly beneath the platysma muscle near the midclavicle. Identify and retract the nerve.

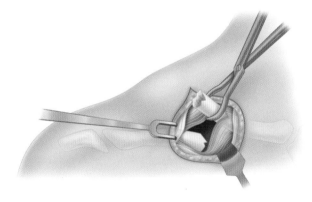

Figure 62-1

- Use a towel clip to elevate the proximal end of the medial clavicle through the incision (Figure 62-1).

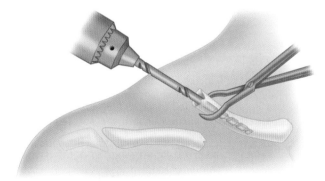

Figure 62-2

- Taking care not to penetrate the anterior cortex, attach the appropriate-sized drill to the ratchet T-handle and drill the medullary canal (Figure 62-2).

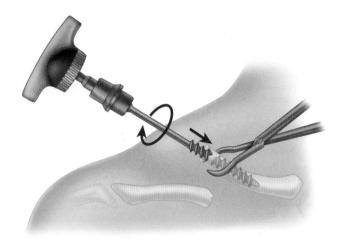

Figure 62-3

- Remove the drill from the medial fragment, attach the appropriate-sized tap to the T-handle, and tap the medullary canal to the anterior cortex. Hand tapping is recommended especially for small patients and smaller-diameter clavicle pins (Figure 62-3).
- Elevate the lateral fragment through the incision; externally rotating the arm and shoulder helps improve exposure.

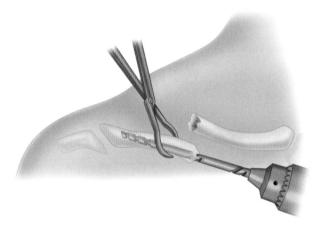

Figure 62-4

- Attach the same-sized drill used in the medial fragment to the ratchet T-handle and drill the medullary canal (Figure 62-4).

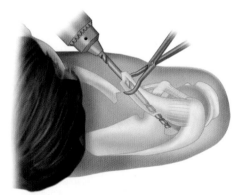

Figure 62-5

- Under C-arm guidance pass the drill out through the posterolateral cortex of the clavicle. The drill position should be posterior and medial to the acromioclavicular joint around the level of the coracoid. Allow the drill to exit no higher than the equator of the posterolateral clavicle (Figure 62-5).

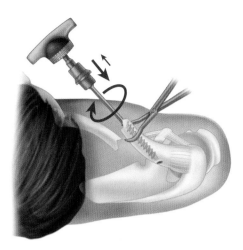

Figure 62-6

- Remove the drill from the lateral fragment, attach the appropriate-sized tap to the T-handle, and tap the medullary canal so that the large threads are advanced fully into the canal. If the tap is a tight fit consider redrilling with the next larger drill size. Again, hand tapping is recommended (Figure 62-6).
- While holding the distal fragment with a bone clamp remove the nuts from the pin assembly and pass the trocar end of the pin into the medullary canal of the distal fragment. The pin should exit through the previously drilled hole in the posterolateral cortex.

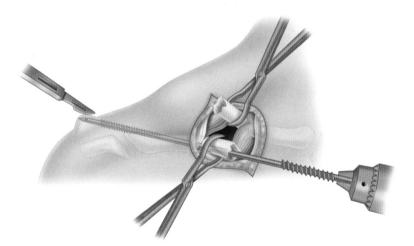

Figure 62-7

- Once the pin exits the clavicle, its tip can be felt subcutaneously. Make a small incision over the palpable tip and spread the subcutaneous tissue with a hemostat. Place the tip of the hemostat under the tip of the clavicle pin to facilitate its passage through the incision. Then drill the pin out laterally until the large medial threads start to engage the cortex (Figure 62-7).

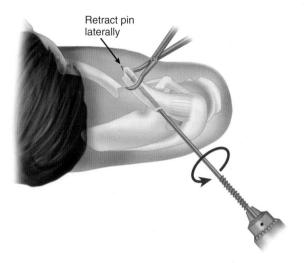

Figure 62-8

- Attach the Jacobs chuck and T-handle to the end of the pin protruding laterally (take care not to place the chuck over the machined threads, both lateral and medial), and carefully retract the pin into the lateral fragment. Ensure that the pin is inserted correctly (Figure 62-8).
- Reduce the fracture and pass the pin into the medial fragment. Advance the pin until all medial threads are across the fracture site. Because the weight of the arm usually pulls the arm down, lifting the shoulder will facilitate pin passage into the medial fragment.
- Place the medial nut on the pin followed by the smaller lateral nut. Cold weld the two nuts together by grasping the medial nut with a needle driver or needle-nose pliers and tightening the lateral nut against the medial nut with the lateral nut wrench. Use the T-handle and wrench on the lateral nut to medially advance the pin down into the medial fragment until it contacts the anterior cortex. Confirm position with fluoroscopy.

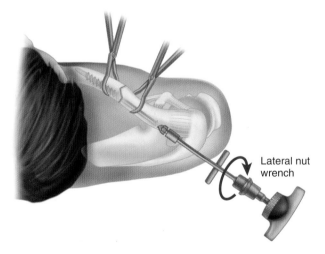

Figure 62-9

- Break the cold weld between the nuts by grasping the medial nut with a needle driver or pliers and quickly turning the lateral nut counterclockwise with the insertion wrench. Advance the medial nut until it against the lateral cortex of the clavicle. Tighten the lateral nut until it engages the medial nut (Figure 62-9).

- Use the medial wrench to back out the pin 1 cm or more to expose the nuts from the soft tissue. Ensure that the clavicle threads are still engaged in the cortical bone of the medial fragment.
- Use a side-cutting pin cutter to cut the pin as close to the lateral nut as possible. Readvance the clavicle pin using the lateral nut wrench.

POSTOPERATIVE CARE 〉

The arm is placed in a standard sling for comfort and gentle pendulum exercises are allowed. At 10 to 14 days sutures are removed and, if healing is seen on radiographs, the sling is discontinued; unrestricted range-of-motion exercises, but no strengthening, resisted exercises, or sports activities are allowed. If radiographs at 6 weeks show union resisted and strengthening activities are begun. Contact sports (e.g., football, hockey) should be avoided for 12 weeks after surgery. If the fracture is healed at 12 weeks the pin can be removed.

INTRAMEDULLARY NAILING OF PROXIMAL HUMERAL FRACTURES

Edward A. Perez

Indications for operative treatment of proximal humeral fractures include displaced two-part surgical neck fractures, displaced (>5 mm) greater tuberosity fractures, displaced three-part fractures, and displaced four-part fractures in young patients. The type of fixation — transosseous suture, percutaneous pin, intramedullary nail, or plate — used depends on the patient's age, activity level, and bone quality; the fracture type and associated fractures; and the surgeon's technical ability. Intramedullary nailing provides more stable fixation than percutaneous pinning, although less than locked plate fixation. Insertion of an intramedullary nail into the proximal humerus violates the rotator cuff, which can lead to postoperative shoulder pain. The advantages of the technique include preservation of the soft tissues and the theoretical biomechanical properties of intramedullary nails. A comminuted lateral cortex or fractures involving the tuberosities may be a contraindication to intramedullary nailing.

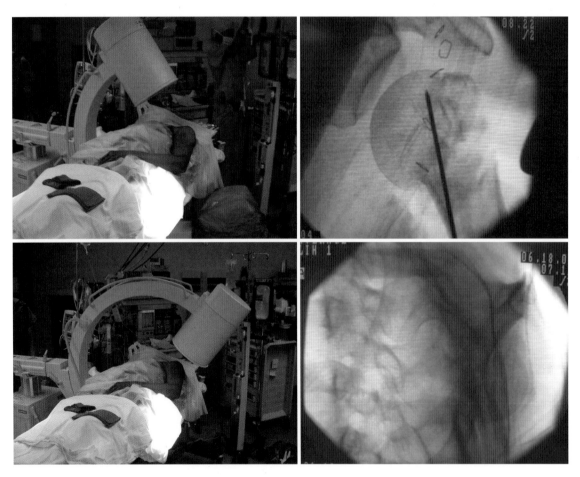

Figure 63-1

- Position the patient on a radiolucent table with the thorax "bumped" 30 to 40 degrees. Place the image intensifier unit on the opposite side of the table from the surgeon; rolling the unit back allows an adequate anteroposterior view, and rolling it forward allows an adequate lateral view of the shoulder and humerus (Figure 63-1).

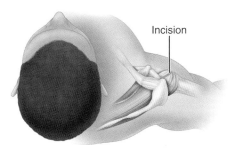
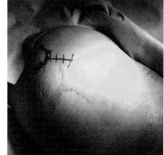
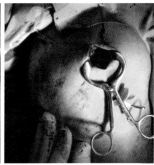

Incision

Figure 63-2

- Make an incision diagonally from the anterolateral corner of the acromion, splitting the deltoid in line with its fibers in the raphe between the anterior and middle thirds of the deltoid. To protect the axillary nerve, avoid splitting the deltoid more than 5 cm distal to the acromion (Figure 63-2).

- Under direct observation, incise the rotator cuff in line with its fibers. Use full-thickness sutures to protect the cuff from damage during reaming of the humeral canal.

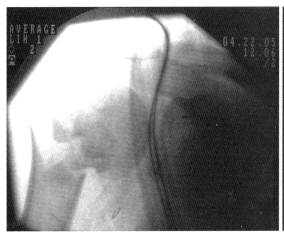
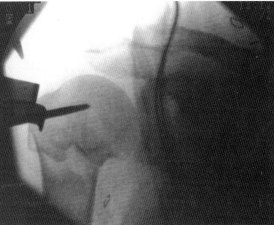

Figure 63-3

- Use a threaded pin as a "joystick" in the posterior humeral head to derotate the head into a reduced position (Figure 63-3).

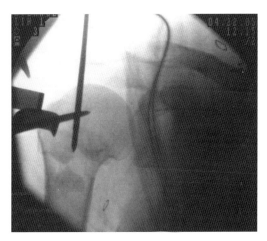

Figure 63-4

- Place the initial guidewire posterior to the biceps tendon and advance it under fluoroscopic guidance into the appropriate position, as shown on the anteroposterior and lateral views (Figure 63-4).

- Carefully advance the proximal reamer, protecting the rotator cuff.
- Use the reduction device to reduce the fracture and pass the bead-tipped guidewire.
- With sequentially larger reamers, ream the humerus to the predetermined diameter, usually 1.0 to 1.5 mm larger than the nail diameter.

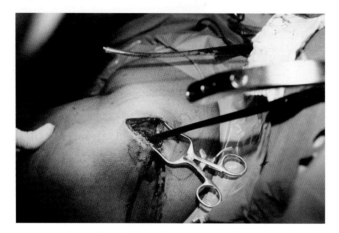

Figure 63-5

- When reaming is completed, pass the nail down the humeral canal, avoiding distraction of the fracture; ensure that the nail is below the articular surface of the humeral head (Figure 63-5).

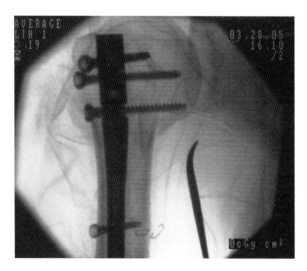

Figure 63-6

- Using the outrigger device, insert the proximal locking bolts. Carefully spread the soft tissues to avoid injury to the axillary nerve (Figure 63-6).

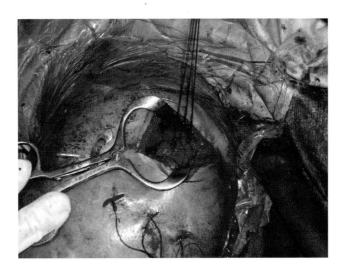

Figure 63-7

- Repair the rotator cuff with full-thickness sutures under direct observation (Figure 63-7).
- Confirm reduction and screw placement and length on anteroposterior and lateral fluoroscopy images.
- Begin an early rehabilitation program with active-assisted range-of-motion exercises.

Our most common indication for operative treatment of humeral shaft fractures in adults is early mobilization of patients with polytrauma. Treatment decisions must take all factors into consideration, tailoring the treatment to the specific patient. Currently, we prefer rigid, locked nails inserted through an antegrade approach when intramedullary nailing is indicated, such as for segmental fractures, proximal-to-middle third junction fractures, pathological fractures, fractures with poor soft tissue coverage, fractures in obese patients, and fractures in certain patients with polytrauma.

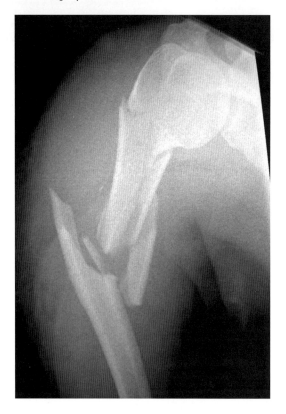

Figure 64-1

- Carefully evaluate preoperative radiographs to ensure that the diaphyseal diameter is adequate to accommodate the intramedullary nail. If the diameter is too small, plate fixation is indicated (Figure 64-1).
- Position the patient on a radiolucent table with the thorax "bumped" 30 to 40 degrees. Place the image intensifier unit on the opposite side of the table from the surgeon; rolling the unit back allows an adequate anteroposterior view, and rolling it forward allows an adequate lateral view of the shoulder and humerus.

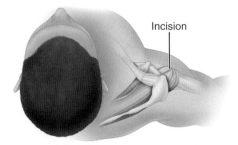

Figure 64-2

- Make an incision diagonally from the anterolateral corner of the acromion, splitting the deltoid in line with its fibers in the raphe between the anterior and middle thirds of the deltoid. To protect the axillary nerve, avoid splitting the deltoid more than 5 cm distal to the acromion (Figure 64-2).

- Under direct observation, incise the rotator cuff in line with its fibers. Use full-thickness sutures to protect the cuff from damage during reaming of the humeral canal.
- Place the initial guidewire posterior to the biceps tendon and advance it under fluoroscopic guidance into the appropriate position, as shown on the anteroposterior and lateral views.
- Carefully advance the proximal reamer, protecting the rotator cuff.

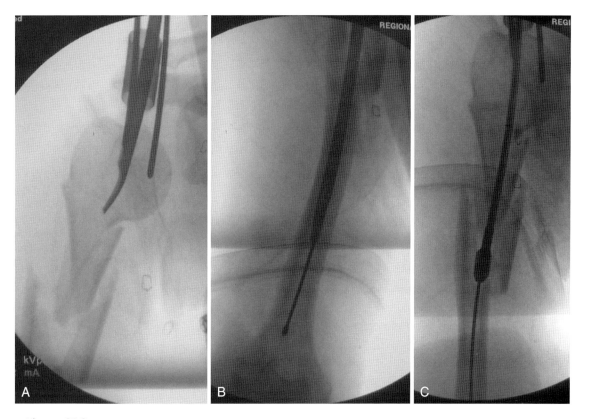

Figure 64-3

- Use the reduction device to reduce the fracture and pass the bead-tipped guidewire (Figure 64-3, A, B). With sequentially larger reamers, ream the humerus to the predetermined diameter, usually 1.0 to 1.5 mm larger than the nail diameter (C). With fractures of the middle third of the shaft, a small incision can be made at the fracture site to ensure manually that the radial nerve is not entrapped in the fracture before reduction and reaming.
- When reaming is complete, pass the nail down the humeral canal, avoiding distraction of the fracture. Ensure that the nail is below the articular surface of the humeral head.

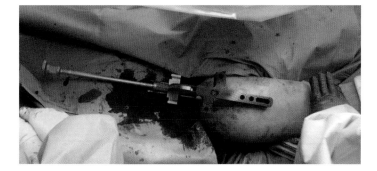

Figure 64-4

- Using the outrigger device, insert the proximal locking bolts. Carefully spread the soft tissues to avoid injury to the axillary nerve (Figure 64-4).

- Place the distal interlocking screws in an anterior-to-posterior direction to avoid the radial nerve. Make a 4- to 5-cm incision anteriorly to expose the biceps musculature; bluntly split the muscle to avoid iatrogenic damage to the brachial artery.
- Repair the rotator cuff with full-thickness sutures.

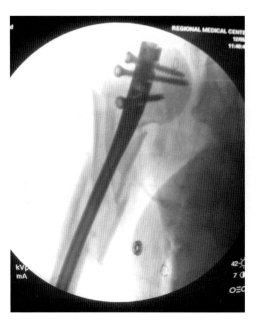

Figure 64-5

- Confirm reduction and screw length on anteroposterior and lateral fluoroscopy images (Figure 64-5).
- Begin an early rehabilitation program with active-assisted range-of-motion exercises.

Edward A. Perez

Most distal humeral fractures in adults must be treated operatively, in contrast to fractures of the proximal humerus or humeral shaft. A variety of approaches have been described for reduction and fixation of distal humeral fractures. Most commonly, a posterior approach with an olecranon osteotomy has been used.

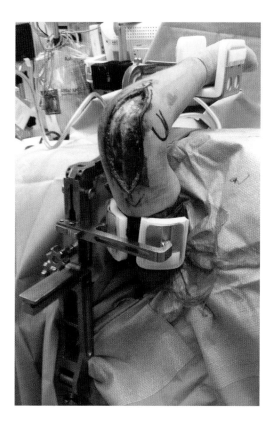

Figure 65-1

- Position the patient in the lateral decubitus position. A prone or supine position is an alternative. An advantage of the supine position is improved anterior exposure of the joint, which is helpful with very low fractures and fractures with anterior comminution. Fixation of the fracture with extension into the shaft can be difficult to reduce with the patient supine. When the supine position is chosen, we use an arm holder (Elbow LOC, Symmetry Medical Inc., Warsaw, IN) to assist with arm positioning (Figure 65-1).

- Prepare and drape the entire forequarter to allow placement of a sterile tourniquet on the proximal arm.

- Make a midline incision, with or without a curve over the tip of the olecranon, and develop full-thickness flaps medially and laterally.

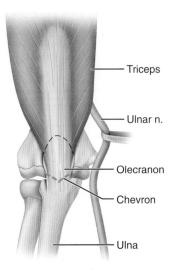

Figure 65-2

- Dissect the ulnar nerve free from the medial edge of the triceps and from the medial epicondyle. Preserve the vascular structures that supply the ulnar nerve (Figure 65-2).
- Laterally, dissect the triceps off the lateral intermuscular septum. Incise the interval between the triceps and anconeus muscles to expose the joint. Alternatively, preserve the anconeus innervation by using the interval between the anconeus and the extensor carpi radialis brevis and elevating the anconeus with the triceps.
- Ensure that the medial and lateral olecranon articular surface can be seen.
- Predrill the holes for olecranon fixation before making the osteotomy. We routinely use plate fixation.

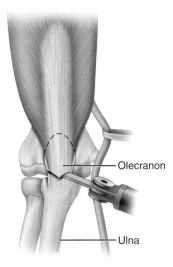

Figure 65-3

- Make a distally-oriented chevron osteotomy with an oscillating saw directed toward the sulcus of the articular surface of the olecranon. Use an osteotome to complete the osteotomy carefully. If the osteotomy is forcefully wedged open with the osteotome, a large cartilaginous flap can be created inadvertently (Figure 65-3).

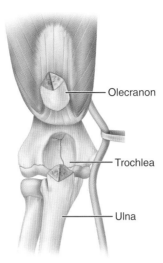

Figure 65-4

- Raise the triceps with the proximal olecranon and direct the triceps musculature off the humerus, preserving the periosteum (Figure 65-4).
- Débride the fracture edges to clean surfaces.
- Use threaded Kirschner wires as joysticks to manipulate the medial and lateral condyles.

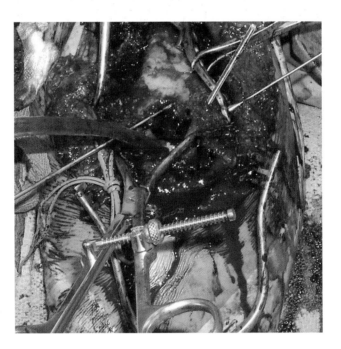

Figure 65-5

- If the articular fracture is simple, reduce the fracture with the joysticks and a Weber clamp and insert Kirschner wires for provisional fixation (Figure 65-5).

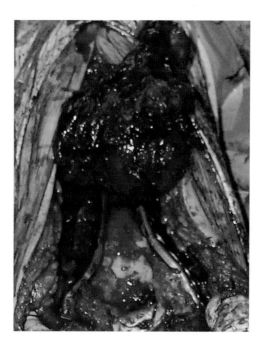

Figure 65-6

- Plate the column with the better key to reduction first, then the opposite column (Figure 65-6).
- If the articular fracture is complex and either the medial or lateral condyle has a good key to reduction with the shaft, reduce the condyle to the shaft. A countersunk mini-fragment (2-mm or 2.4-mm) lag screw can be used for provisional fixation because its low profile does not interfere with plate positioning. Alternatively, a plate can be placed along the column with provisional unicortical screws distally.

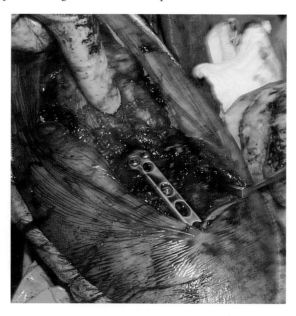

Figure 65-7

- Reconstruct the articular surface "around the clock," provisionally fix the reconstructed fragments, and reduce the remaining condyle to the shaft and apply plate fixation (Figure 65-7).
- Use headless screws, mini-fragment screws, or absorbable screws for fixation of articular comminution.
- Either 90-90 or medial and lateral plates are acceptable.
- Evaluate every screw to ensure that it does not cross the articular surface.
- Repair the olecranon osteotomy, consider transposing the ulnar nerve, and close the incision in layers over closed suction drainage.

POSTOPERATIVE CARE

The elbow is splinted in extension. The drain is removed 2 days after surgery, and range of motion is begun 3 days after surgery. No bracing is used.

OPEN REDUCTION AND INTERNAL FIXATION OF BOTH-BONE FOREARM FRACTURES

Edward A. Perez

See also Video 66-1.

Operative treatment is indicated for almost all both-bone forearm fractures in adults. The goal is to reestablish the anatomical relationship between the radius and ulna with rigid fixation. We routinely use plate fixation for both-bone forearm fractures in adults.

- After evaluation of the radiographs, plan the sequence of fixation:

  If anatomical reduction is possible, begin with fixation of the radius.

  If both fractures are extensively comminuted, begin with fixation of the radius.

  If the radius is comminuted and the ulnar fracture is simpler, reduce and stabilize the ulna first.

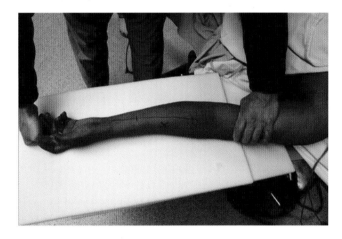

Figure 66-1

- For most fractures, make a volar Henry approach to the distal radius. If a fracture requires fixation proximal to the biceps tuberosity, make a dorsal Thompson approach (Figure 66-1).

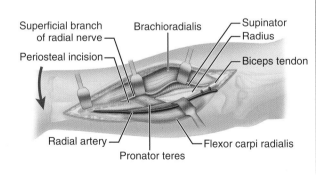
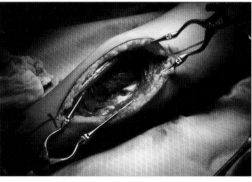

Figure 66-2

- Preserve the periosteum along the proximal and distal segments (Figure 66-2).
- Débride the fracture edges of hematoma and debris.
- Assess the necessity for lengthening; options for attaining length include chemical paralysis, distraction using a screw in the radial shaft and a lamina spreader, and soft tissue releases if the fracture has been in a shortened position for an extended period of time.

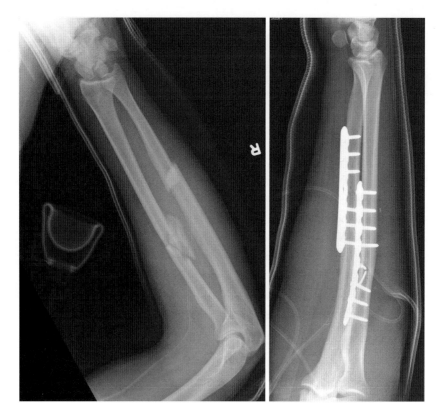

Figure 66-3

- For transverse fractures, apply a 3.5-mm limited-contact compression plate. If there is a butterfly fragment, stabilize it with 2.0- or 2.4-mm lag screws before plate application (Figure 66-3).
- For oblique fractures, reduce the fracture and stabilize it with a 2.0-, 2.4-, or 2.7-mm lag screw, followed by a 3.5-mm limited-contact neutralization plate.
- For extensively comminuted fractures, use a bridge plate at the appropriate length. If the span of the plate is longer than 6 or 7 holes, adding a lateral contour to the plate will help match the radial bow.

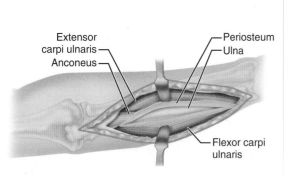
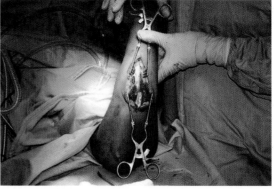

Figure 66-4

- After fixation of the radial fracture, approach the ulna through the interval between the flexor carpi ulnaris and the extensor carpi ulnaris. The plating strategies used for the radius are applicable to the ulnar fracture. We attempt to avoid direct ulnar placement of the plate because of prominent hardware irritation (Figure 66-4).
- The volar or distal aspect of the ulna is chosen for dissection based on which aspect of the ulna has more traumatic dissection. Take care to preserve the periosteum.

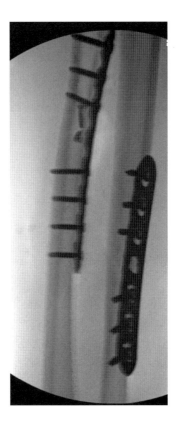

Figure 66-5

- After both the radius and ulna are stabilized, confirm adequate reduction and fixation with fluoroscopy (Figure 66-5).
- Close the wounds in standard fashion.

POSTOPERATIVE CARE

Typically, only a soft dressing is necessary. Splinting is used if the elbow or wrist joint is involved or if fixation is questionable. Range-of-motion exercises are begun 3 to 7 days after surgery; heavy lifting is avoided until fracture healing is evident.

Two techniques for release of the compartments of the lower leg are commonly used: single-incision peri-fibular fasciotomy and double-incision fasciotomy. The single-incision technique may be useful if the soft tissue of the limb is not extensively distorted. Because this rarely is true, the double-incision technique is safe and more effective and generally should be used.

SINGLE-INCISION FASCIOTOMY ⟩

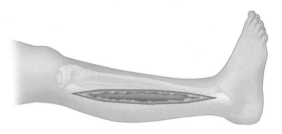

Figure 67-1

- Make a single longitudinal, lateral incision in line with the fibula, extending from just distal to the head of the fibula to 3 to 4 cm proximal to the lateral malleolus (Figure 67-1).
- Undermine the skin anteriorly, and avoid injuring the superficial peroneal nerve.

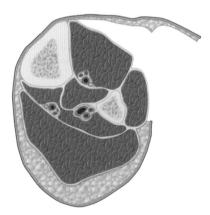

Figure 67-2

- Perform a longitudinal fasciotomy of the anterior and lateral compartments (Figure 67-2).

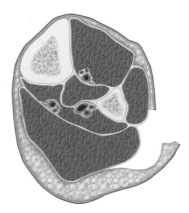

Figure 67-3

- Undermine the skin posteriorly, and perform a fasciotomy of the superficial posterior compartment (Figure 67-3).
- Identify the interval between the superficial and lateral compartments distally, and develop this interval proximally by detaching the soleus from the fibula.
- Subperiosteally dissect the flexor hallucis longus from the fibula.
- Retract the muscle and the peroneal vessels posteriorly.

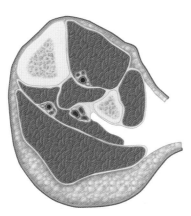

Figure 67-4

- Identify the fascial attachment of the posterior tibial muscle to the fibula, and incise this fascia longitudinally (Figure 67-4).
- Close only the skin over a suction drain or a negative pressure wound device.

DOUBLE-INCISION FASCIOTOMY ⟩

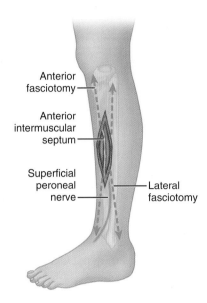

Figure 67-5

- Make a 20- to 25-cm incision in the anterior compartment, centered halfway between the fibular shaft and the crest of the tibia. Use subcutaneous dissection for wide exposure of the fascial compartments (Figure 67-5).
- Make a transverse incision to expose the lateral intermuscular septum, and identify the superficial peroneal nerve just posterior to the septum.
- Using Metzenbaum scissors, release the anterior compartment proximally and distally in line with the anterior tibial muscle.
- Perform a fasciotomy of the lateral compartment proximally and distally in line with the fibular shaft.

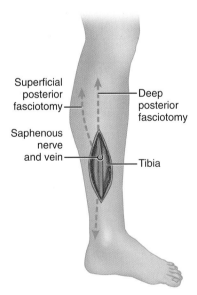

Figure 67-6

- Make a second longitudinal incision 2 cm posterior to the posterior margin of the tibia. Use wide subcutaneous dissection to allow identification of the fascial planes (Figure 67-6).
- Retract the saphenous vein and nerve anteriorly.
- Make a transverse incision to identify the septum between the deep and superficial posterior compartments. Release the fascia over the gastrocnemius-soleus complex for the length of the compartment.

- Make another fascial incision over the flexor digitorum longus muscle, and release the entire deep posterior compartment. As dissection is carried proximally, if the soleus bridge extends more than halfway down the tibia, release this extended origin.

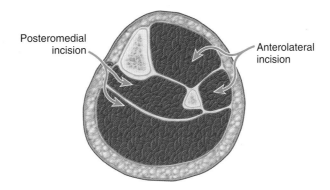

Posteromedial incision

Anterolateral incision

Figure 67-7

- After release of the posterior compartment, identify the deep posterior muscle compartment. If increased tension is evident in this compartment, release it over the extent of the muscle belly (Figure 67-7).
- Pack the wound open, and apply a posterior plaster splint with the foot plantigrade.
- Management of fasciotomy wounds has included primary closure, healing by secondary intention, or split-thickness skin grafting to cover defects, which is necessary in approximately 50% of patients.

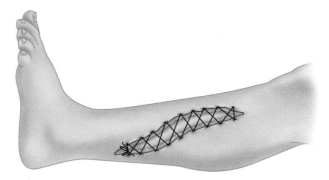

Figure 67-8

- An alternative is a delayed primary closure, which can be accomplished using the vessel loop shoelace technique or commercial closure devices. Vacuum-assisted wound closure can be used to reduce postoperative edema, which may improve wound closure with or without negative pressure therapy (Figure 67-8).

POSTOPERATIVE CARE

At 48 to 72 hours, the patient is returned to the operating room for débridement of any necrotic material. Intravenous fluorescein and a Wood light can be helpful in evaluating muscle viability. If there is no evidence of muscle necrosis, the skin is loosely closed. If closure is not accomplished, the débridement is repeated after another 48- to 72-hour interval, after which skin closure or skin grafting can be done.

Fasciotomy of the forearm should be done in (1) normotensive patients with positive clinical findings and compartment pressures of more than 30 mm Hg and when the duration of the increased pressure is unknown or thought to be longer than 8 hours, (2) uncooperative or unconscious patients with a compartment pressure of more than 30 mm Hg, and (3) patients with low blood pressure and a compartment pressure of more than 20 mm Hg. As a general rule, when in doubt, the compartment should be released.

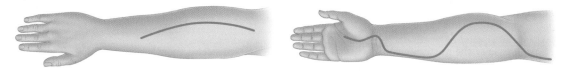

Figure 68-1

- For the volar fasciotomy, make a curvilinear incision similar to McConnell's combined exposure of the median and ulnar nerve neurovascular bundles as described by Henry. Make an anterior curvilinear incision medial to the biceps tendon, crossing the elbow flexion crease at an angle. Carry the incision distally into the palm to allow for a carpal tunnel release, but avoid crossing the wrist flexion crease at a right angle (Figure 68-1).

- Divide the lacertus fibrosus proximally, and evacuate any hematoma.

- In patients with suspected brachial artery injury, expose the brachial artery and determine whether there is a free blood flow. If the flow is unsatisfactory, remove the adventitia to expose any underlying clot, spasm, or intimal tear. Resect the adventitia if necessary, and anastomose or graft the artery.

- Release the superficial volar compartment throughout its length with open scissors, freeing the fascia over the superficial compartment muscles.

- Identify the flexor carpi ulnaris, and retract it with its underlying ulnar neurovascular bundle medially, and retract the flexor digitorum superficialis and median nerve laterally to expose the flexor digitorum profundus in its deep compartment. Check to see if its overlying fascia or epimysium is tight, and incise it longitudinally.

- If the muscle is gray or dusky, the prognosis for recovery may be poor; however, the muscle may still be viable and should be allowed to perfuse.

- Continue the dissection distally by incising the transverse carpal ligament along the ulnar border of the palmaris longus tendon and median nerve.

- In cases of median nerve palsy or paresthesias, observe the median nerve along the entire zone of injury to ensure that it is not severed, contused, or entrapped between the ulnar and humeral head of the pronator teres. If it is, a partial pronator tenotomy is necessary.

- In a patient with a supracondylar fracture, reduce the fracture, pin it with Kirschner wires, and control the bleeding.

- Do not close the skin at this time; anticipate secondary closure later.

- If the median nerve is exposed within the distal forearm, suture the distal radial-based forearm flap loosely over the nerve.

- Check the dorsal compartments clinically, or repeat the pressure measurements. Usually, the volar fasciotomy decompresses the dorsal musculature sufficiently, but if involvement of the dorsal compartments is still suspected, release them also.

- Make the incision distal to the lateral epicondyle between the extensor digitorum communis and extensor carpi radialis brevis, extending approximately 10 cm distally. Gently undermine the subcutaneous tissue, and release the fascia overlying the mobile wad of Henry and the extensor retinaculum.

- Apply a sterile moist dressing and a long-arm splint. The elbow should not be left flexed beyond 90 degrees.

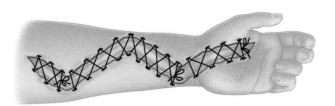

Figure 68-2

- Alternatively, closure of fasciotomy wounds can be accomplished gradually with progressive tension using vessel loops. The vessel loops are tightened progressively postoperatively during dressing changes. Wound closure by this method usually can be accomplished in 2 weeks (Figure 68-2). A vacuum-assisted wound closure system may be used to assist in wound management.

POSTOPERATIVE CARE

The arm is elevated for 24 to 48 hours after surgery. If closure is not possible within 5 days, a split-thickness skin graft should be applied. The splint is worn until sutures are removed or as determined by fracture care.

INTRAMEDULLARY NAILING OF BOTH-BONE FOREARM FRACTURES

S. Terry Canale • James H. Beaty

Operative treatment of both-bone forearm fractures is indicated for (1) open fracture, (2) fracture in an older child, (3) malunion, (4) fracture that is irreducible because of soft tissue interposition, (5) unstable fracture pattern with length or alignment problems, and (6) multiple refractures. Advantages of intramedullary nailing include shorter operative time, minimal soft tissue dissection, ease of hardware removal, early motion after nail removal, and excellent cosmetic results.

- Place the child in the decubitus position with the affected arm on a lateral table and apply a pneumatic tourniquet if open reduction is required but do not inflate it.
- Make a 1-cm longitudinal incision on the lateral side of the distal metaphysis of the less displaced bone.
- With a bradawl, drill a hole in the bone 1 cm proximal to the metaphysis first perpendicularly and then obliquely toward the elbow.

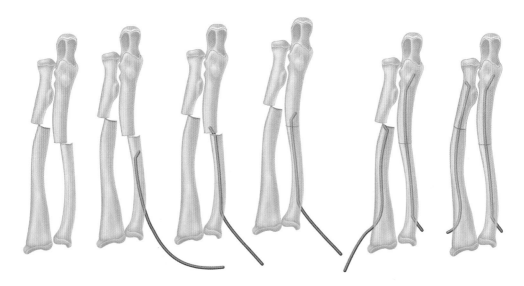

Figure 69-1

- Depending on the diameter of the bone, choose a titanium or stainless steel blunted pin of the appropriate size. The pins range from 2.0 to 4.5 mm and the proximal ends are bent 30 degrees. Introduce the pin into the bone bent side first and push it, with a hammer if necessary, into the fracture site (Figure 69-1).
- Reduce the fracture by external manipulation and fix the pin in the proximal metaphysis. Repeat the procedure for the other bone. Bend the outer tips of the pins and cut them 5 to 10 mm from the bone.
- If necessary perform open reduction of the fracture of the radius or ulna.
- Close all wounds and apply a long-arm, bivalved cast.

POSTOPERATIVE CARE ⟩

After intramedullary pin fixation the cast is removed after 6 weeks. The pins are extracted at 6 months or longer. Participation in sports is avoided for 2 months.

See also Video 70-1.

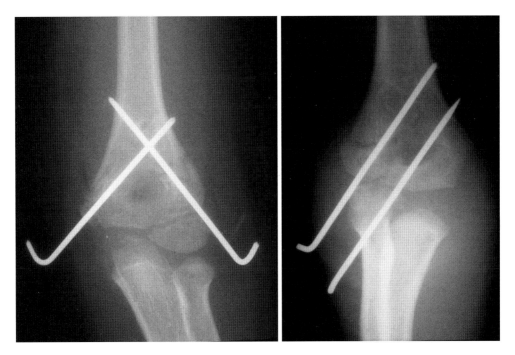

Figure 70-1

Closed reduction and percutaneous pinning (CRPP) has become the treatment of choice for most pediatric supracondylar fractures. Pin configurations include two crossed pins, two lateral pins (three lateral pins can be used if the fracture is unstable with two pins), two lateral "divergent" pins, and two pins laterally and one medially (Figure 70-1). CRPP provides excellent stability of the fracture in any position of the elbow; however, the ultimate result is only as good as the initial reduction.

CROSSED MEDIAL AND LATERAL PINS 〉

- Place the patient prone or supine on a fracture table and prepare and drape the elbow. A radiolucent arm board or the C-arm can be used to support the elbow. Outline the posterior triangle of the elbow joint, the medial and lateral epicondyles, and the olecranon.
- Reduce the fracture by applying longitudinal traction. Extend the fracture and manipulate with the thumbs to correct lateral tilt, medial impaction, or posterior displacement. Flex the elbow to between 90 and 100 degrees. Check anteroposterior and lateral reduction with the aid of an image intensifier.
- Insert a lateral pin across the fracture site and engage the medial cortex. If additional stability is needed insert a second or third lateral pin.
- For fractures with extreme instability a medial pin can be useful. After the two lateral pins are inserted, extend the elbow to 45 degrees of flexion. Make a medial incision to identify the medial epicondyle and ulnar nerve. Insert a medial pin across the fracture site to engage the lateral cortex.
- Cut off the pins outside the skin and bend or cover the pin tips.

TWO LATERAL PINS 〉

- Position the patient supine and use image intensification to determine the direction of displacement and the status of the soft tissues of the injured extremity.

- Supinate and pronate the forearm to tighten the lateral and medial soft tissue hinges. Flex and extend the elbow to tighten the posterior and anterior hinges.
- For the rare flexion supracondylar fracture with anterior displacement of the distal fragment, extend the elbow to obtain satisfactory closed reduction.
- For the more common extension type of supracondylar fracture, with countertraction on the humerus, apply traction to the forearm and examine the fracture with image intensification. Pronate or supinate the forearm to rotate the distal fragment into correct rotational alignment with the proximal fragment. Translate the distal fragment in a similar manner to correct medial or lateral displacement. While maintaining traction and precise forearm rotation, gently flex the elbow. Place gentle pressure on the olecranon as the elbow is flexed to correct posterior displacement of the distal fragment. Maximally flex the elbow and pronate the forearm to lock the posterior and medial soft tissue hinges.
- Confirm the anteroposterior reduction with image intensification by aiming the beam through the forearm and rotating the humerus from medial to lateral. Confirm lateral reduction by externally rotating the shoulder to obtain a lateral view of the elbow.

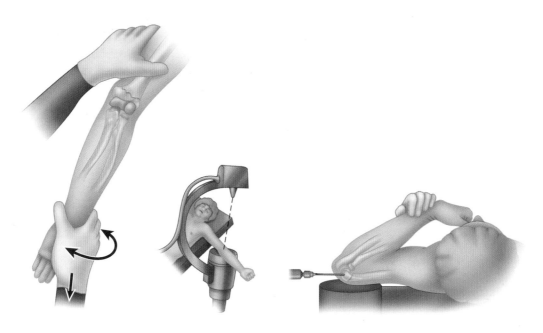

Figure 70-2

- Maintain reduction while performing closed percutaneous pinning with image intensification to verify that the two lateral pins engage both fracture fragments (Figure 70-2).
- After the pins are inserted extend the elbow as far as possible without bending the pins. With the aid of image intensification check the stability of the reduction by rotating and stressing the elbow to determine if a third (medial or lateral) pin is necessary. Compare the carrying angle with that of the normal extremity and obtain true anteroposterior radiographs of both forearms to judge the quality of reduction. Carefully position the arm with the medial and lateral epicondyles parallel to the cassette. Direct the x-ray beam to obtain a true anteroposterior view of the distal humerus. Use the Baumann angle to evaluate the quality of reduction further.

POSTOPERATIVE CARE

A long-arm posterior plaster splint or bivalved cast is worn for 3 weeks. Ulnar, radial, and median nerve function and vascular status should be checked after anesthesia. The pins are removed at 3 to 4 weeks and another posterior splint is applied. At 4 weeks the splint is removed and intermittent active range-of-motion exercises are started at home. These may be taught by the physical therapist to the child and the parent, explaining that the child is to carry out his or her own active range-of-motion program. Passive motion and forceful manipulative motion must be avoided in a child.

Most femoral shaft fractures in children can be stabilized using retrograde fixation. Three points of fixation, established around the fracture or the medullary canal, must be "stacked" with multiple nails at the fracture to prevent angulation. Usually medial and lateral insertion sites are used but a single insertion site, either medial or lateral, can be used in the distal femoral metaphysis. Two divergent C-configuration nails or one C-configuration and one S-configuration nail (bent by the surgeon at a point approximately 5 cm distal to the eyelet) are routine; two straight nails also can be used (Figure 71-1). Additional nails can be added if necessary. Special expertise is needed to stabilize subtrochanteric fractures and fractures of the distal third of the femur. Antegrade insertion commonly is used for the latter.

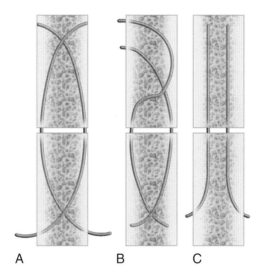

Figure 71-1   A   B   C

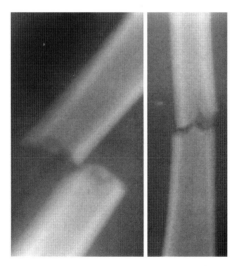

Figure 71-2

- Place the patient on an orthopaedic table and reduce the fracture partially by traction guided by fluoroscopy (Figure 71-2).

- Use blunt-ended nails of quality steel (cold-hammered at 140 degrees) or titanium. The nails should be 45 cm long with diameters of 3.0, 3.5, or 4.0 mm depending on the child's weight and age.
- Prepare the nails preoperatively by angling them at 45 degrees about 2 cm from one end to facilitate penetration of the medullary canal and bend them into an even curve over their entire length.

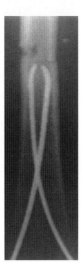

Figure 71-3

- With the help of a T-handle and by rotation movements of the wrist introduce the nails through a longitudinal drill hole, 4 to 5 mm in diameter, made in the distal femoral metaphysis just above the physis. Use two nails, one lateral and one medial, to stabilize the fracture. Carefully push both up the medullary canal to the already reduced fracture site. After touching the opposite internal cortex the nails bend themselves in the direction of the long bone's axis. The nails should cross distal to the fracture site (normally 4 to 6 cm distal) (Figure 71-3).

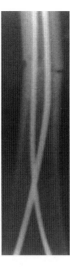

Figure 71-4

- Rotate the T-handle or manipulate the limb to direct the pins into the opposite fragment. If the first is impeded try the second with the aid of an image intensifier. Ensure both nails are in the canal across the fracture site. When they pass the fracture level release traction and push the nails farther, fixing their tips in the spongy tissue of the metaphysis without their passing through the physis. Small distractions can be corrected by rotation of the pins (Figure 71-4).

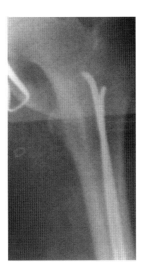

Figure 71-5

- Avoid residual angulation by ensuring that the nails are introduced at the same level so that they have identical curvatures (Figure 71-5).

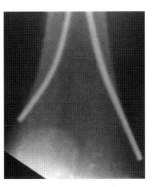

Figure 71-6

- Leave the distal portion of the nails slightly protruding for ease of removal (Figure 71-6).
- If the technique is performed correctly the fracture is finally stabilized by two nails, each with three points of fixation. The fixation is elastic but sufficiently stable to allow automatic small position corrections by limited movements during the limb's loading.

POSTOPERATIVE CARE

Postoperatively, the limb is rested on a pillow. A knee immobilizer may give more comfort. Mobilization using crutches without weight bearing is allowed as soon as the fracture causes no pain. A spica cast can be used if rotation or angulation is evident after the procedure. At the beginning of the third week partial weight bearing is allowed. After the appearance of calcified external callus full weight bearing is allowed. Nails are removed when the surgeon is positive that healing has occurred. Antibiotics are unnecessary after surgery unless infection or inflammation is present.

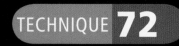
Expose the knee through the distal portion of an anteromedial parapatellar incision. Open the capsule medially to expose the fracture fragments and the defect in the proximal tibia.

- Examine the medial meniscus and with retraction examine the anterior horn of the lateral meniscus to ensure the menisci are not impeding the reduction. Place the knee in extension and reduce the fragment after any clots and cancellous bone have been removed from the defect.

- Drill two holes from distal to proximal through the tibial epiphysis. Take care to drill the holes proximal to the physis. The holes should enter the joint (1) just medial and lateral to the fracture fragments; or (2) into the defect and into the fragment itself if it is large enough.

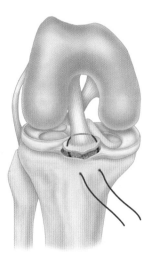

Figure 72-1

- Pass a 19-gauge or 18-gauge wire, or a 1-0 nonabsorbable suture through the most distal portion of the anterior cruciate ligament just proximal to the fracture fragment. With suture carriers pass the ends of the suture through the drill holes and tie them onto themselves after the reduction is satisfactory (Figure 72-1).

- Flex and extend the knee to ensure the reduction is stable. Irrigate and close the wound.

POSTOPERATIVE CARE

A cast is applied with the knee in full extension. At 4 to 6 weeks the cast is removed and range-of-motion exercises are started.

ARTHROSCOPIC REDUCTION OF TIBIAL EMINENCE FRACTURES AND INTERNAL FIXATION WITH BIOABSORBABLE NAILS

S. Terry Canale • James H. Beaty

Arthroscopic techniques can be used for reduction and fixation of tibial eminence fractures. An anterior cruciate ligament guide can be used to secure the reduction and for drill holes and suturing. Antegrade screws and bioabsorbable "smart" screws have been used for bone fixation.

- With a thigh tourniquet applied and inflated, perform standard knee arthroscopic examination through anteromedial and anterolateral portals.
- Remove the ligamentum mucosum and part of the infrapatellar fat pad to better expose the injured area.
- Remove fibrin clots and small fracture fragments from underneath the anterior tibial spine fragment and from the tibial crater.
- If the intermeniscal ligament is trapped in the fracture, interfering with reduction, free it with a probe.

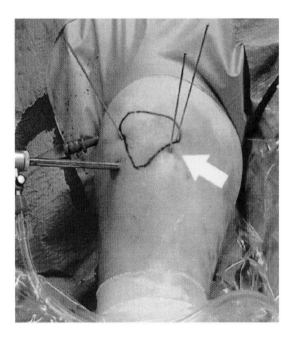

Figure 73-1

- With the knee flexed to 45 degrees, reduce the fragment with a probe and temporarily fix it with a 1.6-mm AO wire introduced through a midpatellar entrance close to the medial margin of the patella (Figure 73-1).
- Keeping as close as possible to the patella and slightly proximal to the AO wire, insert the drill guide into the joint and secure the fragment with bioabsorbable 1.5-mm SmartNails (ConMed Linvatec, Largo, FL). The polylactide polymer SmartNails are constructed proximally with a head and distally with barbs to provide compression during fracture healing.
- Place two or three nails through this entrance. If necessary, reinforce the fixation with one or two nails inserted from the corresponding lateral side of the patella. A total of three or four nails, 20- or 25-mm long, can be used.
- Close the portals in standard fashion and apply a cast with the knee in slight flexion.

POSTOPERATIVE CARE ❭

The cast is worn for 5 weeks, with full weight bearing with crutches allowed. After cast removal, patients complete a 2-month physical therapy program. Regular follow-up is continued until satisfactory knee motion is regained.

S. Terry Canale • James H. Beaty

Proximal tibial physeal fracture is rare and usually occurs in maturing adolescents, especially those engaged in athletics. The radiographs often show little evidence of injury, but the CT scan and tomograms can reveal significant displacement. The radiographs can give a false sense of security in an injury that can produce deformity and disability.

- Prepare the patient and drape the knee in the usual fashion. Inflate the tourniquet.
- Make a long medial or lateral parapatellar incision, depending on the location of the fracture. Carry the soft tissue dissection down to the fracture, and expose the fracture widely.

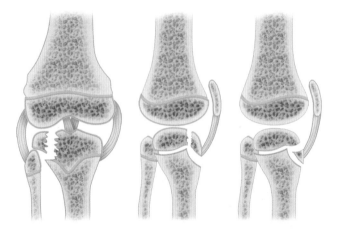

Figure 74-1

- The Salter-Harris type III or IV injury frequently is a tongue-type fracture anteriorly with the entire tibial tuberosity elevated and hinged posteriorly. Dissect medially and laterally into the joint until the physeal fracture is seen. It may be located in the midportion of the joint or posteriorly (Figure 74-1).
- Elevate the entire physeal fragment. Wash out any debris, and remove all soft tissues such as periosteum from the fracture so that the reduction is not impeded.
- Reduce the fracture anatomically. This should be similar to closing a hinge, and if any soft tissue is entrapped, the hinge will not close completely when the knee is extended. After the reduction, observe for joint congruity and reduction of the fracture at its peripheral margins.

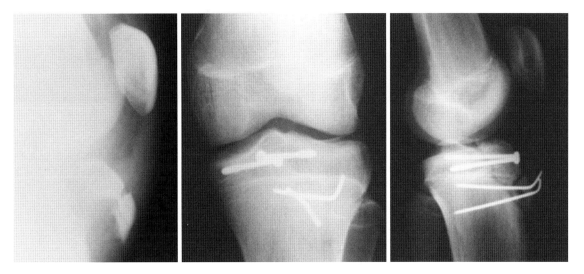

Figure 74-2

- In a vertical fracture, insert transverse pins for fixation. Threaded pins, screws, or cancellous bone screws can be used because the patient is usually an older child. In younger children, use smooth pins transversely or horizontally (Figure 74-2).
- Irrigate the wound copiously with saline, and close the wound in the usual manner. Apply a bent-knee cast.

POSTOPERATIVE CARE

The cast remains in place for 4 to 6 weeks. At 2 weeks, the cast is bivalved for removal of sutures and change of dressing. Gentle mobilization of the knee should be started between 4 and 6 weeks, depending on the age of the child.

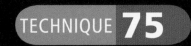

See also Video 75-1.

Currently, percutaneous in situ pinning is the most often used treatment for mild, moderate, and some severe slips of the capital femoral epiphysis. One screw generally is sufficient for stable slips, while unstable slips may require two screws for stable fixation.

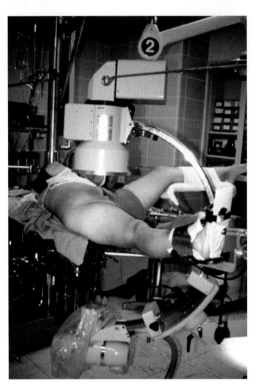

Figure 75-1

- Place the patient supine so that anteroposterior and lateral fluoroscopic views can be obtained without repositioning the patient or the extremity. A fracture table can be used. The entire proximal femoral epiphysis and hip joint space should be clearly visible on both views (Figure 75-1).

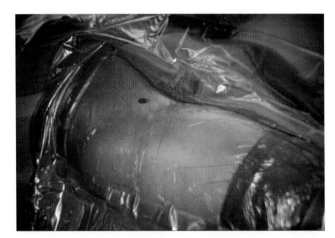

Figure 75-2

- Prepare and drape the extremity to allow free access to the entire anterior surface of the thigh and as far medially as the pubis in the inguinal area (Figure 75-2). A fluoroscopic C-arm is used for an anteroposterior and an exact lateral image. On the lateral view the femoral neck should be parallel to the femoral shaft.

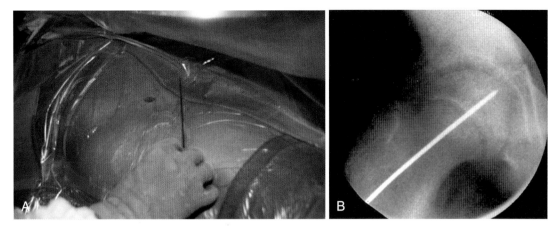

Figure 75-3

- Place a guidewire on the anterior aspect of the thigh (Figure 75-3, **A**) so that the anteroposterior image shows it in the desired varus-valgus position (**B**) and mark the position of the guidewire on the anterior surface of the thigh with a marking pen.

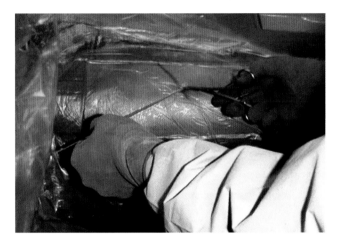

Figure 75-4

- Place the guidewire along the lateral aspect of the thigh so that it is in the correct anteroposterior position on the fluoroscopic image and mark the position of the wire on the skin (Figure 75-4). In SCFE, the epiphysis is displaced posteriorly relative to the femoral neck and this lateral guidewire angles from anterior to posterior and appears on the fluoroscopic image to enter at the anterior femoral neck. The two skin lines should intersect on the anterolateral aspect of the thigh. The greater the degree of the slip (the more posterior the epiphysis) the more anterior the intersection.

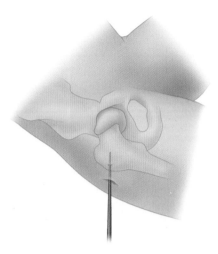

Figure 75-5

- As an alternative, insert a Kirschner wire percutaneously through the anterolateral area of the thigh down to the femoral neck, adjusting the guidwire on the anteroposterior projection to determine the axis of the femoral neck. Obtain a lateral view to determine the amount of posterior inclination necessary (Figure 75-5).

- Place a guidewire, drill, or pin through a small lateral incision or a simple stab (puncture) wound at the intersection of the two skin lines. Monitor proper alignment, position, and depth of insertion in the proximal femoral epiphysis on anteroposterior and lateral fluoroscopic images. Take care not to bend, kink, or notch the guidewire to avoid interosseous breakage.

- When the starting point on the femoral neck and amount of posterior inclination have been estimated, insert the guide assembly through a small puncture wound. Advance the guide assembly to the physis, and confirm placement in the central axis of the femoral head by image intensification. If the position is correct, advance the guide assembly across the plate (if positioning is incorrect, insert a second guide assembly using the first to determine what correction in the starting point or angulation is necessary). When the proper depth is reached (at least 0.5 cm from subchondral bone) remove the cannula and leave the guidewire in the bone.

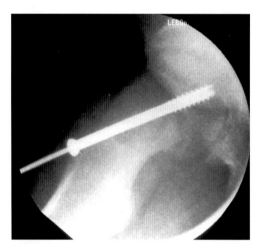

Figure 75-6

- Determine the correct screw length by passing a guidewire of identical length along the one in the bone and measuring the difference. Advance the correct length screw over the guide pin and remove the pin (Figure 75-6).

- Remove the leg from the traction device, and move it in multiple directions using anteroposterior and lateral views to confirm that the screw does not penetrate the joint. If two screws are deemed necessary for an acute slip, the first screw should lie in the central axis of the femoral head and the second below it avoiding the superolateral quadrant. The second screw should stop at least 8 mm from the subchondral bone.

- Close the stab wound with a single subcuticular suture.

POSTOPERATIVE CARE 〉

Range-of-motion exercises should begin the day after surgery. Most patients begin walking with a three-point partial weight-bearing crutch gait on the first day after surgery and are discharged the same day. Crutches are used until all signs of synovitis are gone and motion is free and painless (usually 2 to 3 weeks). For unstable slips partial weight bearing is maintained with crutches for 6 to 8 weeks. All rigorous sports and other activities are limited until the physes have closed. Screw removal is not necessary but the screws can be removed after physeal closure has been shown radiographically. The easiest method of removal is to pass a guidewire into the cannula of the screw under image control to allow the screwdriver to be guided into the head of the screw over the guidewire. Because of surgical problems and complications the screws are not routinely removed.

FLEXOR TENDON REPAIR
David L. Cannon

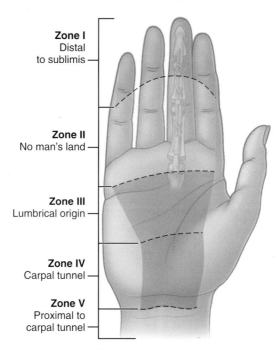

Zone I
Distal
to sublimis

Zone II
No man's land

Zone III
Lumbrical origin

Zone IV
Carpal tunnel

Zone V
Proximal to
carpal tunnel

Figure 76-1

The preparations and techniques for repair of flexor tendons vary from zone to zone (Figure 76-1). As a rule, flexor tendons should be repaired at whatever level they are severed.

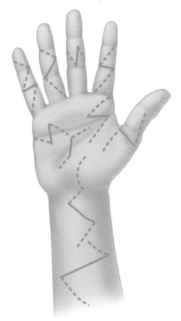

Figure 76-2

- Exposures for primary suture of tendons. Solid lines indicate examples of skin lacerations and broken lines show direction in which they can be enlarged to obtain additional exposure (Figure 76-2).

ZONE I 〉

- When the flexor profundus tendon has been injured in zone I at or near its insertion, approach the distal end of the finger by extending the laceration with an oblique incision into the central portion of the pulp or through a midradial or midulnar incision.
- Avoid injury to the terminal branches of the digital nerve and avoid devascularizing any skin flaps that are elevated. Usually the insertion of the flexor profundus is easily seen. At times the proximal stump of the tendon will have retracted very minimally.

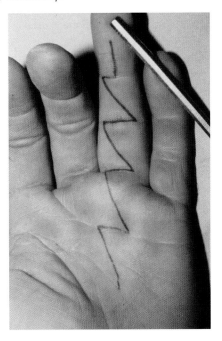

Figure 76-3

- Extend the incision proximally using a volar zigzag (Bruner), midradial, midulnar, or midline oblique incision. Avoid injury to the neurovascular bundles (Figure 76-3).
- Elevate the skin flap by going either dorsal or volar to the neurovascular bundle.

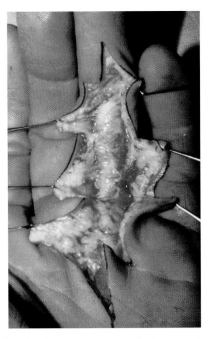

Figure 76-4

- Expose the fibroosseous flexor sheath. If the proximal end of the tendon can be seen, attempt to deliver it into the wound by grasping it with a small forceps such as an Adson or a finer tissue forceps. If the tendon has retracted more proximally, extend the incision as needed in a midradial or a midulnar incision or by extending the skin incision in a volar zigzag or midline oblique incision, avoiding injury to the neurovascular bundle (Figure 76-4).

- Open the thin cruciform portion of the sheath to assist in delivering the tendon. Open the sheath by an L-shaped incision or with a trapdoor with a Z-plasty arrangement to allow easier closure if needed.
- If the tendon has retracted, place a grasping suture in its end using one of the techniques previously described. When opening the flexor sheath over the middle phalanx it is important to preserve the A4 pulley. If the flexor tendon cannot be maintained in such a way that it can be repaired easily, insert a small-gauge (25-gauge or 26-gauge) hypodermic needle, Keith needle, or Bunnell needle through the skin through the tendon, and out the skin on the opposite side of the finger as a temporary tendon retention device. These needles are removed when the tendon repair has been accomplished.
- Although a pull-out wire of the Bunnell type can be attached in such an arrangement it is not always necessary, especially if the antegrade pull-out wire technique is used as opposed to the Bunnell retrograde pull-out technique.
- Using straight needles, pass the suture out through the distal pulp of the finger, usually exiting just palmar to the hyponychium.
- As an alternative, the proximal end of the tendon can be attached distally using a pull-out technique in which a tunnel is drilled in bone and the needles are passed through the tunnel and out through the fingernail or around the distal phalanx. A 4-0 suture is usually used.

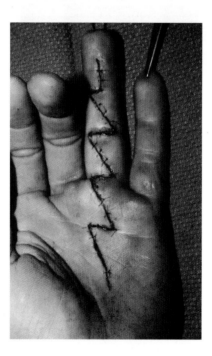

Figure 76-5

- After ascertaining satisfactory rotation and attachment of the tendon, close the wound with fine 4-0 or 5-0 monofilament nylon sutures (Figure 76-5).

ZONE II ⟩

- In zone II the wound must usually be extended with proximal and distal incisions. Regardless of which approach is used, carefully reflect the skin flaps and avoid injury to neurovascular structures during the dissection.
- If digital nerves have been transected gently dissect them and delay their repair until after the tendons are repaired to avoid disruption.

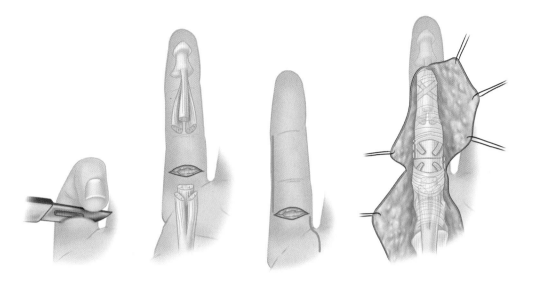

Figure 76-6

- Expose the flexor sheath in the area of injury sufficiently proximal and distal to allow location of the tendon ends. As indicated previously, the distal tendon end can usually be identified easily with passive flexion of the distal interphalangeal joint. Avoid injury to the sheath, particularly the A2 and A4 pulleys (Figure 76-6).

- If opening of the flexor sheath is required, this is best done in the filamentous cruciate areas of the sheath. Small openings in the sheath can be made in the distal tendon insertion, C2 and C3, and C1 areas where the sheath is filamentous. These openings can be made in several configurations. An L-shaped opening allows ease of closure and facilitates passage of the tendon through the sheath (Lister). If several days have passed and the tendon sheaths are contracting, opening the sheath with a Z-lengthening configuration helps to allow partial closure of the sheath in difficult situations.

- Deliver the flexor tendon into the finger by milking the forearm, hand, and wrist and flexing the wrist and fingers to allow the proximal end to be delivered if possible. If it cannot be delivered easily, a transverse incision at the distal palmar crease may be necessary to locate the tendon in the palm.

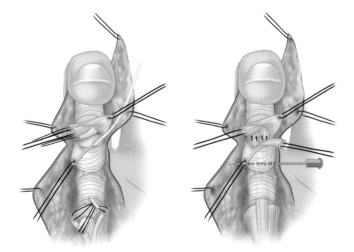

Figure 76-7

- When the proximal end of the tendon has been identified, place a core suture using the definitive suture material in a locking fashion so that the suture material can be used for traction in passing the suture through the sheath (Figure 76-7).

- In a fresh, acute injury, passage of the tendon is usually not difficult. After several days tendon edema and sheath contracture may require additional techniques. The proximal end of the tendon can be passed easily through the sheath and between the slips of the sublimis using a piece of pediatric feeding tubing or plastic intravenous connecting tubing, as recommended by Lister.

- Deliver the tubing into the flexor sheath between the slips of the sublimis.
- Pass the suture into the tubing. Clamp the tubing with the suture within it and "lead" the flexor tendon through the sheath following the plastic tubing and suture.
- As an alternative method, fashion a 20- or 22-gauge wire into a loop and pass it proximally in the sheath to use as a snare for the suture, which is delivered through the sheath followed by the tendon. The tendon also can be sutured to tubing of various types and delivered following the tubing through the sheath as well.
- When the proximal end of the tendon has been delivered to the area of repair secure it in the sheath using a transverse 25- or 26-gauge hypodermic needle for temporary fixation with little or no long-term harmful effects. This is used as a temporary stabilizing device.
- Stabilize the distal end of the tendon in a similar way.
- Introduce the core suture using a four-strand to eight-strand method. Care should be taken at this point to ensure that the profundus tendon is not malrotated. Reference to the vincular attachment and the relationship to the sublimis is helpful in this regard.

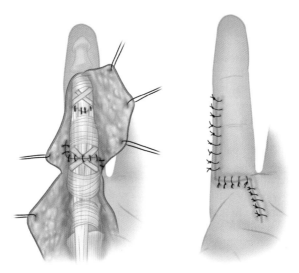

Figure 76-8

- Tie the knots and complete the tendon repair with circumferential 5-0 or 6-0 nylon inverting suture or cross-stitch to minimize exposure of the cut surface of the tendon (Figure 76-8).
- If the flexor sublimis has been transected just proximal to the proximal interphalangeal joint, take care regarding the arrangement of its slips of the sublimis and the so-called flexor digitorum sublimis "spiral". The flexor digitorum sublimis winds around the profundus tendon after it divides at the metacarpophalangeal joint. It inserts into the volar surface of the middle phalanx after decussating. This allows the superficial portion of the sublimis tendon to become deep in the chiasma of Camper. A laceration in this area allows the proximal and distal ends of the sublimis tendons to rotate 90 degrees in opposite directions. The tendon lies in *apparently* satisfactory alignment; however, if it is sutured in this alignment it causes binding of the flexor profundus tendon.
- An additional technical problem can be encountered if the flexor sublimis tendon has been transected more distally, near the proximal interphalangeal joint or its insertion. Here the tendon is quite thin and it is difficult to achieve satisfactory placement of core sutures. Try to place a locked core suture in the tendon because a simple repair with 5-0 or 6-0 nylon would be insufficient to prevent rupture. Use small suture anchors to repair the sublimis if the bone and working space permit secure insertion.
- Sometimes it can be extremely difficult technically to accomplish a flexor sublimis repair. Although most surgeons recommend against sublimis excision, if in the surgeon's judgment sublimis repair cannot be satisfactorily accomplished, or such repair would compromise profundus function, excise the sublimis tendon in the area.
- Usually the sublimis tendon is repaired before the profundus tendon. Tie the knots; use the circumferential 6-0 nylon sutures as needed; and repair the sheath, conditions permitting, with 5-0 or 6-0 nylon.

- Close the wound with interrupted 5-0 nylon and remove the temporary retaining needle.
- Avoid hyperextension of the finger and immobilize the hand in a padded compression dressing with the fingers and the thumb immobilized with a dorsal splint.
- Splint the wrist in 45 to 50 degrees of flexion; splint the fingers in flexion at the metacarpophalangeal joints to 50 to 60 degrees with the proximal and distal interphalangeal joints extended.
- If one or more pulleys are damaged and cannot be repaired they should be reconstructed at the time of primary tendon repair to avoid bowstringing and restriction of motion.
- The flexor sheath/pulley reconstruction can be protected with orthotic thermoplastic rings during postoperative rehabilitation of the flexor tendon and while the patient is regaining motion.

ZONE III ⟩

- In zone III the area between the distal edge of the transverse carpal ligament and the proximal portion of the A1 pulley, perform flexor tendon repair in a manner similar to zone II repair. Incisions that extend the wound proximally and distally may be required. Avoid crossing flexion creases at right angles. Also avoid injuring neurovascular structures and devascularizing the skin flaps.
- Achieve proper orientation of the tendon before repair. At times, if tendons have retracted into the carpal tunnel or more proximally, partial release of the transverse carpal ligament may be required to deliver them distally into the palm.
- Although the flexor sheath is not involved in the palm, be careful in the placement of sutures. It is probably best to use an intratendinous core suture in the palm to avoid exposure of the suture material to adjacent structures. Satisfactory healing and functional results can be expected after repair of the tendons in the palm.
- Apply a compressive, bulky dressing and immobilize the thumb, fingers, and wrist. Immobilize the wrist at about 45 degrees of flexion with the fingers at about 50 to 60 degrees of flexion and the interphalangeal joints extended.

ZONE IV ⟩

- In zone IV, the area of the carpal tunnel, an injury directly to the base of the palm usually also involves the median nerve. If a laceration occurs just proximal to the wrist flexion crease, especially with the fingers flexed, flexor tendon injury in zone IV should be suspected.
- Extend the laceration distally into the palm and proximally into the forearm taking care to cross flexion creases obliquely. If the laceration occurs beneath the transverse carpal ligament, partial or complete release of the transverse carpal ligament may be required.
- Preserve, if possible, a portion of the transverse carpal ligament to avoid bowstringing postoperatively.
- If it cannot be preserved, release it in a Z-lengthening configuration so that it can be repaired and help minimize the risk of postoperative bowstringing.
- Repair the flexor profundus and sublimis tendons in the carpal tunnel; probably the best suture configuration is an intratendinous one with a locking core suture to hold the tendons with minimal exposure of cut surface and suture material.
- In the carpal tunnel ensure proper orientation and location of the individual tendons. The usual arrangement of the flexor sublimis tendons in the carpal tunnel, with the middle and ring finger tendons superficial to the index and small finger tendons, is helpful to recall in this situation. Partial tenosynovectomy may be required to diminish the bulky and edematous tissue that may follow the repair.
- Close the skin with 4-0 nylon and apply the bandage and dorsal splint to maintain the wrist in approximately 45 degrees of flexion.
- If the transverse carpal ligament has been completely released and repair is impossible, bring the wrist to nearly neutral and flex the fingers more acutely to diminish pressure on the volar skin and to minimize bowstringing.
- If the transverse carpal ligament is partially intact or has been repaired, immobilize the wrist in about 45 degrees of flexion with the fingers in 50 to 60 degrees of flexion at the metacarpophalangeal joints and the interphalangeal joints in full extension.

ZONE V ⟩

- In zone V the volar forearm proximal to the transverse carpal ligament, multiple tendons, nerves, and vessels are frequently injured by major lacerations, often from broken glass or in violent altercations with knives. In this area it is important to identify the tendons accurately.

- Because of their common muscle origin, when the sublimis and profundus tendons are divided, particularly at the wrist, they can be delivered into the wound as a group by finding and pulling distally on one tendon.

- Properly match the tendon ends by careful attention to their location and level in the wound, their relation to neighboring structures, their diameters, the shape of their cross sections, and the angle of the cuts through each tendon. Although it is not a disgrace to open an anatomy book in the operating room to be certain of anatomical relationships, it is inexcusable to sew the median nerve to the flexor pollicis longus, the palmaris longus, or some other tendon.

- The proximal and distal ends of the median nerve can usually be identified easily in their appropriate anatomical location and from their more yellowish color and the presence of a volar midline vessel and the nerve fascicles, which can usually be identified in the median nerve's severed ends.

- Although 4-0 sutures usually are used in the palm and more distally, 3-0 nylon may be sufficient for suturing tendons in the distal forearm. Repairs done in the distal forearm do not absolutely require an intra-tendinous repair. A double right-angled or mattress suture may be satisfactory in the forearm.

- Repair nerves and vessels if needed after the tendon repairs in the forearm, working from the repair of deep structures to more superficial structures.

- Close the wounds with 4-0 nylon and immobilize the limb with the wrist flexed approximately 45 degrees and the metacarpophalangeal joints flexed 50 to 60 degrees with the interphalangeal joints in full extension.

POSTOPERATIVE CARE

Excellent results can be achieved using either of two postoperative mobilization techniques. In one (Kleinert), active finger extension is used with passive flexion achieved using a rubber band attached to the fingernail and at the wrist (Figure 76-9). This is subsequently modified with a roller in the palm to alter the line of force of the rubber band.

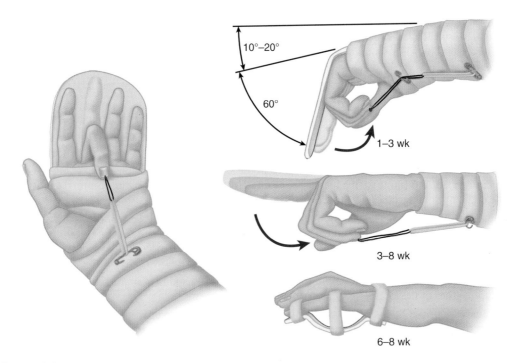

10°–20°

60°

1–3 wk

3–8 wk

6–8 wk

Figure 76-9

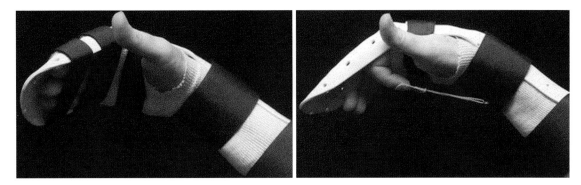

Figure 76-10

The second technique (Duran) involves a controlled passive motion technique with dorsal blocking of the fingers (Figure 76-10). The margin of safety with early passive motion rehabilitation is increased if the tendon repairs have been done with the stronger multistrand techniques (four or more). Multistrand repairs are used if an early active motion program is considered. Children younger than approximately 10 years old and noncompliant patients cannot be entrusted with understanding and following the complexities of either of these techniques, and a more conservative postoperative management routine should be selected, depending on the judgment of the surgeon and the therapist.

James H. Calandruccio

Surgical procedures commonly used in treating Dupuytren contracture are (1) subcutaneous fasciotomy, (2) partial (selective) fasciectomy, (3) complete fasciectomy, (4) fasciectomy with skin grafting, (5) amputation, and (6) joint resection and arthrodesis. The appropriate procedure depends on the degree of contracture, nutritional status of the palmar skin, the presence or absence of bony deformities, and the patient's age, occupation, and general health. The least extensive procedure, subcutaneous fasciotomy, commonly is used for elderly patients who are not concerned with the appearance of the disease or in patients who have poor general health. The results of this procedure are better in the residual phase when dense, mature cords are present than when the lesions are more immature and diffuse. Partial (selective) fasciectomy usually is indicated when only the ulnar one or two fingers are involved.

SUBCUTANEOUS FASCIOTOMY ⟩

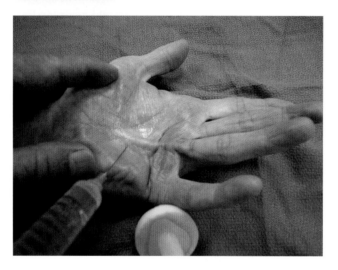

Figure 77-1

- Using a pointed scalpel, make skin puncture wounds on the ulnar side of the diseased palmar fascia at the following levels: (1) just distal to the apex of the palmar fascia between the thenar and hypothenar eminences, (2) at or near the level of the proximal palmar crease, and (3) at the level of the distal palmar crease. Digital nerves are more likely to be cut at the distal palm where they become more superficial and may be intertwined with the diseased tissue (Figure 77-1).

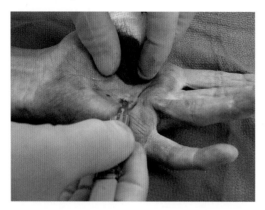

Figure 77-2

- Insert a small tenotomy knife or a fasciotome (Luck) that resembles a myringotome, with its blade parallel with the palm, through each of the puncture wounds. A 15- or 11-blade scalpel works satisfactorily for this purpose. Pass the cutting instrument across the palm beneath the skin but superficial to the fascia (Figure 77-2).

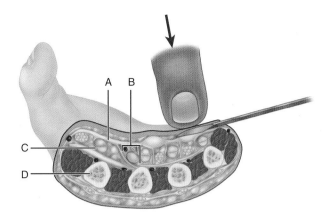

Figure 77-3

- Turn the edge of the blade dorsally toward the palmar fascia, and extend the fingers to tighten the involved tissue. Carefully divide the fascial cords by pressing the blade onto the tense cords with gentle pressure over the blade or at most a gentle rocking motion; never use a sawing motion. Whenever a cord is divided, the sense of gritty, firm resistance disappears, indicating that the blade has passed completely through the diseased fascia. (Figure 77-3; **A**, palmar fascia; **B**, neurovascular bundle; **C**, flexor tendons; **D**, metacarpal.)

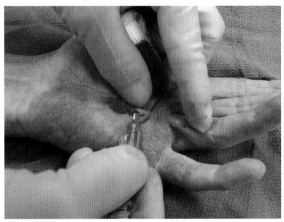 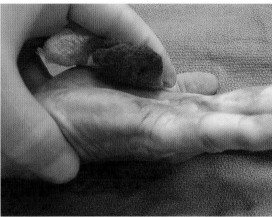

Figure 77-4

- Using the fasciotome or scalpel blade in a plane parallel with the skin, free the latter from the underlying fascia. The corrugated skin, although very thin at times, can be safely undermined and released as necessary with little fear of skin necrosis (Figure 77-4).
- In the fingers, subcutaneous fasciotomy is safe only for a fascial cord located in the midline. Insert the blade through a puncture wound adjacent to the cord, and divide it obliquely.
- For a laterally placed cord, use a short longitudinal incision, and excise or divide the diseased segment under direct vision. Also enucleate larger nodules in both fingers and palm under direct vision.

POSTOPERATIVE CARE ⟩

A pressure dressing is used for 24 hours; then a smaller dressing is applied, and active range of motion of the hand and fingers is encouraged. A night splint that conforms to the contracture correction is worn for 3 months, and progressive extension splinting and a formal physical therapy program often enhance the final result.

PARTIAL FASCIECTOMY ❭

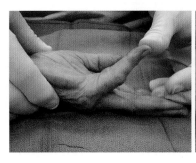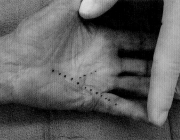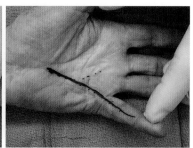

Figure 77-5

- Outline the proposed incision with a marking pen before inflation of the tourniquet. Take into consideration the pits and other areas of skin with diminished vascularity by making an incision over or near these areas, avoiding their presence at the base of a flap. These areas sometimes can be excised when the final rotation of the skin takes place in closure (Figure 77-5).
- Make a vertical or zigzag incision over the deforming pathological structure. Zigzag incisions tend to straighten out, causing tension lines at the creases; however, the flaps created by zigzag incisions may heal more securely. Design the Z-plasty flaps so that a transverse segment is within or near each joint crease.
- Continue the incision proximally into the palm, avoiding crossing the palmar creases at right angles.

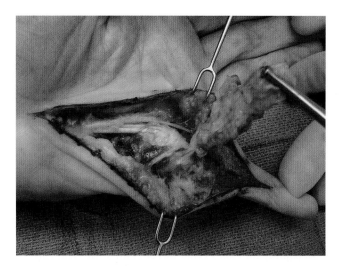

Figure 77-6

- Elevate the skin and underlying normal subcutaneous tissue from the pathological fascia from proximal to distal (Figure 77-6).

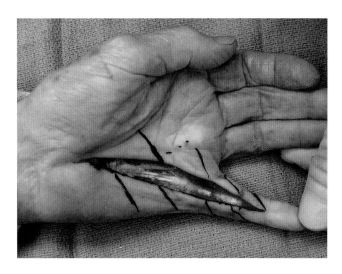

Figure 77-7

- Create the Z-plasty flaps when the wound is ready for closure (Figure 77-7).
- Excise the pathological fascia proximal to distal, taking great care to isolate and protect the neurovascular bundles of each finger. Carefully cauterize small bleeding points. Excision of superficial transverse palmar fascial fibers may be unnecessary. Avoid entering tendon sheaths if possible because bleeding into the flexor tendon sheaths may cause adhesions.
- Carefully excise the pathological fascia by sharp dissection. Avoid cutting displaced digital nerves by locating each nerve in the fatty pad at the level of the metacarpophalangeal joint and following it distally.
- Excise the natatory ligament if it is contracted.
- Follow all the contracted fascial cords to their distal insertions. Insertions may be into tendon sheaths, bone, and skin; occasionally, they are dorsolateral to the proximal interphalangeal joint.
- When excision of the diseased tissue has been completed, all joints should permit full passive extension unless capsular contractures exist.

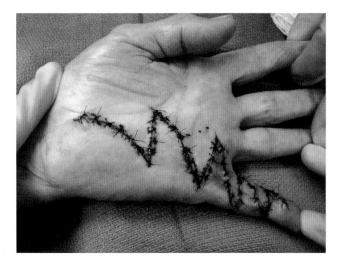

Figure 77-8

- Fashion the skin flaps. If there is any extra skin, the pitted or thinned areas can be excised (Figure 77-8).
- Before closing, elevate the hand, compress the wound, release the tourniquet, hold for 10 minutes, and check for and control bleeding.
- Using skin hooks and with minimal handling of the flaps, suture them in place with 4-0 or 5-0 monofilament nylon. Place few sutures in the palm to allow necessary drainage around a rubber drain.

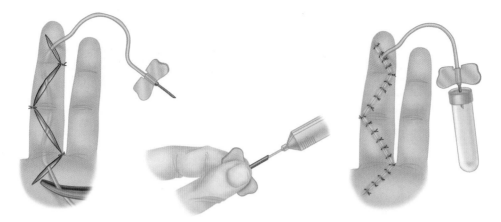

Figure 77-9

- Alternatively, a closed suction drainage system can be constructed with the use of butterfly catheters and Vacutainer tubes. One catheter tube for each operated finger provides adequate and efficient drainage. The likelihood of a flare reaction occurring 4 to 6 weeks postoperatively may be decreased by infusing 15 to 20 mg of betamethasone (Celestone) into the catheters before connecting the Vacutainer tubes. This also seems to decrease the amount of postoperative discomfort, decreasing the need for narcotic analgesics in many patients even after complex fasciectomies (Figure 77-9).
- Apply a layer of nonadherent gauze and a moist dressing compressed gently against the wound to conform to the contours of the palm and fingers. Apply a compression dressing over this, and use a volar plaster splint to maintain the fingers in the degree of extension achieved at surgery.

POSTOPERATIVE CARE

Drains usually are removed within 24 to 48 hours after surgery. The hand is kept elevated for a minimum of 48 hours. Early proximal interphalangeal motion is encouraged. The shoulder is moved actively at intervals during this period to avoid cramping. If there is undue pain in the hand or fever after 48 hours, the wound should be inspected. If a hematoma is found elevating the skin, it should be evacuated and the involved area of the wound should be left open. Otherwise, the first dressing change is done 3 to 5 days after surgery, and range-of-motion exercises are begun. A resting pan splint is fitted with the fingers in maximal extension to be worn at night.

At 2 weeks, the sutures are removed and the hand is left free of all dressings. The patient is warned not to place the hand in a dependent position for rest and not to soak the hand in hot water. Active exercise in warm water is permissible, but no passive stretching is allowed. Moderate use of the hand is permitted at 3 weeks; however, several months of rehabilitation may be necessary. The resting pan splint is worn for 3 months after surgery. Silicone putty may be a valuable adjunct to an exercise program.

Chronic proximal interphalangeal joint contractures of more than 60 degrees may have central slip attenuation. If a tenodesis test is positive (failure of the proximal interphalangeal joint to extend fully with full wrist and metacarpophalangeal joint in full passive flexion), proximal interphalangeal joint splinting for 3 weeks postoperatively may be indicated. During these 3 weeks, distal interphalangeal joint exercises are performed to mobilize the lateral bands dorsally.

Percutaneous pinning after closed reduction is useful for distal radial fractures with metaphyseal instability or simpler intraarticular displacement. An anatomical reduction must be obtained first, and then stability is provided by the Kirschner wires. Usually the first pins are placed from the radial styloid across to the medial radial metaphysis and diaphysis. We generally use at least two pins and confirm adequate reduction on anteroposterior and lateral views. The lunate facet can then pinned into position if needed.

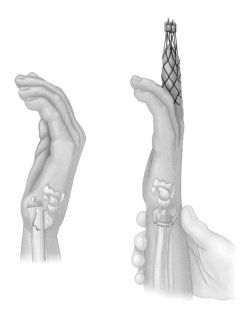

Figure 78-1

- After sterile preparation and draping, place the thumb and index fingers in finger traps for longitudinal traction (typically 10 lb). Manipulate and reduce the fracture (Figure 78-1).
- Evaluate the reduction fluoroscopically; if adequate, proceed with percutaneous pinning. If the reduction is not anatomical or if there is severe comminution, alternative techniques such as an open reduction internal fixation (ORIF) may be indicated.

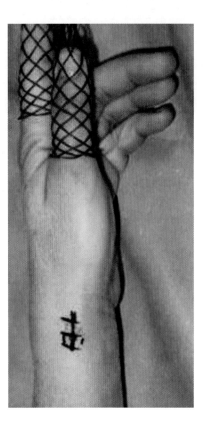

Figure 78-2

- Make a 1.5-cm incision longitudinally beginning at the radial styloid and proceeding distally (Figure 78-2).
- Identify the branches of the superficial radial nerve, mobilize them with blunt dissection, and retract them.
- Identify the first extensor compartment and place two 1.6-mm (0.062-in) Kirschner wires in succession from the radial styloid across the fracture site to engage the ulnar cortex of the radius proximal to the fracture. Place these wires either dorsal or volar to the first extensor compartment depending on fracture pattern and anatomical variations.

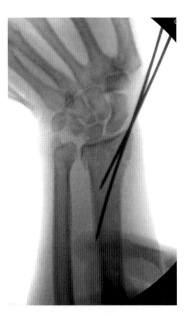

Figure 78-3

- Place one 1.6-mm Kirschner wire percutaneously 90 degrees orthogonally to these wires starting at the dorsal rim of the distal radius just distal to the Lister tubercle. Confirm the correct starting point with fluoroscopy and drive the wire in a proximal and volar direction across the fracture site to engage the volar cortex of the radius proximal to the fracture (Figure 78-3).

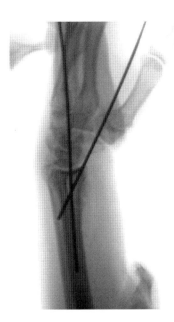

Figure 78-4

- If there is marked dorsal comminution a second dorsal pin can be placed either into the dorsal rim of the distal radius or used as an intrafocal pin. If there is marked radial comminution and prereduction radial translation an additional buttress pin can be placed into the radial aspect of the fracture and driven into the proximal ulnar cortex of the radius. A crossed-pin configuration, in which the pins are placed from the distal ulnar radial cortex and passed to engage the intact cortex radially, also may be helpful (Figure 78-4).
- Place additional wires as necessary to secure additional fracture fragments.
- Bend and cut the wires leaving them superficial to the skin. Close the radial styloid incision with interrupted absorbable sutures. Apply a sugar-tong splint.

POSTOPERATIVE CARE 〉

The splint is worn for 2 weeks to control rotation and minimize irritation at the pin sites and then a soft arm cast is applied. The cast and pins are removed at between 5 and 6 weeks depending on the fracture pattern, the patient's age and bone quality, and the extent of healing seen on radiographs. When healing is confirmed by lack of tenderness over the fracture and radiographic evidence of bridging callus across the fracture, supervised hand therapy is begun, including wound care and 1 to 2 weeks of splinting. As edema and pain decrease, soft tissue and joint mobilization protocols are instituted and active and active-assisted range-of-motion exercises are begun. Functional use and activities are strongly encouraged by 8 to 10 weeks after surgery.

Several clinical studies have reported better functional results with volar plating than with dorsal plating, external fixation, and percutaneous pinning; however, a complication rate of approximately 15% also has been reported with volar plating, primarily problems with tendon ruptures and tenosynovitis from prominent screws. Precise volar plate placement on the metaphyseal area of the distal radius may lessen the problems of flexor tendon irritation and eventual rupture.

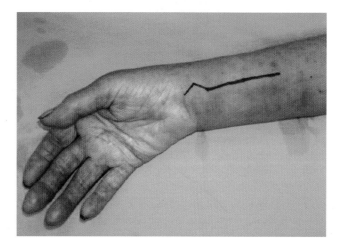

Figure 79-1

- Make an 8-cm incision over the forearm between the radial artery and the flexor carpi radialis. Extension of the incision distally at the wrist crease in a V-shape may provide wider exposure of the fracture and help prevent scar contracture. The distal incision does not need to cross into the palm (Figure 79-1).

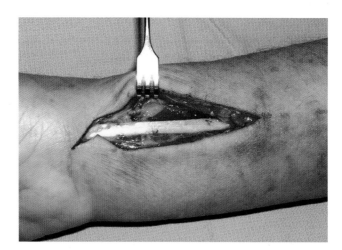

Figure 79-2

- Carry the incision to the sheath of the flexor carpi radialis. Open the sheath and incise the forearm deep fascia to expose the flexor pollicis longus (Figure 79-2).

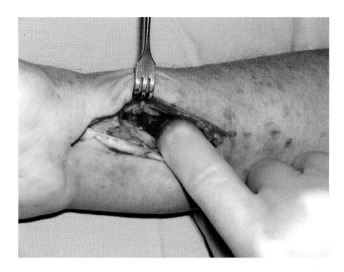

Figure 79-3

- Place an index finger into the wound and gently sweep the flexor pollicis longus ulnarly. Partially detach the flexor pollicis longus muscle belly from the radius to gain full exposure of the pronator quadratus (Figure 79-3).

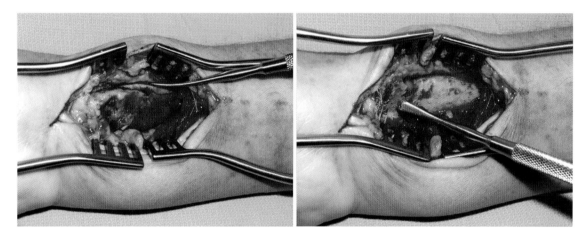

Figure 79-4

- Make an L-shaped incision over the radial styloid along the radial border of the radius to expose the pronator quadratus and use a Freer elevator to elevate it from the radius. The entire fracture line across the distal radius is now fully exposed (Figure 79-4).
- Insert a Freer elevator or small osteotome into the fracture line to serve as a lever to reduce the fracture. Insert the elevator or osteotome across the fracture line all the way to the dorsal cortex to allow disimpaction and reduction of the distal fragment. Apply finger pressure to the dorsal cortex to reduce the dorsal fragments.
- With a displaced radial styloid fracture the brachioradialis may prevent reduction by pulling on the radial styloid. To relieve the deforming force, the brachioradialis can be transected or detached from the distal radius.
- If necessary, use a Kirschner wire to temporarily fix the distal fragment to the proximal fragment. This usually is not necessary because distal traction should maintain reduction while the volar plate is placed.

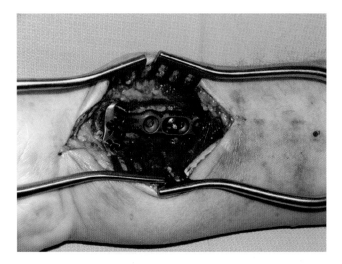

Figure 79-5

- Disimpact and reduce the fracture through capsuloligamentotaxis achieved by an assistant through finger traction. After successful fracture reduction, position the volar plate under fluoroscopic guidance and insert a screw into the oblong or gliding hole first to allow proximal-distal adjustment. Use a 2.5-mm drill bit to drill into the center of the oblong hole and insert a self-tapping 3.5-mm screw (Figure 79-5).
- Confirm proper placement of the volar plate with mini-C-arm fluoroscopy. If necessary, shift the plate proximally or distally to provide the best placement for the distal screws.
- Use a 2.0-mm drill bit to drill the distal holes. Measure the holes for screw length and insert smooth locking screws. Use a screw that is 2 mm shorter than the measured length to avoid having a prominent distal screw perforate the dorsal cortex; typically, 20- to 22-mm screws are optimal, except for screws directed into the radial styloid, which are significantly shorter. Threaded screws may gain better good bone dorsally; pegs may be sufficient when bone quality is poor.

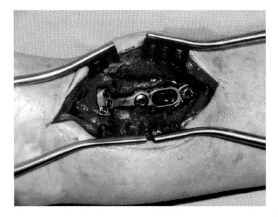

Figure 79-6

- Once the first screw is inserted, distal traction on the fingers can be released because the fracture usually is appropriately reduced and fixed (Figure 79-6).
- Because of the fixed angle design, the screws may perforate into the radiocarpal joint if the plate is placed too far distally. Obtain fluoroscopic views tangential to the subchondral bone in both the coronal sagittal planes to assess for intraarticular penetration. Adjust the plate or screws or both as indicated.

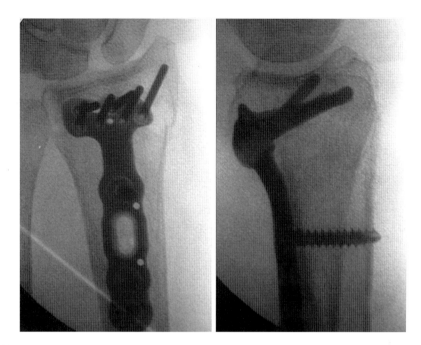

Figure 79-7

- After placement of the distal screws place the remaining proximal screws (Figure 79-7).

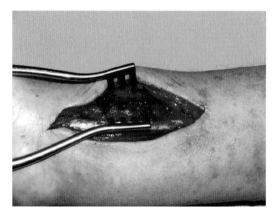

Figure 79-8

- Reattach the pronator quadratus with braided absorbable sutures. Note that the pronator will not be able to cover the entire plate; the distal portion should be covered when possible to reduce flexor tendon-plate contact. For better purchase, the pronator quadratus can be sutured to the edge of the brachioradialis (Figure 79-8).
- If the ulnar styloid is fractured and displaced, making the distal radioulnar joint unstable, fix the styloid with one or two percutaneous Kirschner wires. A volar approach may be helpful to obtain ulnar styloid reduction. Smaller fragments usually do not require surgical management; however, if the distal radioulnar joint is unstable after fixation of the radial fracture, styloid fragments can be excised and the peripheral rim of the triangular fibrocartilage complex anchored to the ulnar styloid base with nonabsorbable braided suture through drill holes or a bone anchor.
- Close the wound in layers and apply a splint.

POSTOPERATIVE CARE 〉

At 1 week, the sutures are removed and active wrist motion is begun when there is confidence in fracture stability. A removable Orthoplast splint is worn for 6 weeks. Most patients are given a home therapy program but elderly patients may require twice-a-week supervised home therapy.

See also Video 80-1.

Treatment of scaphoid fractures is determined by displacement and stability of the fracture. Operative treatment generally is required for displaced, unstable fractures in which the fragments are offset more than 1 mm in the anteroposterior or oblique view, lunocapitate angulation is more than 15 degrees, or the scapholunate angulation is more than 45 degrees in the lateral view (range 30 to 60 degrees). Reduction can be attempted initially by longitudinal traction and slight radial compression of the carpus. If the reduction attempt is successful, percutaneous fixation with a cannulated screw or pins and application of a long-arm thumb spica cast may suffice. Otherwise, open reduction and internal fixation may be required.

ORIF — VOLAR APPROACH 〉

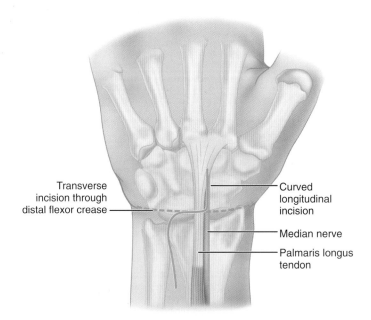

Transverse
incision through
distal flexor crease

Curved
longitudinal
incision

Median nerve

Palmaris longus
tendon

Figure 80-1

- With the patient supine and under suitable anesthesia, prepare the hand and wrist and one iliac crest and inflate a pneumatic tourniquet.
- The volar approach usually gives the best exposure for scaphoid fractures at and distal to the waist. Make a longitudinal skin incision over the palmar surface of the wrist beginning 3 to 4 cm proximal to the wrist flexion crease over the flexor carpi radialis (Figure 80-1).
- Extend the incision distally to the wrist flexion crease and curve it radially toward the scaphotrapezial and trapeziometacarpal joints.
- Protect terminal branches of the palmar cutaneous branch of the median nerve and the superficial radial nerves.
- Reflect skin flaps at the level of the forearm fascia.

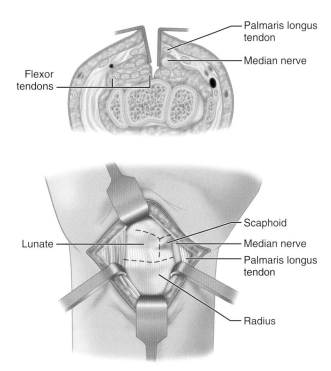

Figure 80-2

- Open the sheath of the flexor carpi radialis, retract the tendon radially, and open the deep surface of its sheath (Figure 80-2).
- Expose the palmar capsule of the joint over the radioscaphoid joint.
- Extend the wrist in ulnar deviation, open the capsule in the longitudinal axis of the scaphoid bone, and obliquely extend the incision toward the scaphotrapezial joint.
- With sharp dissection expose the fracture, incise the long radiolunate and radioscaphocapitate ligaments preserving each leaf of these capsuloligamentous structures for later repair. Inspect the fracture to determine the need for bone grafting.
- If comminution is absent or minimal, reduction and fixation suffice. If comminution is extensive, especially on the palmar surface and with a tendency to flexion of the scaphoid at the fracture, obtain an iliac crest bone graft.
- Kirschner wires placed in the distal and proximal poles as toggle levers ("joysticks") help to manipulate the fragments.
- Reduce the fracture and fix it with Kirschner wires or a screw technique (e.g., cannulated screws), avoiding rotation or angulation. If a cannulated device is used, ensure that the guidewire is centered in the proximal and distal poles. Image intensification with C-arm fluoroscopy is helpful for this step.
- For fractures through the waist and in the distal pole insert the fixation device through a distal portal. Create the distal portal by opening the scaphotrapezial joint with a longitudinal capsular incision.
- Remove a portion of the trapezium with a rongeur to allow placement of the guidewire from distal to proximal.
- Insert the screw until the trailing end (head) is flush with subchondral bone, countersunk beneath the articular cartilage.
- Placement of Kirschner wires down the long axis of the scaphoid is made easier by gentle radial deviation of the wrist aligning the scaphoid vertically. With the wrist in this position direct the wires almost dorsally into the scaphoid.
- After stable reduction and fixation are obtained, check the position and alignment of the reduction and the placement of the internal fixation with image intensification or radiographs.
- Deflate the tourniquet and obtain hemostasis.
- Insert a drain if needed and close the wrist capsule with nonabsorbable sutures or long-lasting absorbable sutures.
- Close the skin and apply a dressing that includes either a sugar-tong splint with a thumb spica extension or a long-arm cast incorporating the thumb.

ORIF — DORSAL APPROACH ⟩

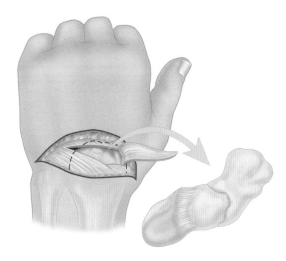

Figure 80-3

- For noncomminuted fractures in the proximal pole of the scaphoid, exposure of the fracture site and placement of internal fixation can be done through a dorsal approach (Figure 80-3).
- Make a dorsal transverse incision 5 to 10 mm distal to the radiocarpal joint. Protect the sensory branches of the radial and ulnar nerves. Preserve, cauterize, or ligate and divide dorsal veins.
- Extend the skin incision from the radial styloid to the ulnar styloid.
- Make parallel incisions in the extensor retinaculum on each side of the extensor digitorum communis tendons. Protect the extensor tendons, especially the extensor pollicis longus tendon as it exits the third dorsal retinacular compartment. Connect the parallel incisions proximally to create a flap to allow access to the dorsal wrist capsule.
- Pass a loop of Penrose drain around the extensor tendons and retract them medially.
- Open the dorsal capsule by creating a radially based flap, incising along the dorsal intercarpal ligament and the dorsal radiotriquetral ligament.
- Retract the capsular flap radially and expose the fracture.
- Insert a Kirschner wire into the proximal fragment parallel to the central axis of the scaphoid. Use this wire as a toggle lever ("joystick") to manipulate the proximal fragment into a reduced position.
- When the fracture is reduced pass the first wire across the fracture for temporary interfragmentary fixation. Insert an additional Kirschner wire, or screw fixation, as the fracture configuration permits.
- If a cannulated screw is used center the guidewire in the proximal and distal poles, monitoring this placement with C-arm fluoroscopy.
- Determine the appropriate length of the screw to be used. Drill and tap the bone according to the device being used and insert the screw of appropriate length. Ensure that the guidewire or screw fixation is placed in the center of the long axis of the proximal and distal poles of the scaphoid using C-arm fluoroscopy. Either leave the initial Kirschner wire as supplemental fixation or remove it if screw fixation has been selected.
- Close the capsular flap and repair the retinacular flap.
- Close the skin and apply a cast or sugar-tong splint that extends from above the elbow to include the thumb.

POSTOPERATIVE CARE ⟩

The sutures are removed and the splint or cast is changed at 2 weeks. Some authors advocate transitioning directly to a removable splint once sutures are removed, whereas others recommend an additional 2 to 4 weeks of short-arm thumb spica cast immobilization. As healing progresses as shown by radiographic examination, a short-arm thumb spica brace is worn until bone healing is ensured. If healing cannot be determined with certainty, CT or MRI can be helpful to evaluate for bridging trabeculae. Finger, thumb, and shoulder motion is encouraged throughout convalescence and, after cast removal, wrist motion and elbow motion are increased gradually followed by strengthening exercises.

PERCUTANEOUS FIXATION OF SCAPHOID FRACTURES ⟩

- The following equipment is needed for this technique: (1) headless cannulated compression screw (standard Acutrak screw), (2) minifluoroscopy unit, (3) Kirschner wires, and (4) equipment for small joint arthroscopy.

- If arthroscopy is to be used to check the fracture reduction and to place internal fixation, have the operating room prepared for wrist arthroscopy.

- Position the patient supine with the upper extremity extended.

- After the induction of appropriate anesthesia and sterile preparation and draping procedures, flex the elbow 90 degrees.

- Use a C-arm fluoroscopic unit or mini C-arm fluoroscope to evaluate the fracture position and alignment and to determine if there are other bone or ligament injuries.

- Use a skin marking pen to indicate the best surface location for a dorsal skin incision and entry of the guidewire, drills, and screw.

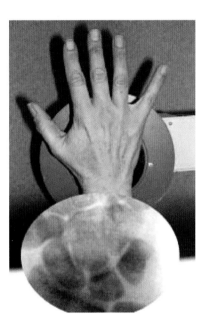

Figure 80-4

- "Target" the scaphoid by locating the central axis of the scaphoid on the posteroanterior view of the reduced scaphoid (Figure 80-4).

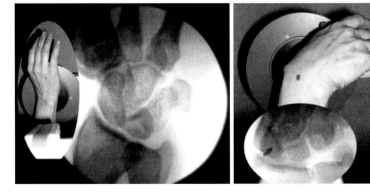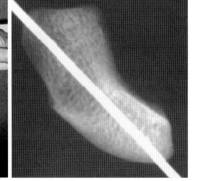

Figure 80-5

- Gently pronate and flex the wrist until the proximal and distal poles of the scaphoid are aligned and confirmed with fluoroscopy. When the poles are aligned, the scaphoid has a "ring" appearance on the fluoroscopic monitor. The center of the "ring" circle is the central axis of the scaphoid, which is the best location for screw placement (Figure 80-5).

- For ease of insertion make a skin incision at the previously marked location to allow blunt dissection to the capsule of the wrist joint.
- With a double-point 0.045-inch (1.14-mm) Kirschner wire in a powered wire driver, insert the wire starting in the proximal pole of the scaphoid under fluoroscopic control.
- If there is uncertainty about wire placement, make the previously mentioned incision distal and medial (ulnar) to the Lister tubercle, opening the dorsal wrist capsule lateral (radial) to the scapholunate interval and exposing the proximal pole of the scaphoid.

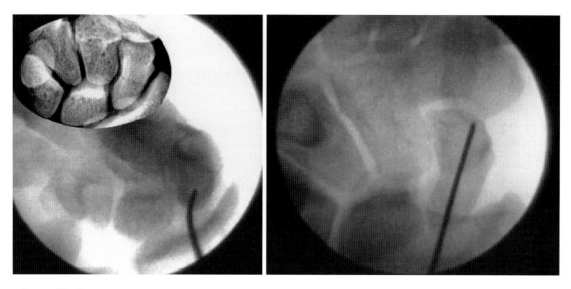

Figure 80-6

- Pass the guidewire from dorsally down the central axis of the scaphoid and out through the trapezium. Use a 12-gauge angiocatheter to assist with positioning of the guidewire. Keep the wrist flexed to avoid bending the guidewire (Figure 80-6).
- Advance the wire through the distal pole out the palmar surface. Check the position of the wire with the fluoroscope.
- Reverse the wire driver to pull the wire far enough distally to allow the dorsal, trailing end of the wire to clear the radiocarpal joint dorsally and to allow full wrist extension.

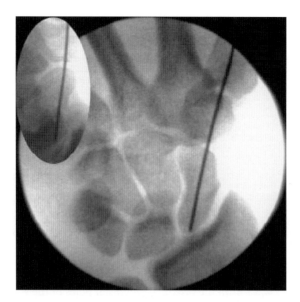

Figure 80-7

- With C-arm fluoroscopy confirm scaphoid fracture alignment and correct positioning of the guidewire (Figure 80-7).

- If a correct path cannot be created with the 0.045-inch wire, use a 0.062-inch (1.57-mm) wire to create the correct path. Exchange the larger wire for the 0.045-inch wire before drilling the scaphoid.

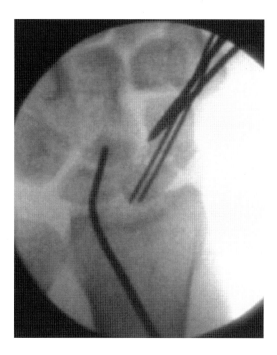

Figure 80-8

- Check for wire position and fracture alignment with the fluoroscope. If the fracture reduction is unsatisfactory, and for displaced fractures, place a 0.062-inch Kirschner wire into each fracture fragment perpendicular to the axis of the scaphoid to act as toggle levers ("joysticks") to manipulate the fracture fragments. If needed place the proximal lever wire in the lunate (Figure 80-8).
- With the wire driver on the distal end of the guidewire, withdraw the wire distally across the fracture site, leaving the wire in the central axis of the distal fragment.
- Align the fracture fragments with the "joysticks."
- Pass the guidewire from distal to proximal across the fracture site to hold the reduction.
- If needed for stability and rotational control insert another 0.045-inch wire, entering the proximal pole of the scaphoid, from dorsal to palmar parallel to the first guidewire to control rotation. Leave the wire levers and the antirotational wire in place during screw insertion.
- Confirm the reduction and wire placement with fluoroscopy.
- If the fracture is difficult to reduce percutaneously insert a small curved hemostat to assist with the reduction.
- If the fracture cannot be reduced, or if the guidewire cannot be properly placed, abandon the percutaneous technique and open the fracture using either the volar or the dorsal approach.

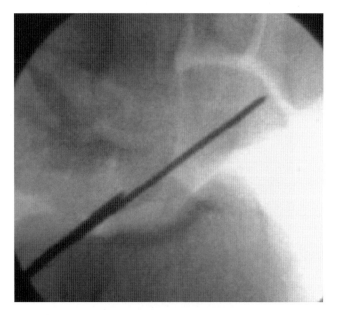

Figure 80-9

- Determine the scaphoid length using two wires. To determine the scaphoid length, adjust the guidewire position so that the distal end is against the distal cortex of the scaphoid. Place a second wire of the same length as the guidewire parallel to the guidewire so the tip of the second wire is against the cortex of the proximal scaphoid pole. The difference in length is the length of the scaphoid (Figure 80-9).
- To allow for countersinking the screw fully within the scaphoid, select a screw length that is 4 mm shorter than the scaphoid length.
- Determine dorsal or palmar insertion of the screw depending on the fracture location. For fractures of the proximal pole, insert the screw dorsally. For fractures of the waist, insert the screw from either the dorsal or the volar side. For fractures of the distal pole, insert the screw from the volar side.

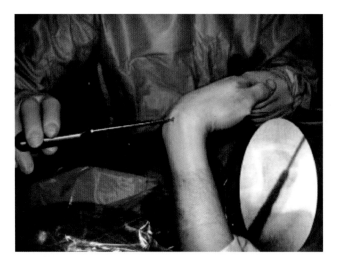

Figure 80-10

- Drill the screw channel 2 mm short of the opposite scaphoid cortex using a cannulated hand drill Always avoid contact with the opposite cortex (Figure 80-10).
- Check the position and depth of the drill with fluoroscopy.

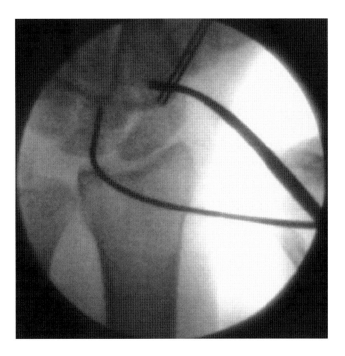

Figure 80-11

- Use a standard Acutrak screw 4 mm shorter than the scaphoid length. Advance the screw, monitoring with fluoroscopy, until the screw is within 1 to 2 mm of the opposite cortex (Figure 80-11).

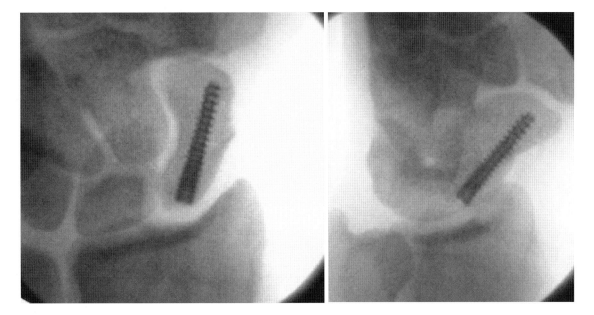

Figure 80-12

- Verify fracture reduction and screw placement with final fluoroscopic images (Figure 80-12).
- If ligament injury or other carpal injuries are suspected add arthroscopic examination to the fracture management.
- Apply longitudinal traction through the fingers.
- Locate the midcarpal and radiocarpal portals with fluoroscopy.
- Insert the arthroscope into the radial midcarpal portal to inspect the fracture reduction.
- Remove clot and synovium with the full radius shaver.

- Examine the scapholunate and lunatotriquetral ligaments.
- Inspect the proximal pole through the 3-4 portal to confirm countersinking of the screw into the proximal pole.
- If ligament tears are encountered treat them with débridement, intercarpal pinning or open dorsal ligament repair.

POSTOPERATIVE CARE

A postoperative splint is applied depending on the extent of soft tissue injury. If no ligament injury is present, a thumb spica splint is applied. If there is ligament injury, a sugar-tong thumb spica splint of the Munster type is applied, extending above the elbow. For fracture management skin sutures are removed at about 2 weeks and the splint changed to a short-arm thumb spica cast. Any remaining pins are removed at 6 to 8 weeks. Casting or removable thumb spica splinting is continued until radiographic healing has occurred, with the cast changed monthly. CT and MRI can help in determining if bridging trabeculae are present. After healing has occurred, a therapist-supervised rehabilitation program is begun.

James H. Calandruccio

Several different methods are commonly used to achieve reduction of proximal interphalangeal joint fracture-dislocations. These techniques rely on coupling distraction and volarly directed forces across the joint. Common to most of these devices is achieving distraction force through pins placed through the rotation axes of the proximal and distal interphalangeal joints. The method by which the volarly directed forces are achieved differs according to the chosen technique.

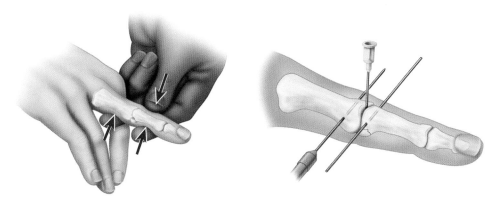

Figure 81-1

- Manually reduce the PIP joint fracture-dislocation. Identify the joint line with a needle and insert Kirschner wires distal and proximal to the joint (Figure 81-1).

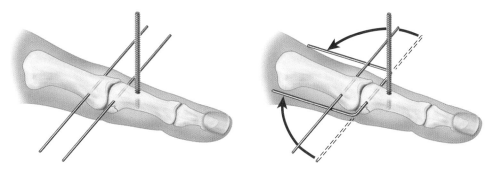

Figure 81-2

- Insert the threaded Kirschner wire dorsal to the palmar cortex in the middle phalanx and bend the distal wire 90 degrees on each side (Figure 81-2).

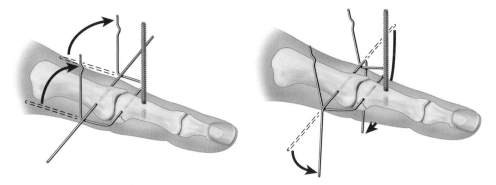

Figure 81-3

- Make a second 90-degree bend in the distal wire and bend a hook into the end of each wire. Bend the proximal wire 90 degrees palmarward on each side (Figure 81-3).

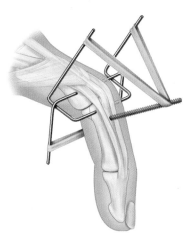

Figure 81-4

- After inserting and forming the Kirschner wires into a mechanical linkage, place a small rubber band with tension adequate to maintain reduction; avoid excessive tension (Figure 81-4).
- When closed reduction is possible, apply the force-couple splint percutaneously, preferably with the patient under digital block anesthesia allowing the patient to demonstrate the joint's active range of motion.
- Determine the quality of joint reduction with anteroposterior and lateral radiographs of the joint in the flexed position.
- Examine the flexion and extension lateral radiographs closely to ensure that the intact dorsal base of the middle phalanx is concentrically reduced, as evidenced by its parallel gliding motion with respect to the head of the proximal phalanx.
- A rocking motion of the middle phalanx on the proximal phalanx should be avoided because it predisposes to high joint surface pressures and secondary traumatic arthritis and recurrent joint subluxation. The force-couple splint maintains joint reduction during bone and soft tissue healing, theoretically minimizing joint stiffness by allowing active range-of-motion exercises. Apply a soft dressing to be worn for 1 or 2 days; then remove all restrictive dressings and apply an antibiotic ointment daily to the pin sites.
- Adjust the smooth Kirschner wire limbs of the device as needed to keep them centered on the finger, avoiding pressure on the skin. The device is maintained for a minimum of 5 weeks, with advancing degrees of comminution and instability requiring 6 to 8 weeks. Obtain interval radiographs until bone and soft tissue healing is judged to be adequate. The effect of the force couple is removed by detaching the rubber band. Obtain flexion-extension lateral radiographs to confirm joint stability before removing the force-couple splint.
- In chronic injuries, perform open reduction through a midlateral incision with the patient under axillary block anesthesia; divide the lateral retinacular ligament along with the dorsal part of the collateral ligament and adjacent joint capsule.

- Frequently, the dorsal side of the opposite collateral ligament must be divided through a separate midlateral incision.
- Use a probe to free the palmar side of the joint and a small, sharp osteotome to mobilize the avulsed fragment from the palmar base of the middle phalanx.
- If portions of the collateral ligaments necessary for adequate stability cannot be maintained, the splint cannot be used because it would convert the dorsal dislocation to a palmar one.
- With adequate reduction of the intact dorsal base of the middle phalanx with respect to the proximal phalanx condyles, apply the force-couple splint, allowing the smooth transverse Kirschner wires to exit through the surgical incision.
- If possible, repair the soft tissues; after hemostasis, repair the skin appropriately.
- Obtain radiographs in anteroposterior, lateral extension, and lateral flexion views to evaluate the adequacy of joint reduction.
- Apply a soft dressing to the finger for several days.

POSTOPERATIVE CARE 〉

To permit active range-of-motion exercises no dressing is used; instead an antibiotic ointment is applied.

Surgery for carpal tunnel syndrome is among the most common hand surgeries. The results are good in 70% to 90% of patients, and benefits seem to last in most patients. Maximal improvement is seen in the first 6 months after carpal tunnel release. The "mini-palm" technique requires only a 1-inch incision, but it still allows a direct view of the area (unlike endoscopy, which is viewed on a monitor). The recovery time with the mini-open approach may be shorter than with the open approach, and results are generally the same.

MINI-PALM OPEN CARPAL TUNNEL RELEASE 〉

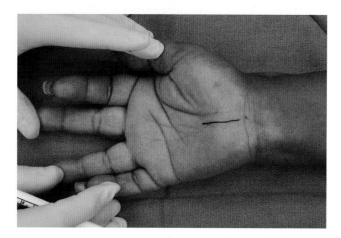

Figure 82-1

- Mark the planned surgical incision with a skin pen so that the longitudinal incision begins just distal to the distal wrist flexion crease and slightly ulnar to the midline of the wrist (center dot reference point) and extends distally 3.0 cm in line with the third web space (Figure 82-1). (*Note:* only rarely is it necessary to extend the incision into the distal forearm.)

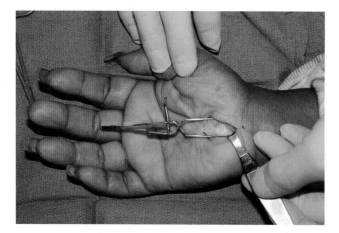

Figure 82-2

- Expose the transverse carpal ligament (TCL) and retract the parallel palmar fascia fibers and hypothenar fat (Figure 82-2).

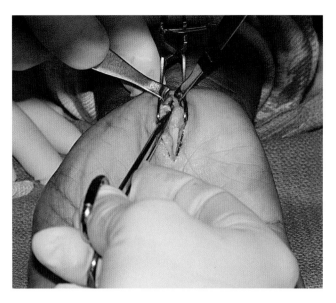

Figure 82-3

▪ Divide the TCL and then the distal 2.0 cm of the antebrachial fascia with Metzenbaum scissors (Figure 82-3).

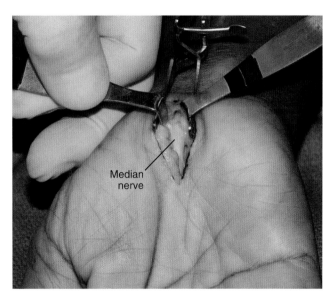

Figure 82-4

▪ If the median nerve is adherent to the divided radial TCL leaf, external neurolysis may be needed (Figure 82-4).

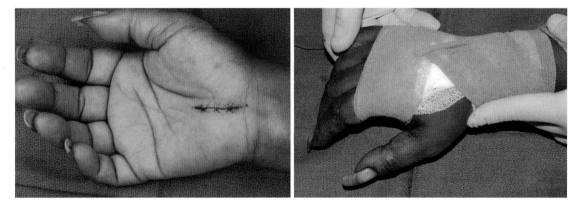

Figure 82-5

▪ Close the incision in routine fashion and apply a compressive dressing (Figure 82-5).

OPEN CARPAL TUNNEL RELEASE ❯

- The thenar crease takes a variable course and palmar incisions should be well ulnar to it to avoid the median nerve palmar cutaneous branch. A curved incision ulnar and parallel to the thenar crease is not advisable because the palmar cutaneous branch of the median nerve proximally may be more at risk of injury. We prefer to use the incision described for the mini-palm technique.

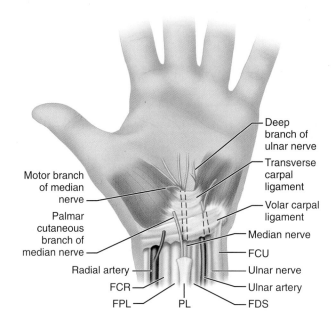

Figure 82-6

- Extend the incision proximally to the flexor crease of the wrist where it can be continued farther proximally if necessary. Angle the incision toward the ulnar side of the wrist to avoid crossing the flexor creases at a right angle but especially to avoid cutting the palmar cutaneous sensory branch, which lies in the interval between the palmaris longus and the flexor carpi radialis tendons. Maintain longitudinal orientation so that the incision is generally to the ulnar side of the long finger axis or radial border of the ring fourth ray. When severed the palmar sensory branch frequently causes a painful neuroma that may later require excision from the scar. Should this nerve be severed, do not attempt to repair it but section it at its origin (Figure 82-6).
- Incise and reflect the skin and subcutaneous tissue.
- Identify the palmar fascia from the wrist flexion crease distally and the distal forearm antebrachial fascia proximally by subcutaneous blunt dissection. Split the palmar fascia and expose the underlying transverse carpal ligament, avoiding the median nerve beneath it.

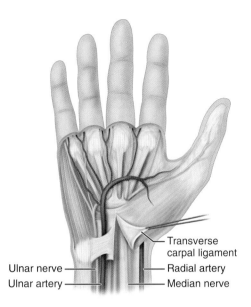

Transverse
carpal ligament
Ulnar nerve ——————— Radial artery
Ulnar artery ——————— Median nerve

Figure 82-7

- Identify the transverse carpal ligament and carefully divide it, avoiding damage to the median nerve and its recurrent branch, which may perforate the ligament and leave the median nerve on the volar side. Fibers of the transverse carpal ligament can extend distally farther than expected (Figure 82-7).
- The flexor retinaculum includes the distal deep fascia of the forearm proximally, the transverse carpal ligament, and the aponeurosis between the thenar and hypothenar muscles. A successful carpal tunnel release usually requires division of all these components.
- Be aware of potential anomalies: connections between the flexor pollicis longus and the index flexor digitorum profundus tendons; anomalous flexor digitorum superficialis; palmaris longus, hypothenar, and lumbrical muscle bellies; and median and ulnar nerve branches and interconnections.
- Avoid injury to the superficial palmar arterial arch, which is 5 to 8 mm distal to the distal margin of the transverse carpal ligament.
- Inspect the flexor tenosynovium. Tenosynovectomy occasionally may be indicated, especially in patients with rheumatoid arthritis.
- Close only the skin and drain the wound as needed.

POSTOPERATIVE CARE 〉

A light compression dressing and a volar splint may be applied. The hand is actively used as soon as possible after surgery but the dependent position is avoided. Usually the dressing can be removed by the patient at home 2 or 3 days after the surgery and then gentle washing and showering of the hand is permitted. Gradual resumption of normal hand use is encouraged. The sutures are removed after 10 to 14 days. A splint may be continued for comfort as needed for 14 to 21 days.

Advocates of endoscopic carpal tunnel release cite less palmar scarring and ulnar "pillar" pain, rapid and complete return of strength, and return to work and activities at least 2 weeks sooner than for open release. The advantages of the endoscopic technique in grip strength and pain relief are realized within the first 12 weeks and seem to benefit those patients not involved in compensable injuries. Anecdotal reports of intraoperative injury to flexor tendons; to median, ulnar, and digital nerves; and to the superficial palmar arterial arch emphasize the need to exercise great care and caution when performing endoscopic release. There are two basic methods of endoscopic carpal tunnel release: single-portal (Agee) and two-portal (Chow) techniques.

ENDOSCOPIC CARPAL TUNNEL RELEASE THROUGH A SINGLE INCISION ⟩

- Ascertain that the operating room setup is satisfactory. Ensure there is an unobstructed view of the patient's hand and the television monitor.
- Use general or regional anesthesia. Although the procedure can be done safely using local anesthesia, the increase in tissue fluid can compromise endoscopic viewing.
- Exsanguinate the limb with an elastic wrap and inflate a pneumatic tourniquet applied over adequate padding. Leave the arm exposed distal to the tourniquet.

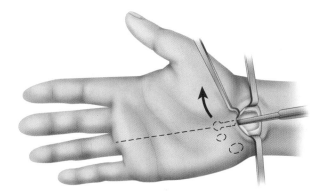

Figure 83-1

- In a patient with two or more wrist flexion creases, make the incision in the more proximal crease between the tendons of the flexor carpi radialis and flexor carpi ulnaris (Figure 83-1).
- Use longitudinal blunt dissection to protect the subcutaneous nerves and expose the forearm fascia.

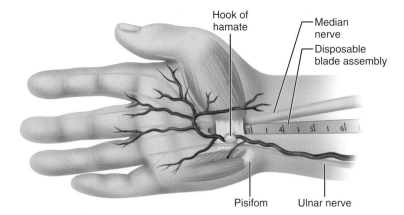

Figure 83-2

- Incise and elevate a U-shaped, distally based flap of forearm fascia, and retract it palmarward to facilitate dissection of the synovium from the deep surface of the ligament creating a mouthlike opening at the proximal end of the carpal tunnel (Figure 83-2).

- When using the tunneling tools and the endoscopic blade assembly keep them aligned with the ring finger, hug the hook of the hamate, and keep the tools snugly apposed to the deep surface of the transverse carpal ligament, maintaining a path between the median and ulnar nerves for the instruments.

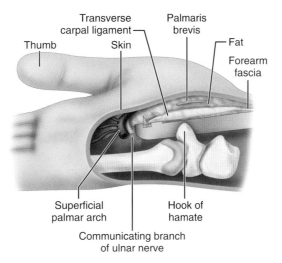

Figure 83-3

- Use the synovium elevator to scrape the synovium from the deep surface of the transverse carpal ligament. Extend the wrist slightly; insert the blade assembly to the carpal tunnel, pressing the viewing window snugly against the deep surface of the transverse carpal ligament. While advancing the blade assembly distally, maintain alignment with the ring finger and hug the hook of the hamate staying to the ulnar side. Make several proximal-to-distal passes to define the distal edge of the transverse carpal ligament with the fat overlying it (Figure 83-3).

- Define the distal edge of the transverse carpal ligament by viewing the video picture, ballottement, and light transilluminated through the skin. Correctly position the blade assembly and touch the distal end of the ligament with the partially elevated blade to judge its entry point for ligament division. Elevate the blade and withdraw the device, incising the ligament.

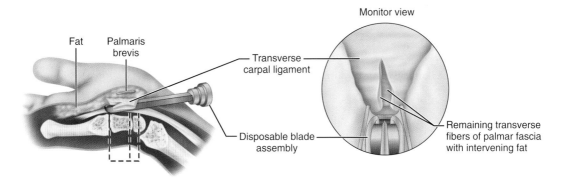

Figure 83-4

- Release distal half to two thirds of transverse carpal ligament completely before making a final pass to release the remainder of the ligament. This prevents fat located superficial to the proximal portion of the ligament from dropping into the wound and compromising the surgeon's endoscopic view of the extent of the ligament division (Figure 83-4).

- Using the unobstructed path for reinsertion of the instrument, accurately complete the distal ligament division with good viewing. Complete proximal ligament division with a final proximal pass of the elevated blade.

- Assess the completeness of ligament division using the following endoscopic observations.

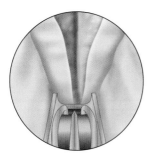
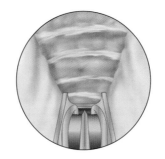
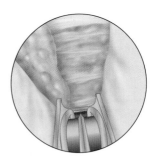

Figure 83-5

- Through the endoscope, note that the partially divided ligament separates on the deep surface creating a V-shaped defect (Figure 83-5).
- Make subsequent cuts viewing the trapezoidal defect created by complete division as the two halves of the ligament spring apart. Through this defect, observe the longitudinal palmar fascia fibers intermingled with fat and muscle. Force these structures to protrude by pressing on the palmar skin.
- Confirm complete division by rotating the blade assembly in radial and ulnar directions, noting that the edges of the ligament abruptly "flop" into the window obstructing the view.
- Palpate the palmar skin over the blade assembly window observing motion between the divided transverse carpal ligament and the more superficial palmar fascia, fat, and muscle.

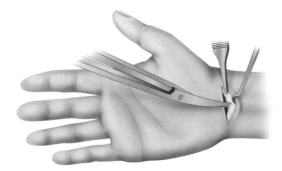

Figure 83-6

- Ensure complete median nerve decompression by releasing the forearm fascia with tenotomy scissors (Figure 83-6).
- Use small right-angle retractors to view the fascia directly avoiding nerve and tendon injury.
- Close the incision with subcuticular or simple stitches.
- Apply a nonadhering dressing. Apply a well-padded volar splint or, in selected patients, leave the wrist unsplinted.

POSTOPERATIVE CARE

The splint and sutures may be removed early or at 10 to 14 days. Active finger motion is allowed early in the postoperative period. Forceful pulling with wrist flexion is discouraged for 4 to 6 weeks to allow maturation of soft tissue healing. Progression of light activities of daily living is allowed at 2 to 3 weeks and more strenuous activities are gradually added in the next 4 to 6 weeks.

ENDOSCOPIC CARPAL TUNNEL RELEASE THROUGH TWO INCISIONS

- Perform the procedure using anesthesia believed most appropriate by the patient, surgeon, and anesthesiologist. Local anesthetic infiltration supplemented with intravenous sedation is commonly used although regional block or even general anesthesia may be more suitable in some situations.
- With the patient supine place the hand and wrist on a hand table. The surgeon usually sits on the axillary side and an assistant should be on the cephalad side of the upper extremity; however, the endoscopic dissection is proximal to distal and the surgeon may elect to be on the cephalad side depending on his or her hand dominance.

- Apply a well-padded pneumatic tourniquet to use if needed.
- At least one television monitor should be placed on the extremity side opposite the surgeon (toward the head of the table) or, as preferred by Chow, two monitors should be used, one for the surgeon and the other for the assistant.

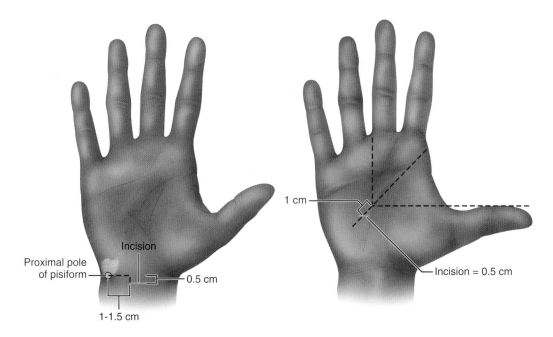

Figure 83-7

- Define the entry and exit portals with a marking pen. Begin at the pisiform proximally and, depending on the size of the hand, draw a line extending 1.0 to 1.5 cm radially. From the end of this line extend a second line 0.5 cm proximally. From the end of the second line draw a third line extending about 1.0 cm radially. The third line is the entry portal. Passively fully abduct the thumb. Draw a line along the distal border of the fully abducted thumb across the palm toward the ulnar border of the hand. Draw another line extending proximally from the web space between the long finger and the ring finger intersecting the line drawn from the thumb. About 1.0 cm proximal to the intersection of these lines draw a third line about 0.5 cm long transverse to the long axis of the hand (Figure 83-7).
- Make an incision in the previously marked entry portal just through the skin and bluntly dissect down to the transverse fibers of the forearm fascia. If a palmaris tendon is present it should remain radial to the dissection field. Gently lift the forearm fascia and make a longitudinal incision through the fascia only. Only the distal 2.0 cm of forearm fascia typically needs to be released. Release the distal forearm fascia distally to the proximal edge of the transverse carpal ligament.
- Gently lift the distal edge of the entry portal incision with a small right-angle retractor revealing the small space between the transverse carpal ligament and the ulnar bursa. Bluntly dissect and develop the space between the transverse carpal ligament and the underlying bursa.
- Use the curved dissector obturator/slotted cannula assembly with the pointed side toward the transverse carpal ligament to enter the space and to push the bursal tissue free from the deep surface of the transverse carpal ligament.
- Use the curved dissector to feel the curved shape of the deep surface of the transverse carpal ligament. Move the dissector back and forth to feel the "washboard" effect of the transverse fibers of the transverse carpal ligament.
- Apply a lifting force to the dissector to test the tightness of the ligament and to ensure that the dissector is deep to the ligament rather than in the tissues superficial to the ligament. Ensure that the dissector and trocar are oriented in the longitudinal axis of the forearm.
- Touch the hook of the hamate with the tip of the assembly; lift the patient's hand above the table extending the wrist and fingers over the hand holder. Gently advance the slotted cannula assembly distally, and direct it toward the exit portal. Palpate the tip of the assembly in the palm.
- Make a second small incision as marked for the exit portal in the palm. Pass the assembly through the exit portal and secure the hand to the hand holder.

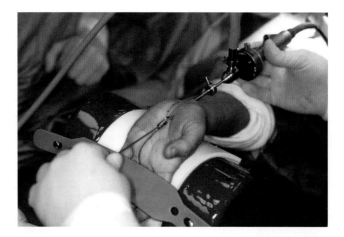

Figure 83-8

■ Insert the endoscope at the proximal opening of the tube (Figure 83-8).

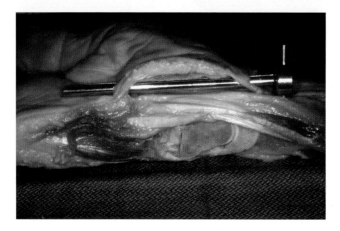

Figure 83-9

■ Examine the entire length of the slotted cannula opening to ensure that there is no other tissue between the slotted cannula and the transverse carpal ligament. If there is any doubt, remove the tube and reevaluate for correct instrumentation placement (Figure 83-9).

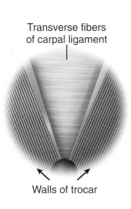

Transverse fibers
of carpal ligament

Walls of trocar

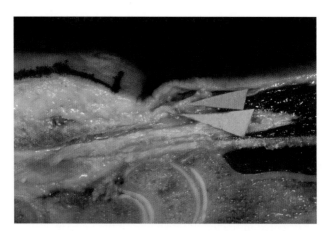

Figure 83-10

■ With the endoscope remaining in the tube, having been inserted from the proximal direction, insert a probe distally and identify the distal edge of the transverse carpal ligament (Figure 83-10).

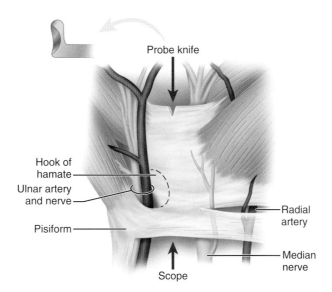

Figure 83-11

- Use the probe knife to cut from distal to proximal to release the distal edge of the ligament (Figure 83-11).

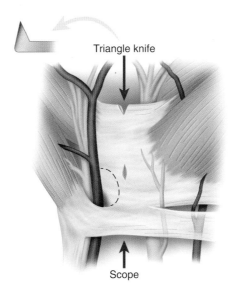

Figure 83-12

- Insert the triangle knife to cut through the midsection of the transverse carpal ligament (Figure 83-12).

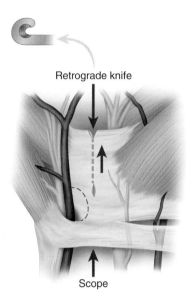

Figure 83-13

- Insert the retrograde knife and position it in the second cut. Draw the retrograde knife distally to join the first cut, completely releasing the distal half of the ligament (Figure 83-13).
- Remove the endoscope from the proximal opening of the open tube and insert the endoscope into the distal opening.
- Insert the instruments from the proximal opening.

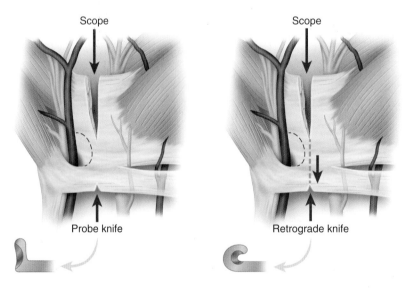

Figure 83-14

- Identify the uncut proximal section of the ligament and use the probe knife to release the proximal edge. Draw the retrograde knife proximally to complete the release of the ligament (Figure 83-14).
- Choose the proper knife to make additional cuts to complete transection of the ligament as needed.
- Reinsert the trocar and remove the slotted cannula from the hand.
- If a tourniquet is used deflate it, and then ascertain hemostasis and that there is no pulsatile or excessive bleeding.
- Suture the incisions and apply a soft dressing.

POSTOPERATIVE CARE 〉

Active movement is encouraged immediately after surgery. The dressing is usually removed by the patient at home 2 to 3 days after the procedure and sutures are removed at 10 to 14 days at the first postoperative visit. Direct pressure to the palm area and heavy lifting should be avoided for 2 to 3 weeks or until discomfort disappears.

Surgical release reliably relieves the problem of trigger finger for most patients: approximately 97% of patients have complete resolution after operative treatment. Persistence of triggering is more common than recurrence. Trigger release should be done with a local block so that the cessation of triggering of a particular finger can be evaluated. Some adjacent finger triggering may become obvious only after a given finger is released; both can be released at the same surgical setting. The safety and effectiveness of percutaneous trigger finger release using a needle or a push knife are documented. Incomplete pulley release and damage to the flexor tendons and digital nerves, especially in the index finger and thumb, remain of some concern with this technique.

OPEN RELEASE OF TRIGGER FINGER ⟩

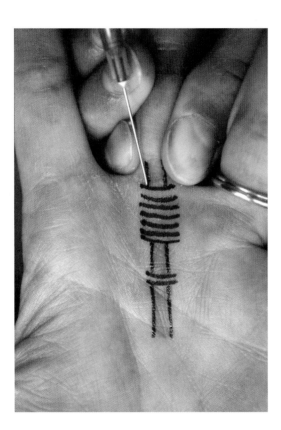

Figure 84-1

- Local anesthetic infiltration in the palm proximal to the incision site is preferred. The use of a pneumatic arm tourniquet may be helpful, although a high forearm Esmarch wrap usually is sufficient (Figure 84-1).

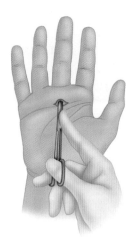

Figure 84-2

- Make a transverse incision about 2 cm long several millimeters distal to the distal palmar crease for middle, ring, and small trigger finger releases and several millimeters distal to the proximal palmar crease for index trigger finger releases. Trigger thumb releases can be done through incisions either distal or proximal to the metacarpophalangeal joint flexion crease. Alternative incisions for the fingers can be made obliquely or longitudinally between the metacarpophalangeal and distal palmar creases and obliquely across the thumb metacarpophalangeal flexion crease (Figure 84-2).
- Avoid the digital nerves, which on the thumb are more palmar and closer to the flexor sheath than might be anticipated. The thumb radial digital nerve is especially vulnerable.
- Identify with a small probe the discrete proximal edge of the first annular pulley of the flexor sheath.

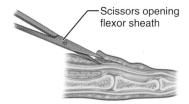

Figure 84-3

- Place a small knife blade or one blade of a pair of slightly opened blunt scissors just under the edge of the sheath and gently push it distally, cutting the first annular pulley. Avoid cutting too far distally and disrupting the oblique pulley. Incise the sheath from proximal to distal, approximately 1 cm, and reassess for triggering. If the finger triggers when the patient actively flexes and extends the digit, either the A1 and palmar pulleys are incompletely released or an alternate site of triggering is present. The distinction between the A1 and A2 pulleys may not be apparent; however, when the distal A1 pulley edge is released the divided pulley leaves are parallel rather than ending in a V-shaped pattern (Figure 84-3).
- Evaluate the distal end of the palmar fascia and the proximal flexor tenosynovium to release all structures proximally that might bind on the tendon. Ensure that all neurovascular structures are retracted out of the way and that all structures to be incised are seen.
- After the tendon sheath has been released, encourage the patient actively to flex and extend the digit to ensure that the release is complete.
- Close the skin and apply a small, dry, compression dressing.

POSTOPERATIVE CARE 〉

The compression dressing is removed after 48 hours. Sutures are removed at 10 to 14 days. Normal use of the finger or thumb is advised after wound healing.

PERCUTANEOUS RELEASE OF TRIGGER FINGER 〉

- Before attempting the percutaneous release it is helpful to have the patient understand that the procedure might fail and that subsequent open release may be necessary.

- Inject local anesthetic into the palmar skin and more deeply proximal to the intended release site (between the proximal and distal palmar creases for the middle, ring, and small fingers and proximal to the proximal palmar crease for the index finger). Maintain an orientation along the flexor tendon sheaths in the midline of the digit being released.
- Use an 18- or 19-gauge needle for the release.

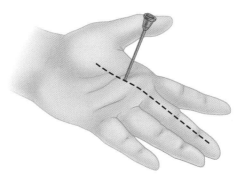

Figure 84-4

- Turn the palm up, resting the hand on a folded towel to permit slight hyperextension of the metacarpophalangeal joint (Figure 84-4).
- Insert the needle into the A1 pulley and orient the bevel of the needle so that it is longitudinally aligned parallel to the flexor tendon.

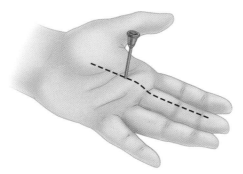

Figure 84-5

- Move the needle proximally and distally in the A1 pulley, pressing firmly proximally and distally. Feel for a scraping or grating sensation as the sheath is incised (Figure 84-5).
- When the grating is eliminated, remove the needle and check for triggering as the patient flexes and extends the digit. Additional needle passes might be needed.
- Injection of corticosteroid is optional.

POSTOPERATIVE CARE 〉

The needle entry site is covered with an adhesive bandage or light nonrestrictive dressing and active hand and finger use is encouraged with stretching exercises.

Arthrodesis may be required for thumb joint deformities caused by rheumatoid arthritis or osteoarthritic processes. Arthrodesis is indicated most often for the metacarpophalangeal joint, which greatly relieves pain and improves strength by rigid stabilization. If adequate bone is present, fixation can be obtained with combinations of Kirschner wires, plates and screws, and wire loops in a tension-band configuration. The more stable and rigid the fixation, the shorter the time required for immobilization. The preferred position for thumb joint arthrodesis is that of the "fist" position: interphalangeal joint in 20 degrees of flexion, metacarpophalangeal joint in 25 degrees of flexion, and carpometacarpal joint in palmar abduction of about 40 degrees with the thumb in opposition.

TENSION BAND ARTHRODESIS OF THE THUMB METACARPOPHALANGEAL JOINT 〉

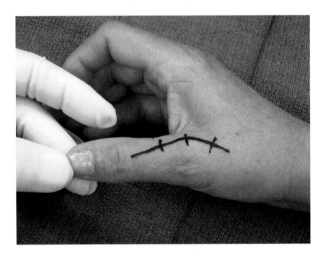

Figure 85-1

- Make a curved dorsal incision to allow safe dissection of sensory nerves from underlying extensor apparatus (Figure 85-1).

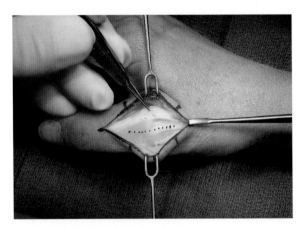

Figure 85-2

- Make an incision through the extensor pollicis brevis tendon and radial aponeurotic fibers to expose the dorsal capsule (Figure 85-2).

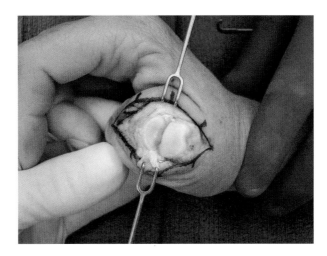

Figure 85-3

- Split the capsule longitudinally to expose the metacarpal head and proximal phalanx base and excise osteophytes, collateral ligaments, and synovitic tissue (Figure 85-3).

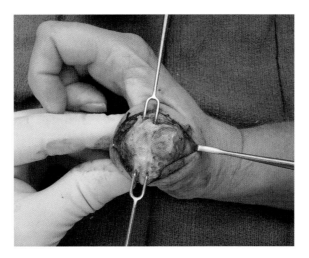

Figure 85-4

- With rongeurs, a coarse-tooth oscillating saw, or congruent reamers, prepare the subchondral bone such that a 20-degree flexion angle is achieved with full contact of the raw cancellous metacarpal and proximal phalangeal surfaces (Figure 85-4).

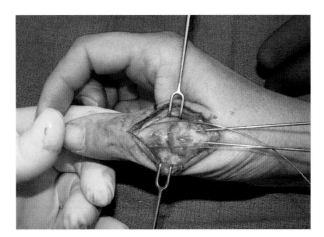

Figure 85-5

- Make a transverse hole with a 0.045-inch Kirschner wire in the distal third of the proximal phalangeal neck to allow a 22-gauge spool wire to pass through this hole (Figure 85-5).

- Hold the metacarpophalangeal joint in the desired position and pass two 0.045-inch Kirschner wires longitudinally across the fusion site and into the proximal phalangeal medullary canal. Verify their position on fluoroscopy before completing the tension band construct.
- Cross the 22-gauge wire and place one limb beneath the Kirschner wires projecting from the metacarpal neck.

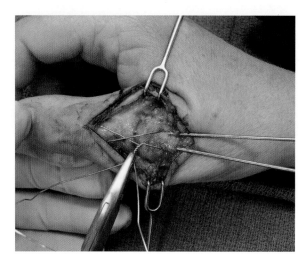

Figure 85-6

- Take the slack out of the 22-gauge wire before twisting the wire and burying the end about the fusion site (Figure 85-6).

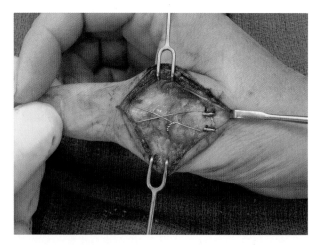

Figure 85-7

- Hold the Kirschner wires and bend the ends with a neurotip sucker so that the hooked ends can be cut and tamped into the metacarpal neck (Figure 85-7).

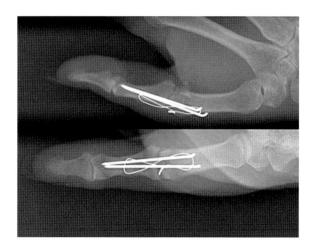

Figure 85-8

- Close the extensor pollicis brevis with a 4-0 nonabsorbable braided suture after the capsule has been closed over the low-profile construct (Figure 85-8).

THUMB METACARPOPHALANGEAL JOINT ARTHRODESIS WITH INTRAMEDULLARY SCREW FIXATION

- Make the skin and capsular exposures as described above.
- With rongeurs, a coarse-tooth oscillating saw, or congruent reamers, prepare the subchondral bone such that a 20-degree flexion angle is achieved with full contact of the raw cancellous metacarpal and proximal phalangeal surfaces (see Fig. 85-4).
- Position the metacarpophalangeal joint at the desired angle with the cancellous surfaces in maximal contact. Verify the guide wire position with fluoroscopy.
- Perform reaming according to the screw diameter.

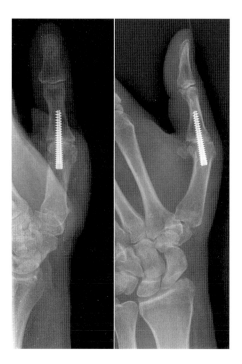

Figure 85-9

- Seat the screw just beneath the metacarpal neck cortex and evaluate the stability of the construct (Figure 85-9).
- Obtain fluoroscopic images to verify position of the arthrodesis before routine wound closure.

METACARPOPHALANGEAL ARTHRODESIS OF THE THUMB 〉

- With an osteotome or oscillating saw, cut across the articular surface of the proximal phalanx in a straight line at 90 degrees to its long axis. The articular surfaces can also be removed in a "cup-and-cone" configuration.
- After the articular surface is resected, place the phalanx at an angle of 15 degrees of flexion with the metacarpal. There is a tendency to osteotomize the distal metacarpal also at 90 degrees; instead, make the osteotomy so that the metacarpophalangeal joint is flexed 15 degrees. This requires removing more bone toward the palmar aspect. The two raw surfaces should fit flush.
- Remove any protruding small edges of bone to smooth the arthrodesis site.
- Fix the arthrodesis with three Kirschner wires inserted longitudinally. Insert them first through the metacarpal and advance them through the phalanx. Ensure that the wires do not pierce the flexor tendon or the distal joint. Cut them off under the skin and approximate the tendons with a small absorbable suture.
- Close the wound and place the hand in a small splint to be replaced later by a cast if indicated.
- When this joint is subluxated shortening of the bone may be required.
- Make a dorsal longitudinal incision over the joint and displace the extensor pollicis longus tendon to the ulnar side.
- On the proximal end of the proximal phalanx, shape a tongue of bone; on the distal end of the first metacarpal, create a V-shaped notch. These should fit like a tongue in a groove. Large surfaces of bone are put in contact but the angle of fusion can be adjusted easily.
- Fix the joint in the proper position with two Kirschner wires that are cut off flush with the bone.
- Pack small fragments of bone into any spaces around the joint margins.
- Close the wound and apply a volar plaster splint that includes the thumb but no other digits.
- In both techniques described here, ensure that the thumb is in appropriate pronation so that the pulp of the thumb can be placed against the other digits. If the first metacarpal is adducted, some of this adduction can be overcome by fusing the joint in slight abduction. This places the thumb in proper position without releasing soft tissues in the palm.

POSTOPERATIVE CARE 〉

For all joints of the thumb the splint and sutures are removed at 10 to 14 days. The thumb is protected in a short-arm thumb spica cast for another 4 weeks. The Kirschner wires are removed at about 6 weeks and a splint is worn another 3 to 4 weeks. Active use of the thumb is resumed gradually despite absence of radiographic evidence of fusion.

James H. Calandruccio

Fingertip amputations vary depending on the amount and configuration of skin lost, as well as depth of the defect. If deep tissues and skin must be replaced after tip amputation, various flaps can be used.

THENAR FLAP 〉

Middle and ring finger coverage can be accomplished by the use of the thenar flap. This technique requires a two-stage procedure but has the advantage of involving only one finger. Donor site tenderness and proximal interphalangeal joint flexion contractures can occur and the flaps should not be left in place for more than 3 weeks.

STAGE 1

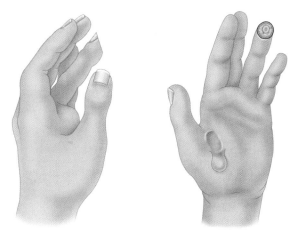

Figure 86-1

- With the thumb held in abduction, flex the injured finger so that its tip touches the middle of the thenar eminence. Outline on the thenar eminence a flap that when raised is large enough to cover the defect and is properly positioned. Pressing the bloody stump of the injured finger against the thenar skin outlines by bloodstain the size of the defect to be covered (Figure 86-1).
- With its base proximal, raise the thenar flap to include most of the underlying fat. Handle the flap with skin hooks to avoid crushing it even with small forceps. Make the flap sufficiently wide so that it is not under tension when sutured to the convex fingertip. Make its length no more than twice its width. By gentle undermining of the skin border at the donor site the defect can be closed directly without resorting to a graft.

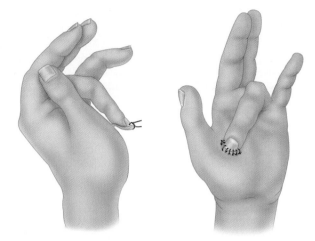

Figure 86-2

- Attach the distal end of the flap to the trimmed edge of the nail by sutures passed through the nail. The lateral edges of the flap should fit the margins of the defect. To avoid impairing circulation in the flap, suture only the most distal parts, if any, to the finger. Prevent the flap from folding back on itself and strangulating its vessels (Figure 86-2).
- Control all bleeding, check the positions of the flap and finger, and apply wet cotton gently compressed to follow the contours of the graft and the fingertip.
- Hold the finger in the proper position by gauze and adhesive tape and splint the wrist.

STAGE 2

At 4 days the graft is dressed again and kept as dry as possible by dressing it every 1 or 2 days and by leaving it partially exposed. At 2 weeks the base of the flap is detached and the free skin edges are sutured in place. The contours of the fingertip and the thenar eminence improve with time.

LOCAL NEUROVASCULAR ISLAND FLAP ⟩

An antegrade neurovascular island graft can provide satisfactory padding and normal sensibility to the most important working surface of the digit.

- Make a midlateral incision on each side of the finger (or thumb) beginning distally at the defect and extending proximally to the level of the proximal interphalangeal joint or thumb interphalangeal joint.

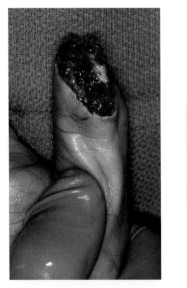
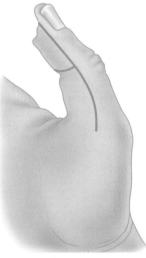

Figure 86-3

- On each side and beginning proximally, carefully dissect the neurovascular bundle distally to the level selected for the proximal margin of the graft (Figure 86-3).

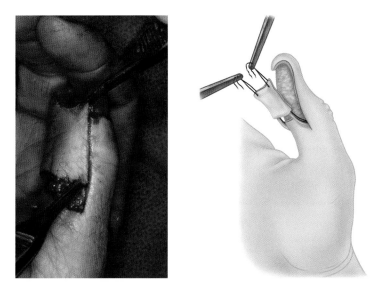

Figure 86-4

- Here make a transverse volar incision through the skin and subcutaneous tissues but carefully protect the neurovascular bundles (Figure 86-4).
- If necessary make another transverse incision at the margin of the defect, freeing a rectangular island of the skin and underlying fat to which are attached the two neurovascular bundles.

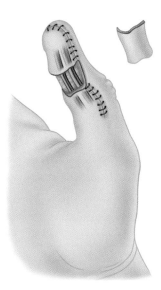

Figure 86-5

- Carefully draw this island or graft distally and place it over the defect. Avoid placing too much tension on the bundles. Should tension compromise the circulation in the graft, dissect the bundles more proximally or flex the distal interphalangeal joint, or both (Figure 86-5).
- Suture the graft in place with interrupted small nonabsorbable sutures.
- Cover the defect created on the volar surface of the finger with a free full-thickness graft.
- Place carefully contoured sterile dressings such as glycerin-soaked cotton balls over the grafts to lessen the likelihood of excess pressure on the neurovascular bundles.
- Apply a compression dressing until suture removal at 10 to 14 days.

POSTOPERATIVE CARE ⟩

Begin digital motion therapy as soon as the wound permits.

ISLAND PEDICLE FLAP 〉

The axial-pattern island pedicle flap may be used to provide sensation or composite soft tissue to adjacent fingers or thumb. The skin paddle size can vary to suit the defect.

- This procedure is performed as outpatient surgery and general anesthesia is preferred.
- Inflate the arm tourniquet after using a skin pen to outline clearly the intended flap design.
- Measure the defect size after appropriate débridement and draw a slightly larger flap onto the donor digit.
- Use a midaxial or a volar zigzag incision to expose the neurovascular bundle of the area of the superficial arch, which is the usual pivot point of the flap.
- If a neurovascular island flap is desired to provide sensation to a given area it is imperative that the ulnar border of the small finger and radial border of the index finger not be used as donors because maintaining or achieving sensation in these areas is desirable. The skin paddle is ideally centered over the neurovascular bundle.
- Under tourniquet control, locate the neurovascular bundle proximally and carefully dissect this to its superficial arch origin. Leave a cuff of soft tissue around the neurovascular bundle because discrete veins are not readily visible but exist in the periarterial tissues. Dissect the bundle deeply and use bipolar cautery well away from the proper digital artery to control perforating vessels entering the flexor sheath.
- Elevate the skin paddle taking care to ensure the vascular bundle is reasonably centered under the flap, and divide the artery distally.
- Use a 5-0 nylon suture to secure the distal vascular bundle to the distal edge of the skin flap.
- Place the paddle over the recipient site to determine the best path for the pedicle because the pedicle should not be under any tension. The skin at the pivot point can be undermined and enlarged by gently but liberally spreading a hemostat in the intended pedicle path. The tunnel must allow easy passage of the flap. Frequently a 2- to 3-cm skin bridge can be left between the proximal donor and recipient incisions. If any doubt remains regarding the pedicle tension or impingement, however, these incisions should be connected.
- Deflate the tourniquet and control bleeding.
- Draw the 5-0 nylon suture gently through the skin bridge taking care not to place shear stress between the pedicle and flap.
- Suture the flap loosely into position, and close the remaining wounds. Ensure the flap remains well vascularized before placing a loose dressing and protective splint.
- When this procedure is performed as a vascular island pedicle flap, the proper digital nerve should be carefully preserved and protected to prevent problematic neuromas. Transient dysesthesias that commonly occur with this technique usually resolve in 6 to 8 weeks.

POSTOPERATIVE CARE 〉

The patient is seen in 5 to 7 days and motion therapy is begun as soon as the wound permits. This is usually 2 to 3 weeks postoperatively.

FOREFOOT BLOCK

E. Greer Richardson

The forefoot block is useful for distal forefoot procedures, including distal first metatarsal osteotomy, sesamoidectomy, or one or two hammer toe procedures.

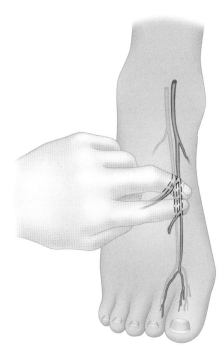

Figure 87-1

- Palpate the dorsalis pedis artery as it reaches the first intermetatarsal space. The deep peroneal nerve to the first web space accompanies this artery (Figure 87-1).
- Using a 25-gauge needle and avoiding the artery, inject 2 to 3 mL of a mixture of short-acting and long-acting local anesthetic agents subcutaneously.

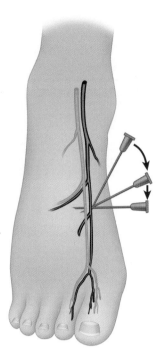

Figure 87-2

- If a second or third hammer toe procedure is planned, direct the needle laterally just beneath the dorsal veins from the same entrance point and block the common digital branches of the superficial peroneal nerve to the second (and if needed, the third) intermetatarsal space. Injection of another 2 to 3 mL should be enough (Figure 87-2).

- Return to the same entrance point but direct the needle medially. Stay immediately beneath the dorsal veins and superficial to the extensor hallucis longus tendon to block the medial hallucal branch of the dorsomedial superficial peroneal nerve. This is the nerve commonly encountered dorsal and medial to the "bunion" during surgery for hallux valgus.

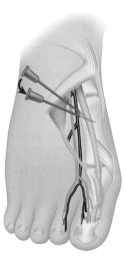

Figure 87-3

- Conclude the dorsal sensory block at the dorsomedial aspect of the forefoot approximately 1 cm distal to the first metatarsomedial cuneiform articulation. By this time, 6 to 8 mL of anesthetic agents has been administered (Figure 87-3).

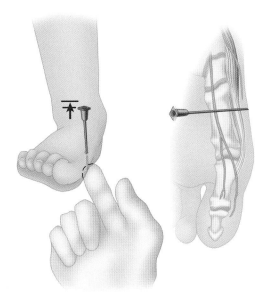

Figure 87-4

- Entering the anesthetized area on the dorsomedial aspect of the forefoot, proceed plantarward in the subcutaneous space superficial to the abductor hallucis muscle until the plantar surface of the medial side of the foot is reached. Inserting a small amount of anesthetic agent as the needle progresses plantarward lessens the discomfort (Figure 87-4).

- The proper plantar branch to the medial side of the hallux is superficial at that level, having penetrated the deep fascia over the abductor hallucis and flexor hallucis brevis at about the level of the first metatarsomedial cuneiform articulation.

- Palpate the tip of the needle subcutaneously and withdraw it 2 to 3 mm. Instill 2 to 3 mL of anesthetic agent.

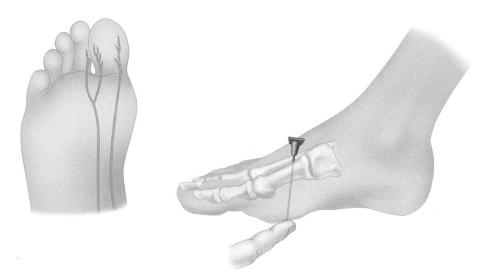

Figure 87-5

- Complete the block by anesthetizing the common digital branch of the medial plantar nerve to the first web space as follows:
  - Return to the dorsal surface of the base of the first intermetatarsal space (Figure 87-5).

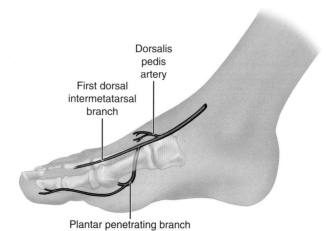

Figure 87-6

- The dorsalis pedis artery bifurcates at this point into the first dorsal intermetatarsal artery and the plantar penetrating branch, which turns immediately plantarward almost at a right angle to its origin to communicate with the deep plantar arch. This is similar to the dorsal branch of the radial artery in the hand. To avoid this arterial bifurcation, move the entrance point distally 1 to 1.5 cm and, angling obliquely 10 to 20 degrees to the skin, pass the 1.5 inch, 25-gauge needle plantarward between the first and second metatarsals until its tip can be felt subcutaneously on the plantar surface of the foot. Instilling a small amount of the anesthetic agent as the needle passes plantarward and moving slowly lessens the discomfort. Withdraw the needle tip 2 to 3 mm and instill 4 to 5 mL of solution (Figure 87-6).

- If a hammer toe procedure is planned, repeat the same technique between the second and third metatarsals. This should provide adequate anesthesia for the third toe if needed. Supplementing the block with 1 mL of anesthetic agent at the base of the third toe near the web space may be necessary.

- The recommended total maximum dose of anesthetic agents should be calculated for each patient. The patient should have no history of allergy to a local anesthetic agent.

ANKLE BLOCK

E. Greer Richardson

Numerous hindfoot procedures can be performed with ankle block anesthesia using a mixture of short-acting and long-acting anesthetic agents. Some of the procedures we perform with the use of regional ankle block anesthesia and a rubber tourniquet are open reduction and internal fixation of tarsometatarsal, midtarsal, and talocalcaneal injuries; osteotomies and arthrodeses distal to the malleoli; tarsal tunnel decompression; and removal of calcific deposits within the Achilles tendon insertion.

SUPERFICIAL PERONEAL NERVE 〉

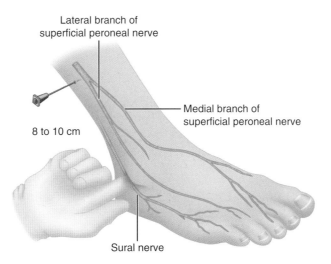

Lateral branch of
superficial peroneal nerve

Medial branch of
superficial peroneal nerve

8 to 10 cm

Figure 88-1

Sural nerve

- Palpate the tip of the lateral malleolus and proceed proximally 8 to 10 cm anterior to the subcutaneous border of the shaft of the fibula (Figure 88-1).
- Instill 5 to 7 mL of local anesthetic agent subcutaneously. The superficial peroneal nerve will have penetrated the deep fascia and lies subcutaneously at this level in most patients. It may have divided into medial and lateral branches but their proximity to one another ensures reaching both with this volume of agent.

DEEP PERONEAL NERVE 〉

- The anterior tibial artery can usually be palpated beneath the superior extensor retinaculum 4 to 5 cm proximal to the distal articular surface of the tibia. This artery and the deep peroneal nerve that accompanies it lie between the tendons of the anterior tibial and the extensor digitorum longus and just lateral to the extensor hallucis longus, which is more deeply situated. The nerve usually lies just lateral to the artery.

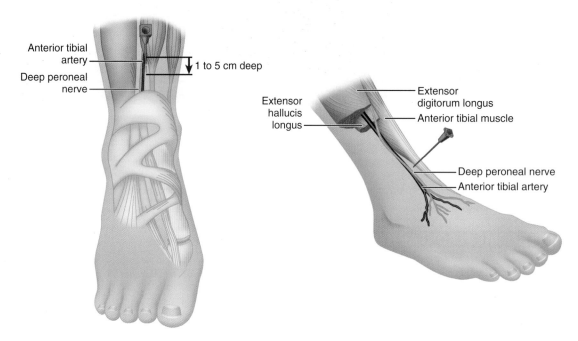

Figure 88-2

- If the artery is not palpable, the tendon of the anterior tibia, which is large and lies adjacent to the subcutaneous border of the tibia, can serve as a landmark. Enter the skin just lateral to this tendon; the nerve is 1 to 1.5 cm deep to the skin (Figure 88-2).
- The anesthetic agent should flow freely. If not, reposition the needle slightly and insert 3 to 5 mL of the agent, being careful to aspirate before the injection.

SAPHENOUS NERVE ⟩

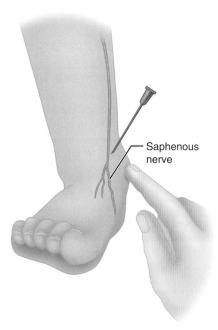

Figure 88-3

- Palpate the tip of the medial malleolus, and 3 to 5 cm proximal to this landmark enter the subcutaneous space, directing the needle anteriorly. The saphenous nerve is just medial or posterior to the saphenous vein and in a slightly deeper plane (Figure 88-3).
- Aspirate and inject 2 mL of the anesthetic agent.

SURAL NERVE 〉

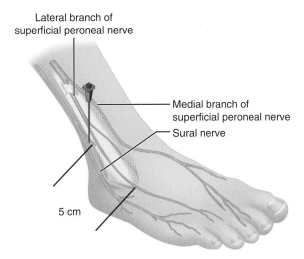

Lateral branch of
superficial peroneal nerve

Medial branch of
superficial peroneal nerve

Sural nerve

5 cm

Figure 88-4

- Palpate the tip of the lateral malleolus and at 5 cm proximal to this point palpate the peroneus longus tendon along the posterior subcutaneous border of the fibula. About half the distance between this tendon and the lateral border of the Achilles tendon passes the sural nerve just anterolateral to the small saphenous vein. These two structures usually cross one another behind the lateral malleolus so that the nerve lies posterior to the vein (Figure 88-4).
- Inject 2 to 3 mL of solution subcutaneously at this point.

TIBIAL NERVE 〉

- The tibial nerve is the most difficult but most important nerve to block to ensure adequate surgical anesthesia.
- Palpate the posteromedial border of the tibia approximately 5 cm proximal to the tip of the medial malleolus. Allow the index and middle fingers to slide over the flexor digitorum longus and (deeper) posterior tibial tendons. At the posterior border of these tendons place a marking pen point of reference.
- Palpate the medial border of the Achilles tendon. At half the distance between these two points lies the tibial artery, which is palpable at this level and serves as a helpful landmark.

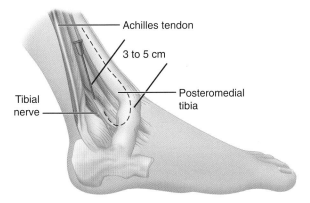

Achilles tendon

3 to 5 cm

Posteromedial
tibia

Tibial
nerve

Figure 88-5

- Point the needle inferiorly at about 60 degrees to the skin, penetrating 1 to 1.5 cm (Figure 88-5).
- Aspirate to ensure the posterior tibial artery or veins have not been entered and then instill 8 to 10 mL of the anesthetic agent.

The usual candidate for soft tissue correction of hallux valgus is a 30- to 50-year-old woman with clinical symptoms and a valgus angle at the metatarsophalangeal joint of 15 to 25 degrees, an intermetatarsal angle of less than 13 degrees, valgus of the interphalangeal joint of less than 15 degrees, no degenerative changes at the metatarsophalangeal joint, and a history of conservative management failure. The modified McBride procedure is successful in properly selected patients.

SKIN AND CAPSULAR INCISION 〉

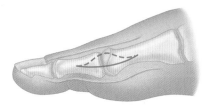

Figure 89-1

- With the patient supine and a tourniquet on the limb, extend a midline, straight, medial incision from the middle of the proximal phalanx to 2 cm proximal to the junction of the medial eminence with the metatarsal shaft. This incision is usually in an internervous plane between the most medial branches of the superficial peroneal nerve dorsally and the medial proper digital branch of the medial plantar nerve plantarward (Figure 89-1). (McBride recommended a single incision beginning at the first web space and extending proximally and medially across the metatarsal, ending on the medial side of the first metatarsal proximal to the exostosis.)

- Mobilize the skin 2 to 3 mm dorsally and plantarward to ensure that no sensory nerve would be injured by the capsular incision.

- Coagulate the superficial veins as encountered to minimize postoperative bleeding.

- Use delicate, two-tooth, retractors and 1.5-mm forceps in this initial dissection to avoid unnecessary skin trauma.

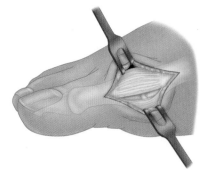

Figure 89-2

- Make a longitudinal capsular incision (the original McBride capsular incision was transverse) 3 to 4 mm plantar to the line of the skin incision (Figure 89-2).

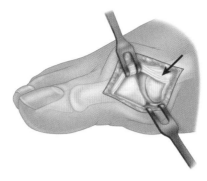

Figure 89-3

- By sharp dissection, raise the periosteum and the capsule dorsally and plantarward from the base of the proximal phalanx to the proximal edge of the medial eminence. At the proximal end of the medial eminence avoid releasing the proximal bony attachments of the medial capsule on the metatarsal neck (especially in the dorsal direction) in an attempt to expose the medial eminence. To ensure adequate exposure without disruption of this proximal attachment a longitudinal capsular incision is suggested (Figure 89-3).
- Elevate the capsule by sharp dissection dorsalward and plantarward to expose the dorsal aspect of the metatarsal head, the entire medial eminence, and the plantar plate. A periosteal elevator is not recommended because of the possibility that the proximal attachments of the capsule may be released.

L-SHAPED CAPSULAR INCISION 〉

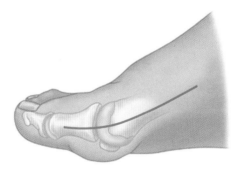

Figure 89-4

- Alternatively, make the capsular incision in an inverted-L shape (Figure 89-4).
- Raise the dorsal flap deep to the nerve and veins until the accessory slip of the extensor hallucis longus tendon is seen in the proximal portion of the incision where it is easier to identify. The tendon can almost always be located with careful searching. If it is not seen at the dorsomedial aspect of the first metatarsal, however, begin the longitudinal limb of the incision at this slope of the metatarsal from dorsal to medial.
- Begin the incision proximally on the dorsomedial side of the first metatarsal shaft and 2 to 3 mm medial to the accessory slip of the extensor hallucis longus tendon. Carry the incision to the bone at the level of the first metatarsal joint, extending proximally 4 to 6 cm.

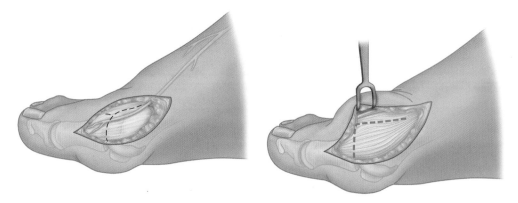

Figure 89-5

- Make the transverse limb of the capsular incision at the level of the joint, stopping 2 to 3 mm from the tibial sesamoid bone; this limb transects the capsular insertion of the abductor hallucis muscle (Figure 89-5).
- Beginning on the plantar aspect of the incision, remove the capsule from the medial eminence from the inside out. Avoid buttonholing the capsule at the junction of the medial eminence and the metatarsal by directing the small-bladed knife down the slope of the eminence.

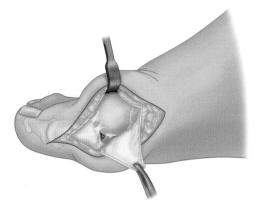

Figure 89-6

- Free the capsule subperiosteally on its dorsomedial surface and retract it proximally and plantarward (Figure 89-6).
- Insert one small Hohmann retractor over the dorsolateral surface of the metatarsal head and another beneath the head at the head and neck junction while distracting and plantar flexing the hallux to expose the articular surface of the metatarsal head for evaluation of its condition and orientation. Reduce the hallux congruently on the metatarsal head.
- If the hallux is in more than 15 degrees of valgus after reduction a distal metatarsal osteotomy is needed.

MEDIAL EMINENCE REMOVAL ⟩

- After inspecting the metatarsophalangeal joint for degenerative changes, loose bodies, or synovial abnormalities, remove the medial eminence by first scoring with an osteotome its proximal edge where the eminence meets the shaft. Always consult the preoperative radiographs to determine how much of the medial eminence should be removed.

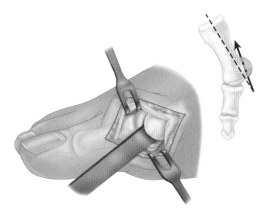

Figure 89-7

- Using the same osteotome or a power saw, begin the exostectomy distally at the parasagittal groove and direct it medially toward the scored area on the metatarsal shaft. If a power saw is used, a 9-mm blade rather than a 4- to 5-mm blade is preferred. The medial direction of the osteotomy prevents splitting of the metatarsal shaft especially if the proximal edge of the osteotomy has been scored as recommended (Figure 89-7).
- After the medial eminence has been removed, use a small rongeur to round off the dorsal and plantar edges of the medial aspect of the metatarsal head. Rasping the raw bone concludes the initial stage of the procedure. Use bone wax on the raw surfaces of bone of the metatarsal head.

ADDUCTOR TENDON AND LATERAL CAPSULAR RELEASE ⟩

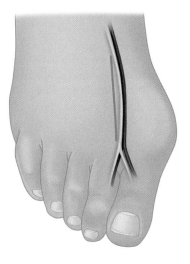

Figure 89-8

- Begin the second stage with a dorsal longitudinal incision beginning 2 to 3 mm proximal to the dorsal aspect of the first web space to avoid web contracture postoperatively; extend it proximally between the first and second metatarsal heads for 3 to 4 cm. This allows adequate exposure of the adductor insertion into the base of the proximal phalanx, the lateral head of the flexor hallucis brevis muscle converging on the fibular sesamoid, and the entire lateral capsule from the extensor hallucis longus muscle to the plantar plate (Figure 89-8).
- Delicate retraction of the skin exposes the dorsal digital branches of the veins, which should be cauterized if they obscure the deeper dissection. The terminal branches of the first dorsal intermetatarsal artery may be encountered at a location adjacent to the proper digital branches of the deep peroneal nerve to the first web space.

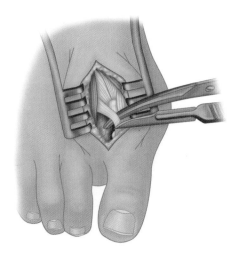

Figure 89-9

- The main portion of the adductor tendon inserts into the base of the proximal phalanx just plantar to the longitudinal axis of the phalanx. It also has a smaller insertion, along with the lateral head of the flexor hallucis brevis muscle, into the fibular sesamoid. The simplest technique to identify the insertion of the adductor hallucis tendon is to place a small, pointed, curved hemostat on the dorsolateral base of the proximal phalanx, slide it firmly plantarward, and lift the hemostat dorsally and laterally; the tip of the instrument usually rests in the axilla of the insertion of the adductor tendon. This is comparable to securing the iliopsoas tendon for tenotomy at the lesser trochanter (Figure 89-9).
- When the primary insertion is released, grasp the tendon with forceps or a hemostat and, with traction, displace it dorsally and laterally toward the second metatarsal so that further dissection is on the medial side of the adductor, or push the sesamoid sling laterally through the previously placed medial incision to aid exposure.
- While spreading the first and second metatarsal heads with a small Inge retractor, heavy-duty two-tooth retractors or a Weitlaner retractor, hold the adductor tendon under tension, which facilitates exposure. The lateral head of the flexor hallucis brevis muscle, the lateral border of the fibular sesamoid, and the slip of the adductor tendon (confluent with the lateral head of the flexor hallucis brevis muscle) come into view in the depths of the wound.

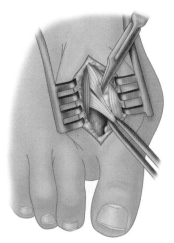

Figure 89-10

- All attachments of the adductor into its conjoined insertion with the lateral head of the flexor hallucis brevis muscle into the fibular sesamoid must be severed; with traction on the adductor, it freely and independently moves without tethering the fibular sesamoid (Figure 89-10).
- This deep transverse intermetatarsal ligament, which lies just plantar to the adductor, may be released by the incision along the lateral border of the sesamoid. If not, release this ligament, carefully preserving the

neurovascular bundle immediately beneath it, and incise the lateral capsule. Mann emphasized that release of the deep transverse metatarsal ligament endangers the neurovascular bundle to the first web space, which lies immediately beneath this ligament. Sliding a small Freer elevator between this ligament and the neurovascular bundle would protect the latter structures.

FIBULAR (LATERAL) SESAMOIDECTOMY: DORSAL APPROACH 〉

- If after complete adductor hallucis release and preferably after a lateral capsular release a fibular sesamoidectomy is needed to correct the valgus deformity of the great toe fully, it should be done at this time.
- Adequately separate the first and second metatarsal heads for exposure.
- Plantar flex the metatarsophalangeal joint 10 to 20 degrees, which reduces tension on the sesamoids.

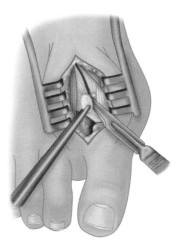

Figure 89-11

- Grasp the fibular sesamoid with a small Kocher clamp or sturdy tissue forceps and pull it laterally into the intermetatarsal space (Figure 89-11).
- Release the intersesamoid ligament. When this ligament has been incised, bring the fibular sesamoid into the intermetatarsal space, where its removal is straightforward. Care must be taken when incising the intersesamoid ligament to avoid severing the flexor hallucis longus tendon immediately plantar to it. If the tendon is severed it probably should not be repaired at this level; loss of the tendon causes little if any functional impairment and repair may result in a fixed flexion contracture of the interphalangeal joint.

FIBULAR SESAMOIDECTOMY: PLANTAR APPROACH 〉

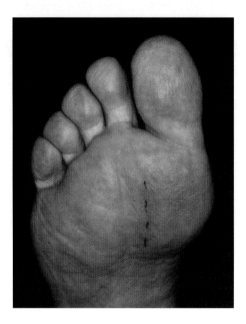

Figure 89-12

- If a plantar approach is chosen for fibular sesamoidectomy, have an assistant hold the ankle dorsiflexed and use a headlight for seeing into the full depth of the wound. Avoid the flexor hallucis longus tendon and the neurovascular bundle to the first web space (Figure 89-12).
- Flex and extend the hallux and inspect the radiograph to locate the sesamoid. Beginning 1.0 to 1.5 cm distal to the metatarsophalangeal joint, make a longitudinal incision in the plantar surface of the foot, extending the incision proximally 3.5 to 4.0 cm between the first and second metatarsals.
- If the fibular sesamoid requires excision it is usually subluxed.
- When the skin and fascial septa within the forefoot pad have been separated, insert a small self-retaining retractor.

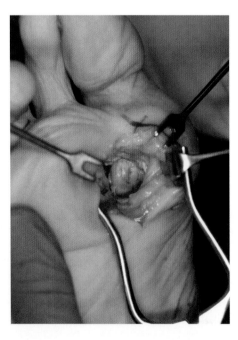

Figure 89-13

- Using small, blunt-tip dissecting scissors, identify the neurovascular bundle to the first web space and retract it laterally or medially depending on the position of the sesamoid (Figure 89-13).

- Palpate the sesamoids and flex and extend the hallux to locate the flexor hallucis longus tendon.
- Open the pulley over the flexor hallucis longus tendon and retract the tendon medially. This maneuver is made easier by having an assistant hold the foot in dorsiflexion at the arch with one hand and flex the metatarsophalangeal joint to relax the flexor hallucis longus tendon with the opposite hand.

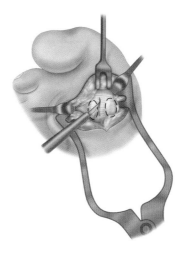

Figure 89-14

- At this point the intersesamoid ligament should come into view; divide it completely. This may require moving the scalpel 1 or 2 mm laterally or medially to find the groove between the sesamoids (Figure 89-14).
- Incise the cleavage plane between the two sesamoids while retracting the flexor hallucis longus muscle medially and the neurovascular bundle laterally.
- Grasp the fibular sesamoid with a strong pick-up or small Kocher clamp and remove the lateral head insertion of the flexor hallucis brevis muscle on the proximal end of the sesamoid using direct vision (loupe magnification makes this easier but is not necessary).
- When the medial and proximal restraints of the sesamoid have been released, sever the attachment of the adductor hallucis muscle to its lateral distal edge close to the bone with a scalpel or scissors.

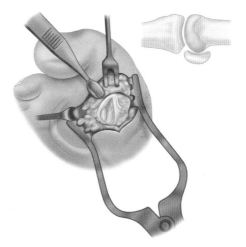

Figure 89-15

- Sever the last attachment of the sesamoid distally where the plantar plate continues its distal insertion into the proximal phalanx (Figure 89-15).
- When the sesamoid has been removed, inspect the wound carefully for any bleeding. Pressing on the edges of the wound helps identify any potential bleeding vessels, which should be cauterized.

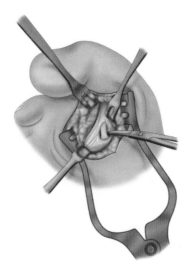

Figure 89-16

- Excising the sesamoid does not release the adductor insertion on the base of the proximal phalanx. This can be released through the plantar incision. Continuing to retract the neurovascular bundle laterally and the flexor hallucis longus muscle medially, and adducting the hallux while the opposite index finger palpates the adductor helps identify the structure (Figure 89-16).

- Using right-angle retractors, expose the adductor, excise a small section of the tendon, and move the hallux medially.

- At the conclusion of this procedure the surgeon should be unable to palpate any restraining structures on the fibular side of the metatarsophalangeal joint. The transverse natatory fibers in the dorsal aspect of the web space should be released manually. All restraints pulling the hallux laterally (except the extrinsic tendons) must be removed.

- Inspect the neurovascular bundle and the flexor hallucis longus tendon.

MEDIAL CAPSULAR IMBRICATION AND WOUND CLOSURE 》

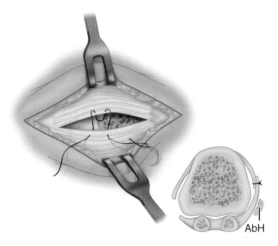

Figure 89-17

- With an assistant holding the metatarsophalangeal joint in a congruously reduced position in the varus-valgus and flexion-extension planes, imbricate the medial capsule in the following manner (Figure 89-17).

- Using absorbable 3-0 or interrupted sutures, place the initial suture through the plantar flap of the capsule at a point 4 to 5 mm medial to the proximal medial border of the medial (tibial) sesamoid and in an outside-to-inside direction.

- Turn the needle on itself and pass it through the dorsal flap at the same level in an outside-to-inside direction. Immediately pass the suture back through the dorsal flap from inside out and finally through the plantar flap from inside out (a swedged-on needle would suffice but a small cutting needle is recommended).
- With the hallux held in the desired position, tie this suture, bringing the plantar flap over the dorsal flap and pulling the plantar-displaced abductor hallucis toward the midline of the longitudinal axis of the proximal phalanx and first metatarsal.
- Allow the toe to rest unassisted to judge its resting posture and the tension on the capsular repair.

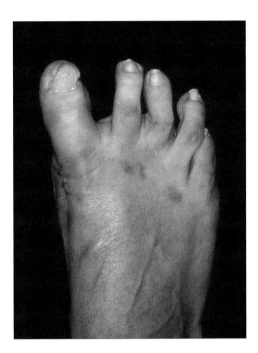

Figure 89-18

- If the fibular sesamoid has been removed do not imbricate the medial capsule to avoid pulling the tibial sesamoid medial to the metatarsal head, which may cause a hallux varus deformity. If a large medial eminence has persisted for many years with increased capsular reaction and redundancy a portion of the dorsal flap may need to be excised before closure (Figure 89-18).

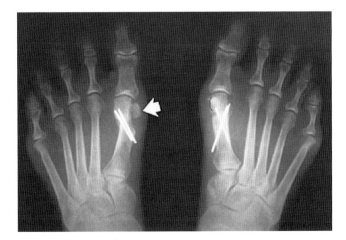

Figure 89-19

- It is imperative to avoid pulling the medial side of the tibial sesamoid medial to the articular surface of the first metatarsal head; do not uncover the tibial sesamoid, because this may cause sesamoid dislocation (Figure 89-19).
- If the resting posture of the hallux is acceptable, close the remaining portion of the capsule with interrupted 2-0 or 3-0 absorbable sutures.

CLOSURE OF THE INVERTED-L CAPSULOTOMY 〉

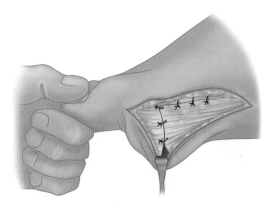

Figure 89-20

- Begin the closure proximally using 3-0 sutures on a small swedged-on needle; bending the needle to increase the curve makes passage easier in a small wound (Figure 89-20).
- While an assistant applies tension distally on the free corner of the capsule, place the most proximal suture in the longitudinal limb of the capsular incision; place two or three sutures at 5-mm intervals. Do *not* place the corner suture.
- Begin to close the transverse limb of the incision at the medial plantar corner.
- Hold the hallux reduced on the metatarsal head while tying all sutures.
- Unless the capsule is redundant, do not imbricate the medial capsule over the area of eminence removal. Close this portion of the transverse limb with side-to-side sutures, and place the imbricating suture in the dorsomedial corner of the capsulotomy.
- Begin this final suture distally on the transverse limb of the inverted L, passing the needle from the outside in.
- Reverse the needle and enter the capsular flap from the outside in on the transverse limb.
- Reverse the needle and reenter the capsular flap from the inside out on the longitudinal limb of the flap.
- Make the final pass of the needle from the inside out on the dorsal side of the longitudinal limb of the incision. Holding the joint in its reduced position, tie the suture.
- If the joint reduction is congruent, but the hallux is still in an unacceptable valgus position, metatarsal osteotomy should be considered.
- If the transverse limb of the capsular repair is too loose, allowing the hallux to slide into valgus, remove the midline medial suture in the transverse limb. While holding the hallux in the proper position, place the suture 2 to 3 mm farther away from the incision or excise more capsule from the proximal portion. Take care in removing any extra capsule because removal of even a small portion results in a significant correction of capsular laxity and may cause varus of the hallux.
- At the conclusion of the procedure the hallux should rest on the metatarsal head in about 5 degrees of valgus and 10 degrees of extension.
- If an elastic wrap has been used as a tourniquet, remove it and have the patient flex and extend the toe (if a local anesthetic has been used) to assess function and congruence of the repositioned hallux.
- Lavage the wound, secure hemostasis, and close the skin with interrupted or simple mattress sutures. If simple sutures are used, ensure that the skin edges are not inverted or overlapped. If everted mattress sutures are used, do not evert the edges so much that they do not approximate evenly.

POSTOPERATIVE CARE 〉

A bulky compression dressing is applied to the forefoot and the foot is placed in a position of maximal elevation for 48 to 72 hours. Bathroom privileges only are allowed and the patient must wear a wooden-soled shoe. Increased ambulation after 72 hours is allowed as tolerated by the patient. The need for crutches or a walker varies, but assisted ambulation is not encouraged unless the patient is unsteady.

At 3 weeks, if the wounds are healed, the sutures are removed and adhesive strips are applied if needed; leaving the sutures in longer has no untoward effect. Some type of immobilizer or toe spacer to hold the toe in proper alignment is used. The wooden-soled shoe is used for 3 to 4 weeks, at which time a deep shoe with a wide toe box is recommended; a jogging shoe is sufficient; an extra-depth orthopaedic shoe with a soft toe box also is permissible. The toe spacer is worn for 6 weeks. At 12 to 14 weeks a reasonably attractive shoe usually can be worn. The period of postoperative edema varies, however, and it may take 4 to 6 months before this type of shoe is tolerated. This is explained to the patient before surgery.

See also Video 90-1.

The Keller procedure combines resection hemiarthroplasty of the first metatarsophalangeal joint with removal of the medial eminence of the first metatarsal (Fig. 90-1). Although removing the base of the proximal phalanx decompresses the joint and mobilizes the hallux, allowing marked correction of valgus, the varus of the first metatarsal is not corrected, thus maintaining correction of the valgus of the hallux is difficult. Other complications of the Keller procedure have been emphasized in the literature to such an extent (with neither the incidence nor the severity of such complications clearly documented) that the indications for this procedure have been limited severely. In our experience however, complications are uncommon if patients are selected carefully. Modifications in the original technique also have allowed expansion of the indications for the Keller bunionectomy.

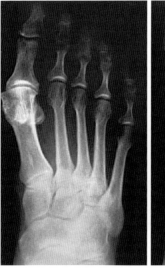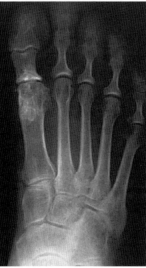

Figure 90-1

Candidates for the Keller procedure are patients older than 50 years with moderate-to-severe hallux valgus (30 to 45 degrees); intermetatarsal angles of 13 degrees or less, indicating mild-to-moderate metatarsus primus varus; and pain over the medial eminence with any shoe worn, so the variety of shoes the patient can wear is severely limited. An incongruous first metatarsophalangeal joint caused by lateral subluxation of the phalanx on the metatarsal head, severe lateral displacement of the sesamoids, and any evidence of degenerative cartilage changes in the joint are all radiographic indications for the Keller procedure.

Two modifications in technique can expand these indications to include patients with more severe deformities (but not to include younger patients): fibular sesamoidectomy and lateral displacement of the first metatarsal. Patients with 50 degrees or more of valgus of the hallux (18 to 20 degrees of varus of the first metatarsal), complete lateral dislocation of the sesamoids, marked degenerative changes, and severe pronation of the hallux may benefit functionally and cosmetically from alterations of the standard technique.

- If pedal pulses are good use an Esmarch wrap tourniquet.
- Use 1% lidocaine (Xylocaine) and 0.5% bupivacaine (Marcaine) in equal portions within standard dose limits for the forefoot block.
- Make a straight midline medial incision 1 cm proximal to the interphalangeal joint of the hallux and extend it proximally to the junction of the distal and middle thirds of the first metatarsal. This lengthy incision is made to avoid excessive traction tension on the skin.

- By blunt dissection, locate the most medial branch of the superficial peroneal nerve at the proximal-dorsal edge of the medial eminence and retract it for protection.
- Carry the dissection to the first metatarsal in the midline medially beginning in the proximal limit of the wound and extending distally across the midline of the medial eminence and along the proximal phalanx to the distal extent of the wound.
- Raise the deep flap of tissue by sharp dissection dorsally beginning at the junction of the medial eminence and shaft of the first metatarsal.
- Raise the periosteum and capsule dorsally up to one third to one half the width of the metatarsal.
- At the joint, continue the capsular elevation along the extensor hallucis brevis insertion until the proximal third of the proximal phalanx is exposed as far laterally as possible under direct vision. To make exposure easier, have an assistant pronate the hallux as the dissection proceeds laterally. Subperiosteal dissection should expose only the portion of the proximal phalanx that is to be removed.
- Plantarly dissect just enough to expose the plantar aspect of the medial eminence proximally, the tibial sesamoid in the center of the wound, and the plantar-medial corner of the proximal phalanx.
- Supinate the proximal phalanx to expose the plantar corner and proximal third of the shaft for the sharp dissection. The proximal phalanx is round on three sides but its plantar surface is flat and even concave in the midline where the flexor hallucis longus tendon passes. This change in contour must be taken into account when dissecting to avoid injury of the flexor hallucis longus tendon.
- By blunt dissection, identify the flexor hallucis longus tendon and retract it plantarward with a small right-angle retractor to protect it throughout the dissection of the proximal phalanx.
- Resect the medial eminence at the sagittal groove beginning dorsally at its distal edge and directing a 9-mm oscillating blade (or osteotome) plantarward and slightly medially (5 to 10 degrees).

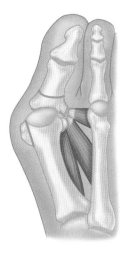 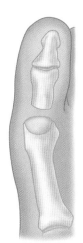 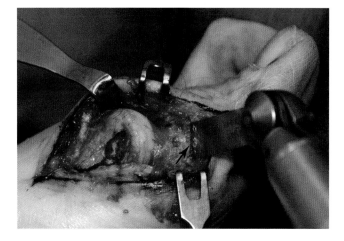

Figure 90-2

- Remove the base of the proximal phalanx at the metaphyseal-diaphyseal junction, which usually constitutes the proximal third of the phalanx. To prevent damage to the flexor hallucis longus and the neurovascular bundles, place a retractor over the bone dorsally and plantarward and rotate the phalanx into view. Also, do not allow the saw blade to exit bone more than 1 to 2 mm (Figure 90-2).

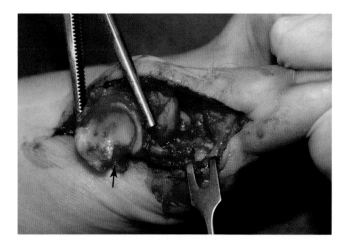

Figure 90-3

- When the osteotomy has been completed, grasp the basilar fragment with a small Kocher clamp or towel clip and rotate the fragment while applying medial pull to excise it. Lift it away from its lateral attachments, which are primarily the lateral collateral ligaments and the adductor muscle tendinous insertion (Figure 90-3).
- With the ankle at 90 degrees, bring the hallux into a corrected position, while manually pushing the first metatarsal as far laterally as possible. Evaluate the alignment, keeping the metatarsal and hallux straight.
- Grasp the hallux in one hand and displace the proximal remnant medially so that, under direct vision, two longitudinal 0.062-inch Kirschner wires can be inserted.
- Hold the interphalangeal joint straight while drilling the wires from proximal to distal, emerging a few millimeters plantar to the nail plate.
- Return the foot to the corrected position and drill the wires into the metatarsal head.
- While holding the metatarsal as far laterally as possible, cross the joint and drive the wires out the plantar cortex just proximal to the head, while holding the hallux in 10 to 15 degrees of extension, neutral abduction, adduction, and rotation and with no translation dorsally or plantarward on the metatarsal head. The wires should penetrate only 2 to 3 mm past the cortex to avoid tenderness over the wires with weight bearing.
- If the Kirschner wires tend to "walk" on the rounded articular surface of the metatarsal head, use a small hemostat snugged up against the wire while it is being drilled to allow accurate placement. Proper placement of the wires and the desired position of the hallux on the metatarsal may require several attempts. The medial aspect of the proximal phalanx should not rest medial to the medial aspect of the metatarsal head.
- Place the hallux in the neutral mediolateral plane and in 10 degrees of extension.
- Before the second wire is driven into the first metatarsal head, place the hallux in proper rotation using the plane of the nail as a guide. The initial length of the hallux is maintained by the wires. Later, collapse occurs when the wires are removed but improved encapsulation of the hemiarthroplasty, by maintaining length for the first few weeks, may help maintain a more desirable position long term.
- Cut the wires 2 to 3 mm distal to the skin edge.
- Remove the tourniquet and secure hemostasis.
- Close the capsule with interrupted 2-0 or 3-0 absorbable sutures. A firm, complete capsular closure is imperative. A box stitch is recommended. Increasing the curve of the needle manually is helpful.
- Starting proximal and plantarward, pass the suture through the capsule from the outside in.
- The second pass of the suture is from the inside out through substantial soft tissue on the plantar-medial aspect of the phalangeal base.
- Reenter the soft tissue at the base of the proximal phalangeal remnant dorsomedially for the third pass. Move the suture back and forth to ensure uninhibited excursion.
- Make the fourth pass from inside out through the dorsal capsule in line with the initial plantar capsular suture. Have an assistant grasp the ends of the capsule, pulling them together, while the tie is completed. This is basically a four-corner box stitch, which may leave a small area of capsule in the middle that cannot be approximated, but this is of no consequence.
- Intersperse interrupted sutures as needed to complete a firm closure.

- Release the tourniquet and close the skin with nonabsorbable 4-0 sutures.
- Apply a compression forefoot dressing extending just distal to the tarsonavicular tuberosity so that only the toenails are exposed and no loose edges of gauze are raised above the dressing. A snug but nonconstricting, layered, contoured forefoot dressing is vital to reduce edema.
- Cover the tips of the wires with circular adhesive bandages or commercially available "pin balls."

Several modifications of the Keller technique can expand the indications for its use with more severe deformities.

REMOVAL OF THE FIBULAR SESAMOID 〉

- When the medial eminence and phalangeal base have been excised, remove the fibular sesamoid.

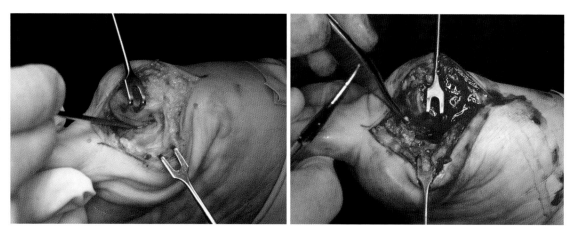

Figure 90-4

- Place a sturdy two-toothed retractor beneath the metatarsal head and have an assistant lift it dorsally. Using a Freer elevator or a small osteotome for its strength, mobilize the fibular sesamoid. This may be difficult in elderly patients with significant deformity and adherence of the sesamoid to the metatarsal head. When mobilization of fibular sesamoid is complete, the entire sesamoid is visible for excision (Figure 90-4).

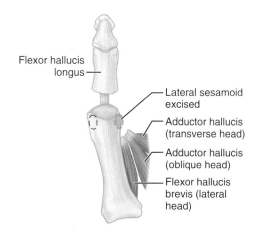

Figure 90-5

- By excising the fibular sesamoid, the valgus moment of conjoined tendon of the flexor hallucis brevis and adductor hallucis no longer pulls the flexor hallucis longus tendon laterally (carrying the hallux with it) through the capsulosesamoid plantar plate and pulley system (Figure 90-5).

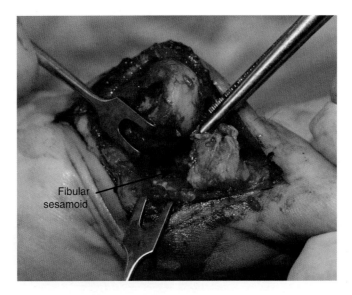

Figure 90-6

- Lift the metatarsal dorsally for exposure (Figure 90-6).
- When the sesamoid is mobile, identify the flexor hallucis longus tendon by placing traction on the hallux and flexing and extending the interphalangeal joint of the hallux. The tendon is visible just distal to and in alignment with the sesamoids, which straddle it.
- Identify and expose the lateral neurovascular bundle just lateral to the tendon by blunt dissection.
- Pull the plantar-medial capsule medially. This requires a firm grasp on the capsule. The medial traction brings the intersesamoid "ligament" into better view.
- Incise the intersesamoid ligament longitudinally with a no. 67 Beaver or no. 15 Bard-Parker blade. If tenotomy scissors are used, place one arm of the scissors under the ligament (this arm rests on the dorsal side of the flexor hallucis longus) and the other arm dorsal to the ligament.
- When the intersesamoid ligament is incised, grasp the sesamoid firmly with forceps or a small Kocher clamp, flex the toe at the interphalangeal and metatarsophalangeal joints to relax the flexor hallucis longus tendon, and pull the fibular sesamoid distally and medially.
- With release of the intersesamoid ligament the medial surface of the fibular sesamoid is free from soft tissue. Distally the sesamoid is free because of resection of the base of the proximal phalanx. This leaves two sides of the sesamoid, distal and medial, free of soft tissue.
- While pulling the sesamoid distally and medially use a small blade to incise along the lateral margin of the sesamoid under direct vision. Keep pulling the head of the metatarsal dorsally and holding the hallux distracted and in flexion. This greatly aids in identification of the margins of the fibular sesamoid, particularly laterally and proximally.
- The most difficult part of the sesamoidectomy and that which should be done last is release of the proximal lateral corner of the sesamoid where the flexor hallucis brevis lateral head inserts. While incising the lateral capsular attachments to the sesamoid do not bury the blade of the knife because the neurovascular bundle to the lateral side of the hallux is just lateral to the capsule.
- Now all attachments to the fibular sesamoid have been removed except the lateral head of the flexor hallucis brevis, which inserts on the proximal lateral margin of the sesamoid. This is a difficult section to remove; however, this section can be released under direct vision by pulling the sesamoid distally and medially and lifting the metatarsal head dorsally with a strong two-toothed retractor.

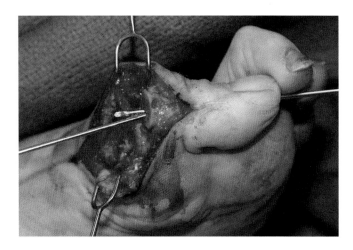

Figure 90-7

- When the sesamoid has been removed, insert two 0.062-inch Kirschner wires retrograde from the tip of the toe 2 to 3 mm plantar to the nail bed, leaving about 5 to 7 mm of the pins exposed at the base of the phalangeal remnant to help align the phalanx on the metatarsal before antegrade passage of the pins into the metatarsal (Figure 90-7).

LATERAL DISPLACEMENT OF THE FIRST METATARSAL

- Push the metatarsal laterally several times. Occasionally, this does not move the metatarsal, but some lateral mobility is usually present.
- While standing next to the patient looking distally at the dorsum of the foot, dorsiflex the ankle to neutral.
- Viewing the foot as the patient would, hold the first metatarsal firmly and move its distal end laterally. Hold this position with one hand and use the other hand to place the hallux on the metatarsal head and out to length.

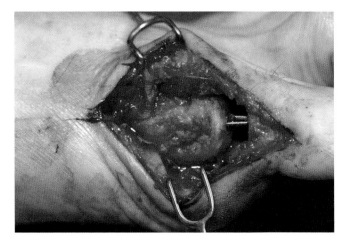

Figure 90-8

- While holding the first ray straight with the foot vertical, have an assistant insert the wires from distal to proximal. Often these wires, which run through the first metatarsal and hallux, hold the first ray straight and most of this correction is maintained after the wires have been removed (Figure 90-8).

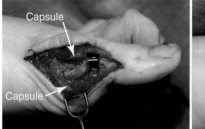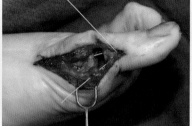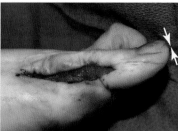

Figure 90-9

- Close the capsule with a purse-string suture (Figure 90-9).

Presumably, the laterally displaced fibular sesamoid, when pulled proximally by the lateral head of the relaxed flexor hallucis brevis, pulls the flexor hallucis longus laterally through the sesamoid apparatus, which encases it and contributes to recurrent hallux valgus. In addition, while reoperating after a failed Keller procedure, we observed a strong, linear, fibrous attachment of the fibular sesamoid to the proximal phalangeal remnant (Figure 90-10), which pulled the hallux into valgus when tension was applied to it. For these reasons, when the deformity is severe, the hallux and first metatarsal maintain better alignment if excision of the fibular sesamoid and lateral displacement of the metatarsal are added to the procedure.

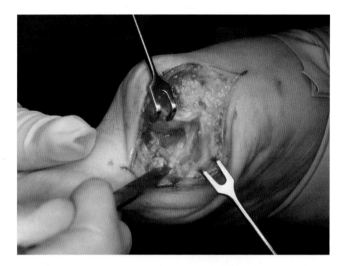

Figure 90-10

POSTOPERATIVE CARE

A firm-soled, postoperative shoe is worn, and weight bearing is allowed to tolerance with or without the assistance of crutches or a walker. Bathroom privileges only are allowed for the first 72 hours. The foot is elevated except during meals and bathroom visits. After this period the patient may be up and about as symptoms allow. Taking more pain medication to allow increased activity is discouraged. For 7 to 10 days after surgery the foot should be elevated when the patient is sitting.

The dressing is changed at 19 to 23 days and the wires remain in place for 21 to 28 days. If the hallux migrates proximally on the wires and the wires protrude too far before time to remove them, the tips are cut 1 to 2 mm distal to the skin edge. The Kirschner wires are removed in the office by placing a large or medium-sized needle holder longitudinally over the tip of the wire, rotating it back and forth gently and pulling with gentle traction. To prevent excessive bleeding, the foot is elevated for 5 minutes after the wires have been removed. A good method of elevation is to place the patient supine with the unoperated knee flexed 90 degrees and the foot flat on the table and then to place the ankle of the operated foot on the flexed knee. A small plastic strip bandage is placed over the holes when the bleeding has stopped.

A small or medium-sized toe spacer (commercially available) is worn in the first web for an additional 4 to 6 weeks; this spacer is removed only for bathing. A wide, soft shoe is allowed after the pins have been removed. Dress shoes are allowed only after most of the edema has resolved, which may take 3 to 4 months. The expected results are a satisfactorily well-aligned hallux with 40 to 50 degrees of motion at the metatarsophalangeal joint, relief of pain, and some improvement in the variety of shoes that can be worn.

See also Video 91-1.

MODIFIED CHEVRON DISTAL METATARSAL OSTEOTOMY ⟩

The modified chevron osteotomy is simply a more proximal placement of the apex of the osteotomy in the metatarsal head. Potential problems of this modification of the chevron osteotomy are instability of the osteotomy and insufficient metaphyseal bony contact. Proper placement of the osteotomy cuts is mandatory. The metatarsal osteotomy must be internally fixed. With some modifications, however, the chevron osteotomy can be used for more severe deformities (up to 35 degrees of hallux valgus and up to 15 degrees of first to second intermetatarsal diversion). As an alternative, the valgus appearance of the hallux can be corrected by an additional few degrees with an additional osteotomy of the proximal phalanx. This phalangeal osteotomy augments cosmetic correction only if the metatarsophalangeal joint has been rendered congruent in the corrected position. Also, a basal osteotomy of the proximal phalanx adjacent to the distal metatarsal osteotomy may cause more limitation of motion of the first metatarsophalangeal joint than a single osteotomy. The patient should be informed of this possibility.

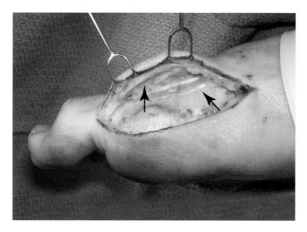

Figure 91-1

- Make a medial midline incision, protecting the dorsal veins and dorsal and plantar sensory nerves to the medial side of the hallux (Figure 91-1).
- When the capsule is exposed, make a longitudinal incision along the dorsomedial aspect of the first metatarsal.

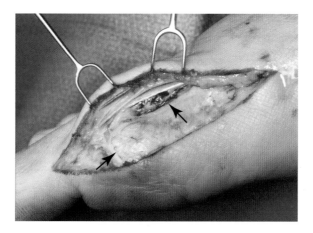

Figure 91-2

- Begin the second limb of the capsulotomy 1 to 2 mm proximal to the base of the proximal phalanx and in a coronal plane at right angles to the first limb of the capsulotomy (Figure 91-2).

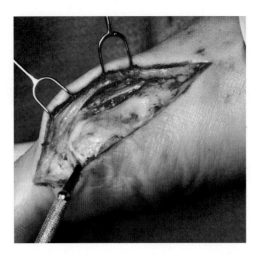

Figure 91-3

- Extend the coronal incision plantarward 1 to 2 mm proximal to the junction with the tibial sesamoid (Figure 91-3).

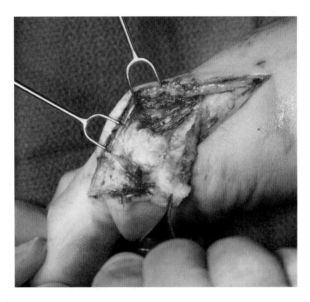

Figure 91-4

- Raise the capsule, beginning medially and plantarward, by sharply dissecting it from the inside out and off the most prominent part of the medial eminence until its dorsal aspect is reached (Figure 91-4).
- Maintain the incision close to bone, curving over the medial eminence as the contour demands, and take a full-thickness piece of capsule from the medial eminence and proximally along the metatarsal shaft for 3 to 4 cm. This should leave the fascial attachment of the abductor hallucis in continuity with the periosteum and fascial covering of the first metatarsal shaft.
- Ensure that the plantar aspect of the metatarsal head where it meets with the shaft is adequately exposed so that the plantar osteotomy cut can be made under direct vision. Remove the medial eminence.

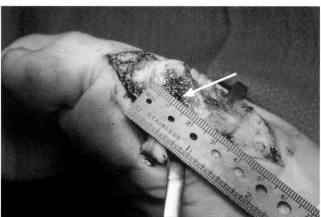
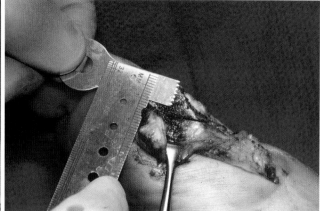

Figure 91-5

- Using a 0.062-inch Kirschner wire and starting 1.0 to 1.3 cm proximal to the subchondral bone and in the center of the first metatarsal head, drill a hole from medial to lateral marking the apex of the intended osteotomy (Figure 91-5).
- Mark the limbs of the osteotomy with a sharp osteotome or a marking pen and begin the osteotomy with the dorsal cut. Avoid pushing the saw blade in and out of the bone; slowly glide the blade across the head-neck fragment with gentle back-and-forth rather than in-and-out movements.
- When there is no further resistance to the blade laterally, extract it and return to the centering hole. Ensure that the dorsal and lateral aspects of the cortical bone have been incised.

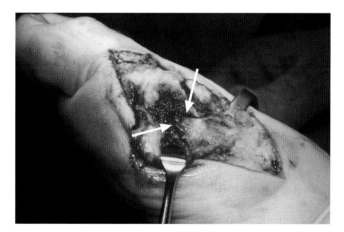

Figure 91-6

- Begin the plantar limb of the osteotomy at a point approximately 30 degrees from the midline or 60 degrees from the original dorsal osteotomy. Make this cut slowly and deliberately at right angles to the bone, exiting plantarward 2 to 3 mm proximal to where the articular surface of the metatarsal head meets the shaft. A small, right-angle retractor pulling the capsule plantarward increases exposure (Figure 91-6).
- If the osteotomy cuts have been made appropriately the capital fragment usually displaces laterally with minimal lateral pressure. If this is not the case, either the osteotomy cuts are not parallel, or the plantar cortex, dorsal cortex, or both have not been penetrated laterally.
- If gentle pressure on the head fragment does not displace it laterally while the shaft fragment is held stable, reposition the saw blade, being careful not to start the saw until the blade is in the depths of the osteotomy cut.

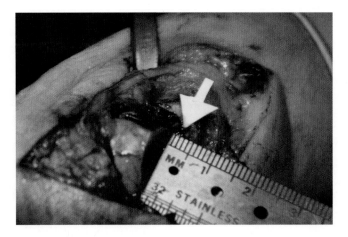

Figure 91-7

- When the capital fragment has been freed from the proximal fragment, shift it laterally 4 to 5 mm (Figure 91-7).
- Impact the head fragment on the shaft by applying gentle pressure to the hallux.

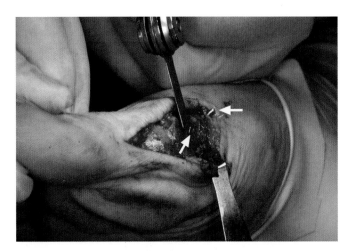

Figure 91-8

- While holding the capital fragment straight on the metatarsal shaft, internally fix the osteotomy. Insert one or two 0.062-inch Kirschner wires obliquely across the osteotomy site (Figure 91-8).
- Begin inserting the first wire dorsomedially and far enough proximally in the shaft to leave cortical bone between the pin and the cancellous portion of the distal-medial shaft when the overhanging ridge of bone is made flush with the capital fragment. Direct the wire so that it reaches the lateral aspect of the capital fragment.
- Insert the second wire into the metatarsal head at a point 3 to 4 mm plantar and parallel to the first.
- Test the osteotomy for stability and gently open the metatarsophalangeal joint by pushing the toe laterally.
- Examine the entire surface of the metatarsal head with a small Freer elevator to locate any Kirschner wire points. If the joint has been entered, retract the wire slightly so that it rests in subchondral bone. Because the entrance of the wire into subchondral bone and its exit through the cartilage of the head usually can be felt while drilling, withdrawing the wire about 2 mm usually places it in the proper position.
- Circumduct the hallux on the first metatarsal head; if any catching occurs, reinspect the joint for wire points. If there is any doubt, obtain radiographs.

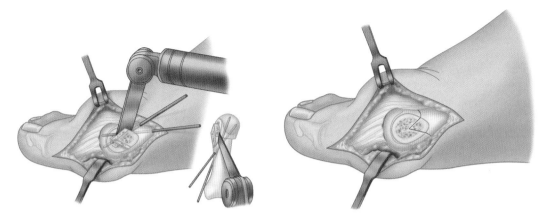

Figure 91-9

- Incise the overhanging segment on the medial side of the proximal fragment and with a rasp smooth it flush with the capital fragment (Figure 91-9).

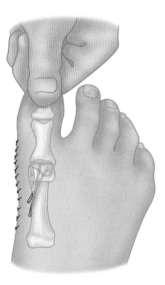

Figure 91-10

- Place the hallux on the metatarsal head in a congruous position, which can be determined by flexing, extending, abducting, adducting, and rotating the hallux on the first metatarsal head and observing the foot from the top (Figure 91-10).
- While an assistant holds the toe reduced, close the capsular incision by first closing its proximal part with two or three interrupted 2-0 or 3-0 absorbable sutures.
- Dorsally, pass the needle through the periosteum and deep fascia, over the metatarsal shaft, and through the accessory extensor hallucis longus tendon.
- Plantarward, the strong tissue is the deep, investing fascia over the abductor hallucis and the tendinous edge of this muscle; anchoring the capsular repair proximally before beginning the distal repair is important. Close the plantar-medial corner of the capsule with one or two interrupted sutures.
- The most important sutures, which hold the hallux congruously on the metatarsal head, form a pants-over-vest closure as follows. Enter the transverse limb of the capsular incision 2 to 3 mm plantar to the apex of the incision from the outside in; turn the needle 180 degrees and reenter the corner of the capsule from the outside in. Reverse the needle 180 degrees and reenter it from the inside out, still on the proximal part of the capsule. Place the final pass of the stitch through the distal capsule on the dorsal side of the apex of the incision. Pull the capsule into the corner in a pants-over-vest manner and suture it. During capsular closure, observe the dorsal aspect of the foot while an assistant externally rotates the foot slightly to judge the proper alignment of the hallux.

- To obtain more correction of the valgus deformity carefully imbricate the transverse or coronal limb of the capsulotomy. Do not attempt to correct hallux valgus interphalangeus by pulling the hallux into a more varus position at the metatarsophalangeal joint with imbricating sutures during capsular repair because hallux varus can develop if the imbrication is too tight. In most instances, close the transverse limb by approximating the edges, unless the capsule is so redundant that it requires partial excision. Finish closing the capsule at any weak points.

- The hallux should be in neutral to 5 degrees of valgus at completion of the capsulorrhaphy. Correct any varus by removing capsular sutures one at a time and observing the position of the hallux. Begin by removing one or more transverse limb sutures. If necessary, remove all of the distal capsular repair and start over.

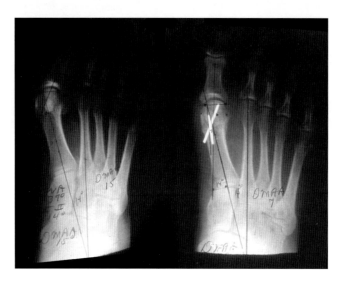

Figure 91-11

- Secure hemostasis and close the wound in layers. Apply a forefoot dressing with the hallux taped in the proper position (Figure 91-11).

POSTOPERATIVE CARE ❯

The dressing and sutures are removed at 19 to 23 days and a toe spacer is worn to hold the hallux in the proper position. A wooden-soled shoe is worn for 4 weeks and then a deep, wide jogging shoe is worn with a toe spacer for the next 6 to 8 weeks. Usually by the third or fourth month a reasonably attractive shoe can be worn, but this varies. A short-leg walking cast worn for 4 weeks after surgery is an alternative but it is not routinely recommended except in adolescents. The Kirschner wires can be removed at 3 months or earlier if they cause symptoms, or they may be left if the patient is asymptomatic.

JOHNSON MODIFIED CHEVRON OSTEOTOMY ❯

Johnson, who popularized the chevron osteotomy, also modified it by changing the length and position of the limbs of the osteotomy in the metatarsal head, which extended the indications for the osteotomy to severe deformities with intermetatarsal angles of 15 or 16 degrees. A 2.7-mm screw is used for internal fixation. Johnson did not recommend this osteotomy for patients older than 60 years or for patients who had previous hallux valgus surgery or diminished joint mobility with crepitance.

- Make a midline, longitudinal, medial capsular incision, and expose the medial eminence.

- Expose the metatarsal head dorsally and plantarward just enough to see the dorsal and plantar limbs of the osteotomy, laterally enough to place a 2.7-mm screw. Avoid excessive stripping of the capsule.

- Using a power saw with a 9-mm blade, remove the medial eminence at an angle that is parallel to the medial border of the foot as opposed to the medial border of the cortical shaft or metatarsal.

- Begin the inferior or plantar limb of the osteotomy 5 or 6 mm proximal to the medial articular surface of the first metatarsal and midway between the superior and inferior margins of the metatarsal head in its center portion. This plantar extension of the osteotomy exits extracapsularly at the inferior aspect of the metatarsal head and neck junction or just proximal to that.

- The lateral portion of this osteotomy cut can be difficult so ensure it is completely through the bone before attempting to shift the metatarsal head laterally.

- Make the second limb of the osteotomy from the apex or distal extension of the first osteotomy and direct it dorsally at an approximate angle of 70 degrees to the first limb of the osteotomy. Exit this limb of the osteotomy dorsally just proximal to the dorsal border of the articular surface of the head of the metatarsal.

- Stabilize the metatarsal shaft proximally with a manual grip or a towel clip while the capital fragment is displaced laterally 4 to 6 mm without any tilting or opening of the osteotomy site medially, laterally, superiorly, or inferiorly.

- Compress the great toe longitudinally on the head of the metatarsal shaft fragment to impact the osteotomy site.

- For insertion of a 2.7-mm screw use a 2-mm bit to drill a hole in the dorsal surface of the distal shaft of the metatarsal just proximal to the dorsal limb of the osteotomy. Leave an approximately 3-mm ledge of bone between the drill hole and the superior arm of the osteotomy.

- Direct the drill bit from proximal to distal at about a 10-degree angle and 10 to 15 degrees lateralward to place the screw in the substance of the transposed capital fragment.

- Pass the 2-mm drill bit through the dorsal cortex of the distal shaft of the metatarsal and then through the cancellous bone of the capital fragment into subchondral bone of the fragment.

- Ream the proximal aspect of the hole with a 2.7-mm drill bit to create a lag effect at the osteotomy and then measure the screw length (usually 16 to 18 mm) with a depth gauge.

- Tap the drill hole with a 2.7-mm tap. Insert the 2.7-mm screw and tighten it to close the osteotomy. Do not allow the screw to exit through the articular surface of the metatarsal head because it may impair sesamoid glide.

- Use a power saw to contour the overhang of the medial aspect of the distal metatarsal that resulted from lateral shift of the capital fragment with the medial aspect of the first metatarsal shaft. Do not skive laterally into the center of the shaft of the metatarsal. Use a small rongeur to smooth the dorsomedial aspect of the metatarsal head.

- Overlap the capsule while holding the hallux in neutral flexion and extension and about 10 degrees of varus, and excise any excess capsule (usually 3 to 5 mm). Close the capsule with multiple 2-0 or 3-0 nonabsorbable sutures.

- After capsular closure is completed, the hallux should rest in a straight position with the medial aspect of the proximal phalanx resting against the medial aspect of the displaced capital fragment.

- Apply the dressing in such a way as to hold the hallux in proper position and to take some of the pressure off the medial capsular repair (see Fig. 91-10).

POSTOPERATIVE CARE

The patient is allowed partial weight bearing with crutches for the first 3 to 4 days then the dressing is changed and a short-leg walking cast is applied. The cast, which should extend distal to the great toe for gentle support, is primarily for comfort and patient mobility, allowing ambulation without crutches or a walker. It is removed approximately 1 week later and gentle exercises of the great toe are begun. A hallux valgus night splint is applied to protect the medial capsular repair and a stiff-soled postoperative shoe is worn for approximately 3 weeks; after this a deep, wide, soft shoe can be worn.

PROXIMAL CRESCENTIC OSTEOTOMY WITH A DISTAL SOFT TISSUE PROCEDURE 〉

Most hallux valgus deformities that require a distal soft tissue procedure also require a proximal osteotomy. This procedure is not recommended if excessive valgus posturing (>15 degrees) of the distal metatarsal articular angle is present on the weight-bearing radiograph or in patients with moderate-to-severe degenerative arthritic changes of the metatarsophalangeal joint. The decision to perform an osteotomy should be made at the time of surgery by passively reducing the intermetatarsal angle. If the first metatarsal does not move laterally, or if it springs back quickly into varus after the laterally directed pressure is released, a basilar osteotomy should be done.

- This procedure is performed through three incisions. The first incision is made dorsally in the intermetatarsal space to release the adductor hallucis, the deep transverse intermetatarsal ligament and the lateral capsule of the first metatarsophalangeal joint. The second incision is made midline-medial over the medial eminence to remove the medial eminence and perform a capsulorrhaphy. The third incision is made dorsally over the proximal end of the first metatarsal and extends a few millimeters over the medial cuneiform.

- Make the first incision in the first intermetatarsal space beginning at the proximal end of the web space and extending proximally 3 to 4 cm.

- Dissect the soft tissue with scissors to identify the branches of the deep peroneal nerve and be sure to protect them.

- Place a Weitlaner retractor in the first intermetatarsal space and widen this space to expose the adductor hallucis.

- Use a sponge to clear away the soft tissue in the first web space.

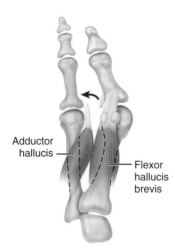

Adductor hallucis

Flexor hallucis brevis

Figure 92-1

- The adductor hallucis approaches the base of the proximal phalanx in an oblique direction. When it has been identified, release it completely from the base of the proximal phalanx and from the lateral edge of the fibular sesamoid (Figure 92-1).

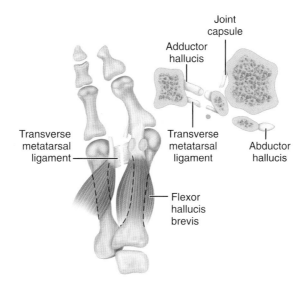

Figure 92-2

- Release the deep transverse intermetatarsal ligament that is plantar to this tendon. Because the neurovascular bundle to the first web space is immediately plantar to the transverse intermetatarsal ligament, use just the tip of the blade to release this. Placing a small Freer elevator on the plantar surface of this ligament helps avoid the neurovascular bundle as the incision is made (Figure 92-2).
- Make multiple small stab wounds in the lateral capsule.
- Complete the capsular release by manually forcing the hallux into 25 to 30 degrees of varus and pushing the first metatarsal lateralward.
- When the lateral release has been completed, release the deep transverse intermetatarsal ligament that attaches to the fibular sesamoid. Releasing the deep transverse intermetatarsal ligament prevents its deforming force on the fibulosesamoid from pulling the sesamoid apparatus laterally from under the metatarsal head.

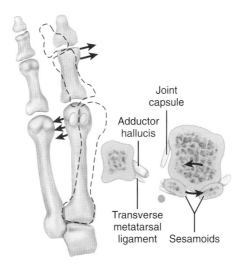

Figure 92-3

- Push the first metatarsal head laterally. If it tends to rest in that position, an osteotomy is not necessary; however, if it springs back to the varus position, an osteotomy should be performed (Figure 92-3).
- Return to the adductor hallucis, which is completely freed, and lift it up into the wound from the bottom of the foot.
- Pass three absorbable 2-0 sutures first through the lateral capsule on the first metatarsal head just proximal to the lateral capsular release. Make the second throw of the suture through the adductor hallucis tendon and the third throw through the capsuloligamentous intrinsic tendinous tissue on the medial side of the second metatarsal head. Do not tie these sutures but hold them with hemostats and allow them to fall into the first web space.

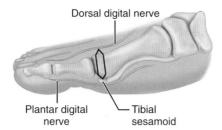

Figure 92-4

- Make a second midline incision, avoiding the dorsal sensory branch of the superficial peroneal nerve dorsalward and the proper branch of the medial plantar nerve to the medial side of the hallux plantarward. Continue this incision down to the capsule and raise the dorsal flap deep to the dorsal sensory nerve (Figure 92-4).
- Raise the plantar flap on the capsule until the plantar aspect of the abductor hallucis muscle is reached, which is just a few millimeters from the tibial sesamoid. This is best done with the hallux in about 30 degrees of flexion, which relaxes the digital nerve just plantar to the dissection.
- Make a vertical incision in the capsule 2 to 3 mm proximal to the base of the proximal phalanx extending from a few millimeters medial to the extensor hallucis longus tendon in a plantar direction through the medial capsule and through the thickened portion of the capsule plantarward, which is actually the abductor hallucis tendon capsule junction. This vertical limb ends 2 mm medial to the tibial sesamoid. The most inferior portion of this vertical limb is best made from plantar to dorsal to avoid the digital nerve.
- Depending on the enlargement of the medial eminence and the subsequent redundancy and stretching of the medial capsule, remove an elliptical wedge of capsule measuring 4 to 8 mm wide at its widest section. Dorsally and plantarward, taper this incision into a V shape and excise the elliptical wedge of capsule.
- Extend the capsular incision proximally beginning at the dorsal edge of the vertical limb. This limb of the incision (an inverted L) should end 2 to 3 mm proximal to the junction of the medial eminence with the metatarsal shaft.
- Raise this capsular flap from dorsal distal to plantar proximal to expose the entire medial eminence.

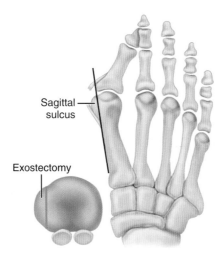

Figure 92-5

- Remove the medial eminence. Do this in a plane parallel to the shaft of the first metatarsal and begin just medial to the sagittal groove (Figure 92-5).
- Begin a third incision on the dorsal aspect of the proximal third of the metatarsal. Extend this incision proximally over the dorsal surface of the medial cuneiform. Avoid the superficial peroneal nerve sensory branch to the hallux. Retract or ligate the dorsal venous arch.
- Identify the metatarsocuneiform joint and incise the periosteum of the first metatarsal and medial cuneiform longitudinally medial to the extensor hallucis longus tendon.

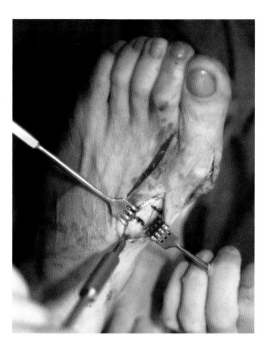

Figure 92-6

- Score the dorsal aspect of the metatarsal transversely at 1- and 2-cm levels distal to the metatarsocuneiform articulation. The first scored mark represents the osteotomy site and the second represents the area for placement of the screw for internal fixation of the osteotomy (Figure 92-6).
- Release the soft tissue dorsally, medially, and laterally, being careful to avoid the penetrating branch of the dorsalis pedis artery in the proximal part of the first intermetatarsal space.
- If a screw is to be used for fixation, make a glide hole. This is much easier to do at this point than when the metatarsal becomes less stable after the osteotomy.
- Drill a 3.5-mm hole 1 cm distal to the osteotomy site in the center of the metatarsal shaft and direct it proximally 45 degrees to the metatarsal shaft, penetrating only the dorsal cortex.
- Use a countersink to enlarge the entrance hole. It is important to enlarge this at its most distal extension rather than at the proximal edge of the drill hole because it gives the screw head a place to sit and does not permit it to rise dorsally, which might crack the cortical bridge into the osteotomy site as the screw is tightened.
- If a 5/16-inch smooth Steinmann pin is to be placed in an oblique direction from distal medial to proximal lateral, drill the hole in the medial aspect of the metatarsal before the osteotomy.
- Using a 1/16-inch drill bit, drill a hole in the medial aspect of the metatarsal in an oblique direction, crossing the osteotomy site.

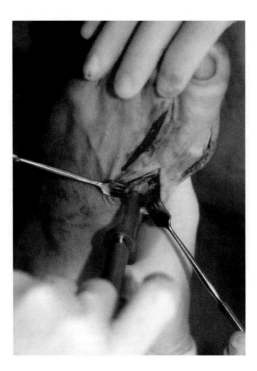

Figure 92-7

- Using an oscillating saw with a crescent-shaped saw blade placed convex distally, begin the osteotomy on the most proximal scored mark (Figure 92-7).
- The initial cut should just be a deeper scoring. Place the saw blade gently into the first metatarsal base without oscillation or manual turning of the blade.
- When this superficial scoring has been performed with the crescentic blade, evaluate the angle of the osteotomy carefully. It should not be perpendicular to the first metatarsal shaft and it should not be perpendicular to the sole of the foot but should bisect that angle.
- Drop the handle of the saw 10 to 15 degrees proximally to direct the osteotomy correctly.
- When the dorsal cortex has been scored, complete the osteotomy by gently rocking the blade medially and laterally. Mann emphasized that the lateral aspect of the blade must exit the lateral side of the metatarsal shaft. It is not as important that the blade exit the medial side because a small osteotome can be used to complete that part of the osteotomy.

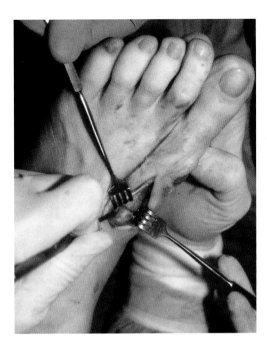

Figure 92-8

- When the osteotomy is completed, use a Freer elevator to ensure that there are no periosteal attachments medially or laterally that would prevent displacement of the osteotomy (Figure 92-8).

The following steps are crucial:

- Displace the proximal fragment medially and hold with a Freer elevator or some other instrument.
- While holding the proximal fragment medially displaced, rotate the distal fragment around the osteotomy site (usually 2 to 4 mm of lateral displacement or rotation of the distal fragment).
- Do not let the distal fragment slide dorsally or plantarward.
- Have an assistant complete the drilling, tapping, and placing of the screw while the surgeon holds the osteotomy in the corrected position.
- With the osteotomy held reduced, enter the initial hole with a centering device, sometimes referred to as a "golf tee" or "mushroom," which guides the 2.0- or 2.5-mm drill bit into the basilar fragment.
- Use a 4.0-mm tap and insert a 4.0-mm fully threaded cancellous screw (usually 26 mm long).

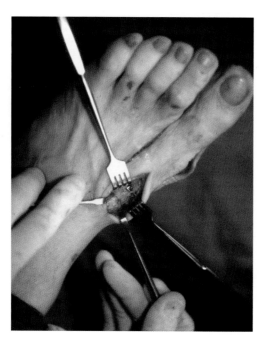

Figure 92-9

- Be careful on the last few turns of the screw that the head of the screw does not rise dorsally on the cortex because this would fracture the intervening cortical bridge. If this appears to be happening, remove the screw and countersink deeper so that part of the head of the screw would rest just plantar to the cortex (Figure 92-9).
- According to Mann, making the osteotomy convex distally should prevent overcorrection of the intermetatarsal angle.

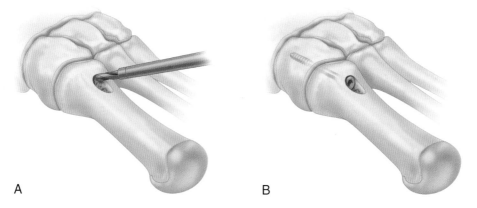

A　　　　　　　　　　B

Figure 92-10

- A useful technical tip is to use the countersink in the drill hole before placing the screw. This gently removes bone from the distal part of the screw hole, allowing the screw to sit firmly in the metatarsal (Figure 92-10, **A**). If this is not done, as the screw is placed the screw head abuts this bone distally and the screw displaces dorsally. This causes the fragile dorsal lip of bone between the screw hole and the osteotomy to break and lose the ability to achieve stable fixation with a screw. Because the screw is placed at an angle to the cortex a true countersinking is not actually done but a pathway for the screw head to travel is created (**B**); a small burr can be used for this.
- After completing screw or pin fixation of the osteotomy, return to the dorsal wound in the first intermetatarsal space and tie the three sutures to bind the adductor hallucis and the first and second metatarsal heads together. The first ray should rest in a corrected position.
- Close the medial capsule to hold it in place. Excise only the capsular overlap. Mann emphasized the importance of passing the sutures through the abductor hallucis tendon and capsule toward the plantar aspect of the vertical limb of the capsulotomy. Place the hallux in about 5 degrees of varus while the sutures are tied. It is unnecessary to close the dorsal proximal limb of the inverted-L capsulotomy.
- Apply a bulky compression dressing and remove the tourniquet.

The major complications of this procedure have been hallux varus, dorsiflexion malunion of the osteotomy site with transfer metatarsalgia, and limitation of motion of the first metatarsophalangeal joint; however, these complications are infrequent and most patients are satisfied with their outcomes.

PROXIMAL CHEVRON FIRST METATARSAL OSTEOTOMY 〉

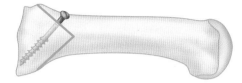

Figure 92-11

The proximal chevron metatarsal osteotomy has been described for correction of moderate-to-severe deformities. The primary benefit of this configuration of the osteotomy is the increased stability at the osteotomy site, although it must be internally fixed with a pin or screw (Figure 92-11).

- After standard preparation and draping, make a 6-cm curvilinear incision beginning at the proximal phalanx medially, curving plantarward beneath the bunion just above the sole and continuing proximally along the medial first metatarsal shaft to a point 1 cm distal to the metatarsocuneiform joint. Divide the deep tissues in line with the skin incision.
- Elevate the metatarsophalangeal capsule sharply from the medial condyle of the first metatarsal and resect redundancy from the dorsal flap.
- Remove the exostosis 1 mm medial to the sulcus on the distal metatarsal articular surface in line with the medial cortex of the metatarsal shaft with an oscillating microsaw.
- Release the proximal plantar capsular attachment at the metatarsal neck to mobilize the sesamoids.
- Apply longitudinal traction to the great toe while it is flexed slightly plantarward.
- Elevate the first metatarsal neck with a small bone hook and expose the fibular sesamoid.
- Working beneath the metatarsal head and neck, retract the lateral border of the fibular sesamoid by pulling it medially with a skin hook.

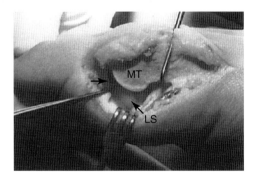

Figure 92-12

- Using sharp dissection, carefully detach the fibular sesamoid-metatarsal ligament and the conjoined tendon of the adductor hallucis muscle from the lateral aspect of the sesamoid. Cut the fibers of the conjoined tendon under direct vision as they come into view (Figure 92-12).
- Medial traction on the sesamoid pulls the capsule and tendon away from the neurovascular bundle in the first web space.
- Release the fibers of the conjoined tendon longitudinally from the fibular sesamoid-phalangeal ligament and from their attachment to the proximal phalanx.
- Do not divide the transverse metatarsal ligament.
- Extend the incision dorsally to release the lateral capsule.
- Manipulate the hallux to ensure that all tight lateral structures have been released.

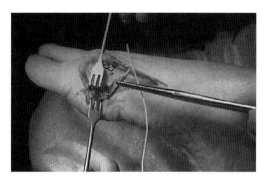

Figure 92-13

- With a cutting needle, percutaneously pass a large Dacron braided polyester suture around the second metatarsal neck. The needle emerges beneath the first metatarsal into the wound (Figure 92-13).
- Pass a curved hemostat over the first and second metatarsal necks and beneath the toe extensor tendons to exit through the needle puncture wound. Grasp the free end of the suture with the hemostat and pull it beneath the skin and tendons to emerge over the first metatarsal through the wound medially.
- Using a suture passer, pass the deep leg of the suture through a 2-mm transverse hole drilled in the dorsal half of the first metatarsal head-neck junction.

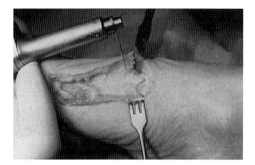

Figure 92-14

- Make a transverse chevron osteotomy with an angle of 45 degrees and with the apex directed distally at the diaphyseal-metaphyseal junction of the first metatarsal. The proximal arm of the osteotomy should end 1.5 cm from the metatarsocuneiform joint (Figure 92-14).
- After rotating the distal fragment of the osteotomy laterally to correct the metatarsus primus varus, hold the osteotomy in the corrected position with a guide pin and check the position with radiographs.
- Insert a 4-mm screw (usually 34 mm long). The screw should not cross the tarsometatarsal joint. Use a countersink to ensure that the cortex does not split when the screw is inserted. Insert the screw from the plantar aspect of the distal fragment and direct it laterally and dorsally across the osteotomy into the proximal fragment.
- Before final tightening of the screw, tie the large Dacron "lashing" suture.
- Use image intensification to confirm proper positioning of the screw. At this point, the alignment of the sesamoids is partially corrected.
- To correct the hallux valgus and reduce the sesamoids, close the medial capsule with 2-0 absorbable mattress sutures placed from dorsal distal to plantar proximal. The capsular closure holds the sesamoids beneath the first metatarsal head and corrects the hallux valgus.
- Close the skin incision with a subcuticular 4-0 absorbable skin suture. Apply a compression dressing and provide the patient with a postoperative wooden clog.

POSTOPERATIVE CARE

The bulky compression dressing holding the hallux in a corrected position is changed the following day and at weekly intervals for 6 to 8 weeks, holding the hallux in the corrected position. Weight bearing to tolerance is allowed the day of surgery. The patient usually prefers to walk on the lateral border of the foot or to use crutches for a few days.

The use of endoscopy for plantar fascia release is based on limited release of the central cord of the fascia. Although earlier reports in the orthopaedic literature emphasized complications of this procedure, more recent studies have reported that endoscopic plantar fasciotomy is an effective procedure with reproducible results, a low complication rate, and little risk of iatrogenic nerve injury. Anatomical dissections have shown that, if properly performed, endoscopic plantar fascia release appears to be a reasonably safe procedure.

TWO-PORTAL ENDOSCOPIC PLANTAR FASCIA RELEASE 〉

- After administration of an intravenous sedative and local anesthesia, prepare and drape the patient in the usual manner. Exsanguinate the foot and inflate a pneumatic ankle tourniquet.
- Make a reference point for incision immediately anterior and inferior to the inferior aspect of the medial calcaneal tubercle, as viewed on a non–weight-bearing lateral projection.

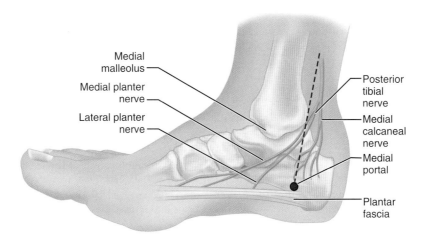

Figure 93-1

- Make a 5-mm vertical stab incision and bluntly dissect to the level of the plantar fascia. Because direct observation through this small incision is impossible, palpation is necessary (Figure 93-1).
- The Endotrac (Instratek, Houston, TX) consists of a fascial elevator, hook probe, slotted obturator-cannula system, and two blade handles for disposable hook and triangle blades.
- Palpate the medial investment of the plantar fascia with the fascial elevator.

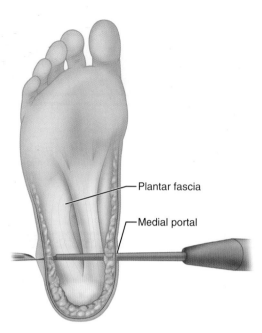

Plantar fascia

Medial portal

Figure 93-2

- Create a channel immediately inferior to the plantar fascia with the fascial elevator. Introduce the obturator-cannula system into this channel and advance it across the inferior surface of the plantar fascia to the lateral aspect of the foot (Figure 93-2).
- Palpate the obturator and make a 5-mm vertical incision over its tip, allowing the obturator-cannula to be passed through the skin.
- Remove the obturator from the slotted cannula, leaving the cannula in place.
- Introduce the endoscope medially and the fascial probe laterally.
- Using the endoscope, view the entire inferior surface of the plantar fascia on the monitor. Double marks on the interior wall of the cannula indicate the approximate location of the medial plantar fascia investment. Proceeding laterally, a single mark indicates the approximate location of the medial intermuscular septum. The first two marks are 9 mm and 11 mm from the medial dermis, respectively, whereas the third mark is 13.5 mm from the midpoint of the first two marks. These marks correspond to average dermal and medial band widths obtained from cadaver dissections and should be used only as guides.

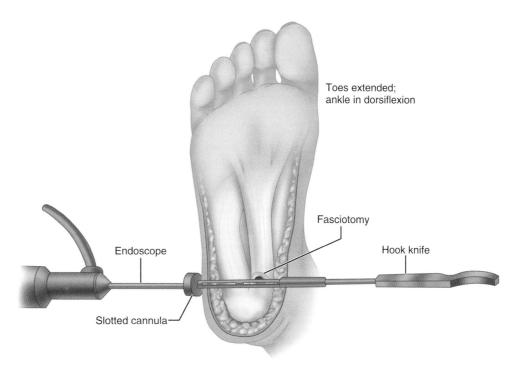

Figure 93-3

- While viewing the medial investment of the plantar fascia through the endoscope, use the probe to palpate its fibers. Introduce the retrograde knife to this anatomical reference point and sever the medial band of the plantar fascia (Figure 93-3).

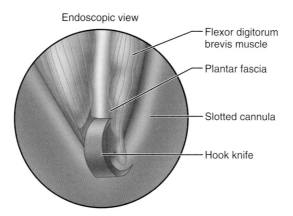

Figure 93-4

- Insert the endoscope laterally and the fascial probe medially to allow a 180-degree perspective. If any remaining plantar fascial fibers are palpated, introduce the triangle blade medially to release them. It is important to see the complete thickness of the plantar fascia on the video monitor to ensure a proper release (Figure 93-4).
- After fasciotomy, irrigate the area with sterile saline and remove the slotted cannula.
- Approximate the two incisions with two 5-0 Prolene sutures and infiltrate the area with 0.5% bupivacaine and 1 mL of dexamethasone to decrease postoperative discomfort. Apply a sterile compressive gauze dressing and deflate the tourniquet.

POSTOPERATIVE CARE ⟩

Patients are allowed full weight bearing immediately after surgery but should avoid excessive ambulation. The dressings are removed on the third day after surgery and sterile cloth adhesive bandages are applied. The patient may return to regular shoes fitted with an orthotic appliance as soon as tolerated.

SINGLE-PORTAL ENDOSCOPIC PLANTAR FASCIA RELEASE 〉

- Make an incision on the medial aspect of the foot 1 cm distal to the medial tubercle of the calcaneus just above the junction of the plantar skin. Dorsiflex the hallux to identify the medial portion of the plantar fascia and make the incision within the slightly oblique skin lines that run dorsal-proximal to plantar-distal.

- Use a hemostat to bluntly dissect down to the plantar fascia.

- Use a fascial elevator to separate the subcutaneous layer from the plantar fascia on the inferior heel and introduce an obturator cannula from medial to lateral in the pathway created by the fascial elevator.

- Remove the obturator and place a 30-degree 4.0-mm endoscope within the cannula to view the plantar fascia superiorly.

- Remove the endoscope and apply the cannulated depth gauge with a stop device. Reintroduce the endoscope with the depth gauge from medial to lateral.

- Identify the medial half of the central plantar fascia band by rotating the cannula 180 degrees and viewing this location externally by transillumination on the inferior heel.

- Note the measurement corresponding to the appropriate level of transection, usually 7 to 8 on the depth gauge.

- Withdraw the endoscope, remove the depth gauge, and attach a disposable cannulated knife with the stop device at the appropriate number to allow transection of the medial half of the central plantar fascia. Reinsert the endoscope and use the knife to transect the fascia. Dorsiflexing the toes can aid in the transection.

- After transection, examine the cut ends of the plantar fascia as well as the first plantar muscle layer. When appropriate fasciotomy is confirmed, remove all instrumentation and irrigate the surgical site.

- Use small scissors to transect any palpable taut fibers of the medial band under direct vision.

- Close the incision with one or two horizontal mattress sutures.

POSTOPERATIVE CARE 〉

A short below-knee cast boot is worn for 4 weeks with the sutures removed at about 2 weeks. Patients are kept non–weight bearing on crutches for the first 2 weeks and are advised to use a foot orthosis during initiation of weight bearing. Physical therapy, consisting of stretching, massage, ultrasound, and gradual strengthening is begun at 4 weeks. Running is resumed when the patient can tolerate 30 to 40 minutes of continuous walking and has no daily symptoms.

CREDITS

Figures 93-1 through 93-4 redrawn from Ferkel RD, Hommen JP: Arthroscopy of the ankle and foot. In Coughlin MJ, Manna RA, Saltzman CL, eds: Surgery of the Foot and Ankle, ed 8, Philadelphia, 2007, Elsevier.

Chronic degenerative Achilles tendinosis may produce calcification that is visible on lateral standing radiographs. Patients with extensive disease on clinical examination or MRI or for whom surgical treatment has failed may be candidates for flexor hallucis longus transfer. It is our procedure of choice in this group as opposed to complete detachment and repair.

- Place the patient prone on the operating table after administering a satisfactory general anesthetic.

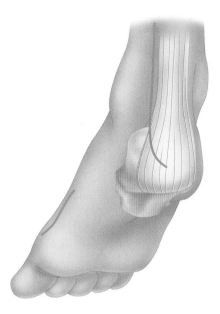

Figure 94-1

- Make an incision just medial to the Achilles tendon for a total length of approximately 10 cm centered over the diseased section of tendon (Figure 94-1).
- Carefully incise the paratenon and remove any inflammatory peritendinitis with a rongeur.

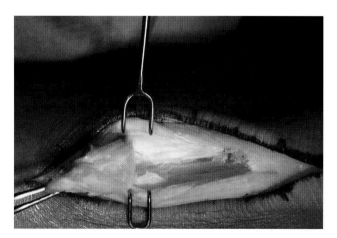

Figure 94-2

- Retract the medial border of the tendon posteriorly with a double skin hook retractor for access to the deep involved portion of the tendon (Figure 94-2).

- Débride the area of degeneration sharply until normal tendon is present. If less than 50% of the tendon is involved, close the wound with interrupted 2-0 braided, nonabsorbable suture. Do not excessively strip the vascular supply of the mesotenon on the deep surface of the Achilles tendon. If substantially more than 50% of the tendon is involved, flexor hallucis longus transfer may be indicated.

- Make a longitudinal incision just deep to the Achilles tendon. Numerous small veins are present in the area and must be cauterized.

- Develop the interval between the flexor hallucis longus and peroneal tendons. Take care to avoid the neurovascular structures by staying at or lateral to the flexor hallucis longus tendon.

- After identifying the flexor hallucis longus tendon, make a longitudinal incision over the medial aspect of the dorsal arch of the abductor hallucis muscle. Deepen the incision with plantar retraction of the abductor hallucis muscle.

- Identify the master knot of Henry proximally. Avoid the medial plantar nerve and artery, which generally lie just deep and lateral to the flexor hallucis longus tendon.

- Dissect distally to allow sufficient harvest of the tendon depending on how much will be needed to augment the repair. If the entire insertion of the Achilles tendon is removed, a longer tendon graft will be needed.

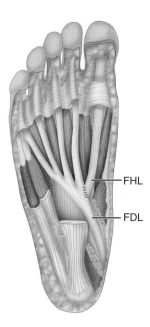

FHL

FDL

Figure 94-3

- With the toes in flexion, suture the flexor digitorum longus tendon and flexor hallucis longus tendon together with interrupted 2-0 Vicryl suture (Figure 94-3).

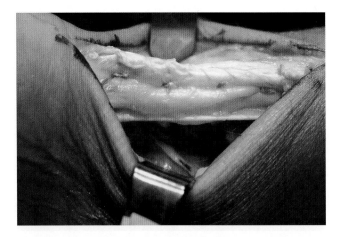

Figure 94-4

- Harvest the flexor hallucis longus tendon. Release all connections between the flexor hallucis longus and the flexor digitorum longus and deliver the flexor hallucis longus into the posterior calf incision (Figure 94-4).

- For noninsertional Achilles tendinosis débridement, sew the flexor hallucis longus muscle belly and tendon into the defect created by the débridement.
- Use successively larger drill bits to drill a tunnel from medial to lateral in the tuberosity of the calcaneus. Generally a 3/8-inch tunnel is satisfactory to allow passage of the tendon with ease.

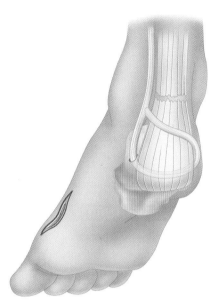

Figure 94-5

- For insertional Achilles tendinosis, after complete débridement of the Achilles tendon insertion, weave (Pulvertaft) the flexor hallucis longus tendon through the Achilles tendon and then pass it through the bone tunnel and suture it onto itself with interrupted no. 2 Ethibond or nonabsorbable sutures (Figure 94-5).
- If complete débridement of the Achilles tendon has been done, tension the graft with the ankle in moderate equinus provided that the ankle can be brought to neutral after final suturing of the graft. This helps to provide sufficient push-off power postoperatively.
- Alternatively, an interference-type absorbable screw can be used in the bone tunnel to secure the flexor hallucis longus tendon to the calcaneus.
- Close the paratenon with interrupted 2-0 absorbable sutures and close the skin in a routine fashion.

POSTOPERATIVE CARE 〉

A non–weight-bearing cast is worn for 4 weeks in slight equinus. After 4 weeks a prefabricated walking brace is applied with multiple heel lifts approximately $2\frac{1}{2}$ to 3 inches in total height. One wedge of heel lift is removed each week as the patient begins bearing weight on the foot. The ankle is in neutral in the prefabricated walking boot until about 8 weeks. At this point, general calf stretching and range-of-motion exercises are started. Gradual return to activities is delayed until $3\frac{1}{2}$ months.

See also Video 95-1.

For open reduction techniques, either patients are operated on within the first 12 to 24 hours, or, more commonly, surgery is delayed 10 to 14 days to allow soft tissue swelling to resolve enough for the skin to wrinkle. After 3 weeks, open reduction becomes more difficult, but it is possible up to 4 to 5 weeks. Advantages of a lateral exposure include wide exposure of the subtalar joint allowing more accurate reduction of the facet fragments, ability to decompress the lateral wall, exposure of the calcaneocuboid joint, and sufficient area laterally for plate fixation. Disadvantages include inability to assess reduction of the medial wall directly and inability to restore height and length of the calcaneus accurately; because of the extensive soft tissue dissection, wound problems and skin necrosis can occur with this exposure.

OPEN REDUCTION OF CALCANEAL FRACTURE 〉

- Administer preoperative antibiotics and apply a tourniquet.
- Place the patient in a true lateral position and use the lateral approach.

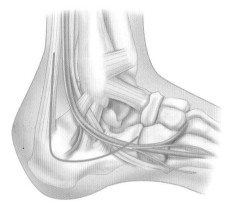

Figure 95-1

- Carry the incision directly down to the periosteum of the lateral wall with no blunt soft tissue dissection in the midportion of the wound. The sural nerve may cross the incision at its proximal and its distal end, so soft tissue dissection should be done in these areas to avoid cutting the nerve (Figure 95-1).

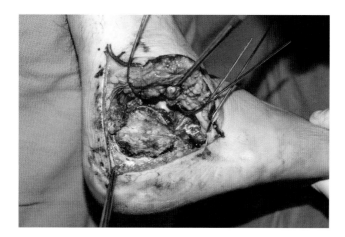

Figure 95-2

- Gently retract the flap while performing subperiosteal dissection along the lateral wall. It is essential to follow the contours of the blown-out lateral wall and not stray into the soft tissues to avoid damage to the peroneal tendons. These tendons should be contained in the flap. Elevate the entire flap in one piece and hold it out of the way with a Kirschner wire placed longitudinally into the fibula, one from lateral to medial in the talus, and one into the cuboid. Bend these wires back to retract the flap, which does not need to be touched again for the remainder of the procedure (Figure 95-2).

- Expose the entire lateral wall of the calcaneus distally to the calcaneocuboid joint.

- Carry the dissection above and below the peroneal tendons at the level of the calcaneocuboid joint if necessary. This extensile lateral approach exposes the lateral wall of the calcaneocuboid joint and posterior facet. Reduction of the tuber-sustentacular fragment is done indirectly.

- When the exposure is completed, remove the lateral wall and place it in a secure place on the back table for later replacement because this fragment blocks direct observation of the posterior facet. Do not reduce the posterior facet immediately because room for the piece must first be created.

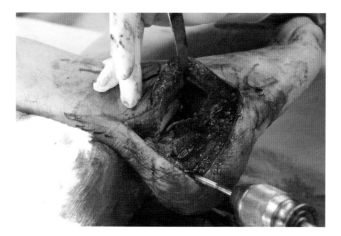

Figure 95-3

- When a fracture line separates the anterior process from the sustentacular fragment, reduce this part first to allow better exposure of the relationship between the medial part containing the sustentacular fragment and the lateral part with the posterior facet and tuberosity (Figure 95-3).

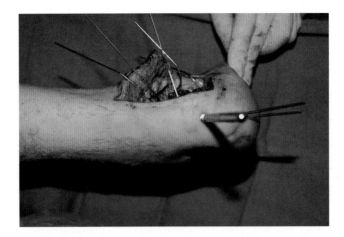

Figure 95-4

- Reduce the tuberosity to the sustentacular fragment with manipulation of a large threaded Steinmann pin placed into the tuberosity fragment from either lateral to medial or directed posteriorly to correct the varus and loss of height and length; perform a provisional fixation using axially directed Kirschner wires introduced from the heel into the sustentacular fragment (Figure 95-4).

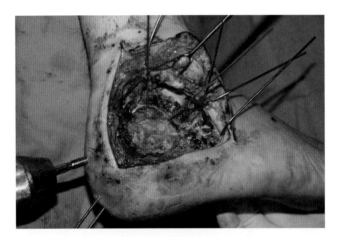

Figure 95-5

- With the bone now out to length from these two reduction maneuvers, turn attention to the depression of the posterior facet, reducing it to the intact medial piece and holding it with provisional fixation (Figure 95-5).
- Obtain intraoperative radiographs to assess overall reduction.
- A large defect often remains in the substance of the calcaneus beneath the reduced posterior facet. If good stability of the fracture and secure internal fixation are obtained, this defect may be accepted, or bone graft or bone cement can be used to fill the void.
- Reduce the lateral wall along the outer edge of the posterior facet and perform fixation, which should take advantage of the known anatomy. The thickened bone in the thalamic portion, which supports the posterior facet, provides the most reliable fixation in most instances.

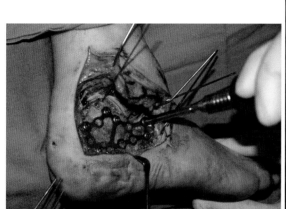
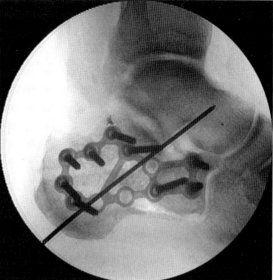

Figure 95-6

- Insert small cortical lag screws (3.5 mm) into the sustentacular fragment to maintain the reduction of the posterior facet. Apply a lateral plate that extends from the anterior process of the calcaneus into the most posterior aspect of the tuberosity. The plate helps to maintain a neutral alignment of the calcaneus. When contouring the plate, be careful not to fix the heel in varus. Obtain an intraoperative axial view to confirm neutral alignment before application of the plate (Figure 95-6).

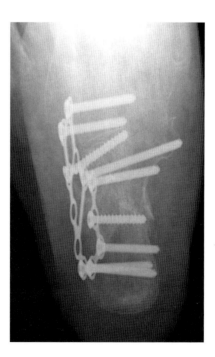

Figure 95-7

- When possible, direct screws from the plate into the sustentacular fragment for maximal fixation. Place the most anterior screw into the subchondral bone supporting the calcaneocuboid articular surface. Place the most posterior screw into the thickened bone at the posterior aspect of the calcaneus. Contour the plate into a "frown" shape (concave plantarly), and fill the remaining holes (Figure 95-7).
- Close the flap over a deep drain. Apply a short-leg splint.

POSTOPERATIVE CARE ⟩

Closed suction drainage is used for 24 to 48 hours. Strict icing and elevation protocols should be maintained to minimize swelling and pain. At the second postoperative week, active range of motion of the ankle and subtalar joint is instituted if the flap shows uncomplicated healing and the wound is sealed. Patients learn to draw the alphabet with the hallux of their injured limb or make progressively larger circles with their feet. No weight bearing is allowed for 12 weeks. Protection is provided by the use of a removable posterior splint. Weight bearing is instituted at 10 to 12 weeks, extensive physical therapy is started, and hardware can be removed if the injury is symptomatic at 1 year.

To minimize wound complications, closed reduction and percutaneous fixation of calcaneal fractures has become popular. The disadvantage of this approach is an inaccurate reduction of the posterior facet, and therefore it should be attempted only by those who have enough experience and a thorough knowledge of the anatomy to gain the appropriate reduction and fixation. This technique may not be appropriate in patients with more severe fractures. It is helpful to perform the surgery as soon as feasible after the injury, before the fracture becomes "sticky," thus making reduction more difficult. The patient should be counseled on the possible need to convert to an open procedure if the fracture cannot be reduced through indirect means.

PERCUTANEOUS REDUCTION AND FIXATION OF CALCANEAL FRACTURE ⟩

- Place the patient in the lateral decubitus position with a thigh tourniquet in place.
- Place a large threaded Steinmann pin into the tuberosity fragment for traction and manipulation of the fragment.
- If necessary, use an external fixator for traction.

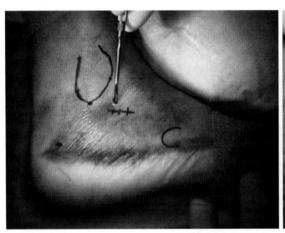 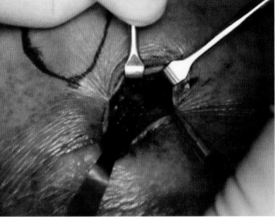

Figure 95-8

- Reduce the posterior facet with an elevator placed through a small stab incision under fluoroscopic guidance. Arthroscopy can be helpful in evaluating the reduction, especially in Sanders types IIA and IIB fractures (Figure 95-8).

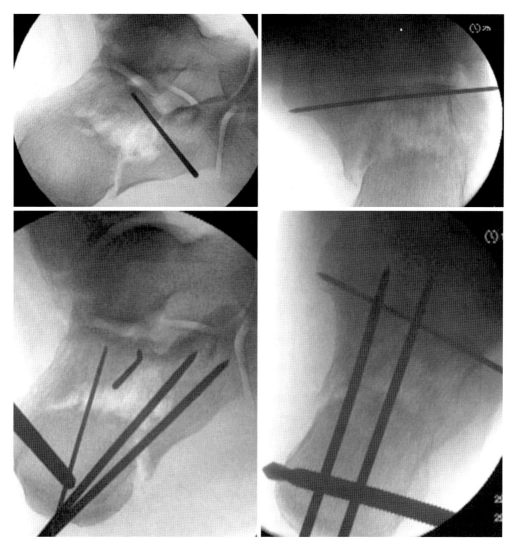

Figure 95-9

- After fracture reduction is obtained, insert Kirschner wires for provisional fixation (Figure 95-9).

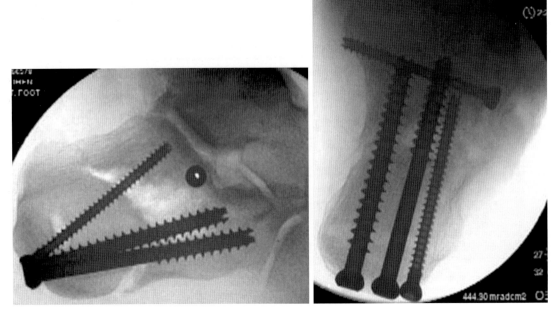

Figure 95-10

- Place percutaneous screws for fixation as needed depending on the fracture pattern. This usually consists of 3.5-mm cortical screws placed from lateral to medial, holding the posterior facet to the sustentacular fragment. Additionally, place fully-threaded screws parallel to the Steinmann pin to maintain the tuberosity position (Figure 95-10).

CREDITS

Figures 95-6, 95-7 from DeOrio M, Easley ME: Intra-articular calcaneus fractures. In Pfeffer G, Easley M, Frey C, et al, editors: Operative techniques: foot and ankle surgery, Philadelphia, 2009, Saunders.

Figure 95-8 from Lawrence SJ: Open calcaneal fractures: assessment and management, Foot Ankle Clin North Am 10:491, 2005.

SCREW FIXATION OF FIFTH METATARSAL FRACTURES

Susan N. Ishikawa

A great deal of attention has been directed toward the treatment of fractures of the proximal portion of the fifth metatarsal because of the potentially poor healing in this bone secondary to a watershed area of the blood supply. Three fracture zones have been described (Figure 96-1). Surgery should be considered for zone II and III fractures that are not healing clinically at 8 to 12 weeks and for acute fractures in competitive athletes and others whose occupational demands do not allow prolonged non–weight-bearing immobilization.

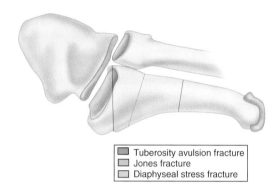

▨	Tuberosity avulsion fracture
▢	Jones fracture
▧	Diaphyseal stress fracture

Figure 96-1

- Expose the base of the fifth metatarsal on its dorsolateral surface. The sural nerve, in particular the dorsolateral branch, lies very close to the insertion point of the screw. Sufficient exposure must be obtained to identify and protect this cutaneous nerve branch.
- Incise the skin only, and observe and protect the two branches of the sural nerve — one dorsal and one straight lateral—that are vulnerable. If the peroneus brevis obscures the portal for the drill, raise a portion of it from the bone.
- Use a guidewire to find the medullary canal. This can be difficult, and the drill must lie almost parallel to the hindfoot. Starting slightly dorsal and medial to what appears to be the center of the bone also helps.

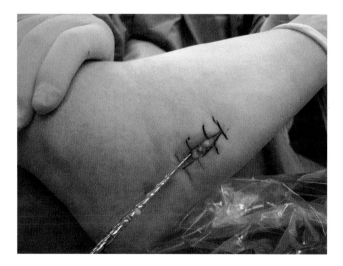

Figure 96-2

- Drive a drill bit into the medullary canal, and confirm its location by anteroposterior and lateral radiographs (Figure 96-2).

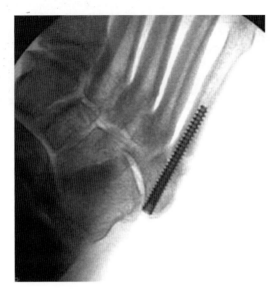

Figure 96-3

- Estimate the length of the screw from the intraoperative radiographs and place the screw over the guide-wire, making sure that the head of the screw is buried (Figure 96-3).

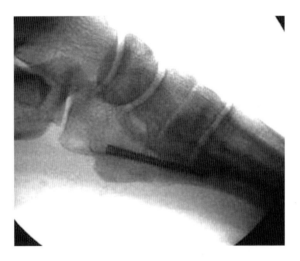

Figure 96-4

- Verify screw placement with radiographs, and close the wound (Figure 96-4).
- Exposing a nonunion and applying a small cancellous bone graft may or may not enhance union; but if cortical thickening and sclerosis are present, we usually do so.

POSTOPERATIVE CARE

A well-padded, short-leg, non-walking cast, extending to the toes, is applied. Weight bearing in a cast may be started 2 weeks postoperatively. Return to competitive sports is discouraged until the fracture has healed clinically and radiographically, which usually takes 10 to 12 weeks.

LATERAL REPAIR OF CHRONIC INSTABILITY: MODIFIED BROSTRÖM

David R. Richardson

Chronic instability of the ankle from an earlier rupture of a ligament should initially be treated conservatively. When disabling pain and instability persist, reconstruction of the lateral ligament should be considered. We have obtained good results with the modified Broström procedure in patients with moderate or severe instability; it reliably produces good results with few complications.

- After administration of general or spinal anesthesia, place the patient on his or her side, apply a tourniquet to the thigh, and exsanguinate the extremity.

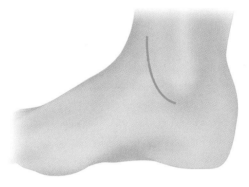

Figure 97-1

- Make a curvilinear incision along the inferior border of the lateral malleolus, ending when the peroneal tendons are encountered (Figure 97-1).

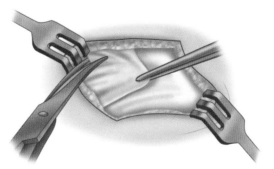

Figure 97-2

- Divide and ligate the lesser saphenous vein, which usually crosses the field. Avoid the intermediate dorsal cutaneous nerve (the lateral branch of the superficial peroneal nerve), which often lies near the talar end of the anterior talofibular ligament, and the sural nerve lying over the peroneal tendons. Identify the lateral portion of the extensor retinaculum, and mobilize it for attachment to the distal fibula at the end of the procedure (Figure 97-2).

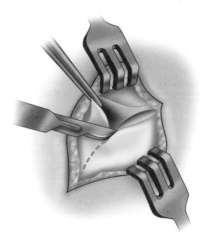

Figure 97-3

- Make a capsular incision along the anterior border of the fibula, leaving a small cuff (3 to 4 mm) on the fibula for reattachment (Figure 97-3).

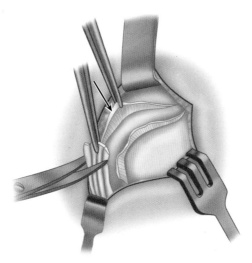

Figure 97-4

- Identify the attenuated anterior talofibular ligament, which usually is a thickening in the anterior capsule (Figure 97-4).
- Find the calcaneofibular ligament in the distal portion of the wound under the tip of the fibula, running deep to the peroneal tendons. The calcaneofibular ligament usually is attenuated or avulsed from the fibula. It may be torn from the calcaneus rather than from the fibula, making repair more difficult. Inspect the talofibular and tibiotalar joints for loose bodies, soft tissue entrapment, and articular damage, such as traumatic osteochondritis dissecans.
- Place the ankle in valgus and the foot in eversion-abduction, and have an assistant hold this position for the rest of the procedure.

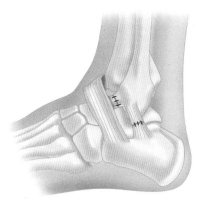

Figure 97-5

- With the foot in position, trim any redundancy in the calcaneofibular and anterior talofibular ligaments, and repair the ligaments with permanent sutures by excision and end-to-end repair, a "vest-over-pants" technique, or through drill holes in the bone (Figure 97-5).
- Gently test ankle stability with anterior drawer and talar tilt tests. Move the ankle through a full range of motion in plantar flexion and dorsiflexion to ensure that these motions have not been compromised by the repair.

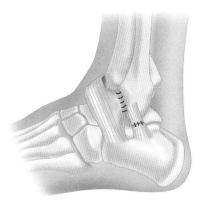

Figure 97-6

- Pull the previously identified retinaculum tightly over the distal fibula to limit inversion and stabilize the subtalar joint; suture the retinaculum in place with 2-0 chromic sutures (Figure 97-6).
- The foot should now be limited in inversion and adduction to just past neutral. Move the ankle again through a full range of plantar flexion and dorsiflexion, and check dorsal tilt and talar tilt.
- If an ossicle has been avulsed with one of the ligaments, instability may exist between the ossicle and the fibula. If the ossicle is large, freshen the bone and reattach the ossicle with a screw. If the ossicle is small, it can be used as a guide to suture the ligament in its anatomical location; it can be left in place or excised.
- Irrigate the wound with bacitracin and with 0.25% bupivacaine for postoperative pain relief.
- Close the wound in layers, and approximate the skin with an absorbable subcutaneous stitch and adhesive strips while the ankle is held in neutral dorsiflexion. Place the ankle in anteroposterior plaster splints.

POSTOPERATIVE CARE ❯

Crutches are used for the first 4 to 7 days, until swelling subsides and then a short-leg non-walking cast is applied with the ankle in neutral. The cast is removed at 4 weeks, and an air splint is worn 2 to 4 more weeks for protection. At 6 weeks after surgery, gentle range-of-motion exercises and isometric peroneal strengthening are begun. At 8 to 12 weeks after surgery, the patient is encouraged to return to dancing or sports if peroneal strength is normal. Complete rehabilitation of the peroneal tendons is essential.

David R. Richardson

Reconstructive methods for large osteochondral lesions (>5 mm) of the talus may involve transplantation of osteochondral autografts or allografts into the defect. A single plug of bone is obtained in the osteochondral autograft or allograft transplantation (OATS) procedure; mosaicplasty refers to harvesting and transplanting multiple smaller plugs.

- With the patient under general anesthesia, prepare the affected lower extremity from the ankle to the knee. Examine the ankle arthroscopically to delineate the chondral lesion further.

- Harvesters are made for lesions 5 to 11 mm (larger sizes also are available).

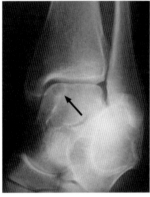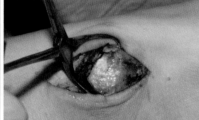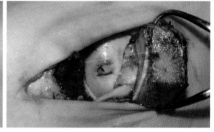

Figure 98-1

- Approach lateral lesions through an anterior sagittal incision, and perform a medial malleolar osteotomy for medial lesions. Rarely, a lateral malleolar osteotomy is needed to access posterolateral lesions (Figure 98-1).

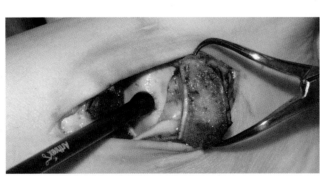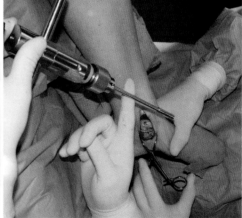

Figure 98-2

- Use a commercially available recipient sizer and harvester to create a recipient hole for the donor osteochondral plug. Extract the plug to a depth of 10 mm (Figure 98-2).

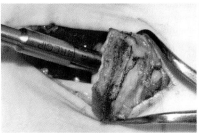
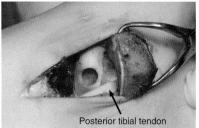
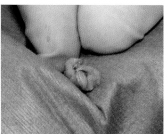

Posterior tibial tendon

Figure 98-3

- Place the harvester perpendicular for dome lesions and at 45 degrees for talar shoulder lesions (Figure 98-3).

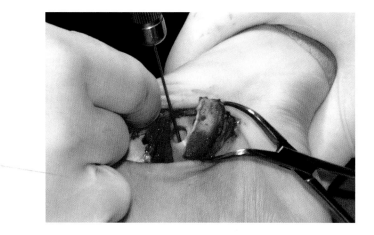

Figure 98-4

- Drill multiple holes into the subchondral bone of the recipient hole (Figure 98-4).

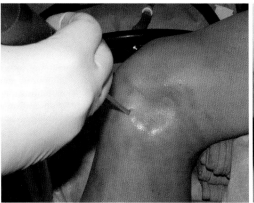
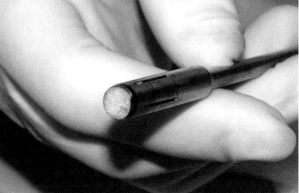

Figure 98-5

- Obtain a graft from the ipsilateral knee, arthroscopically from the medial femoral condyle, or from the lateral femoral condyle through a small incision. For talar shoulder lesions, obtain a graft from the lateral trochlea (Figure 98-5).
- Use the specially designed donor harvester to obtain osteochondral grafts that measure 5 to 11 mm in diameter and 10 to 12 mm in depth (slightly deeper than the recipient hole).

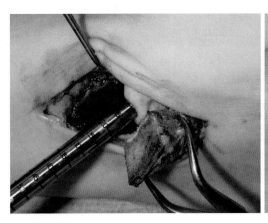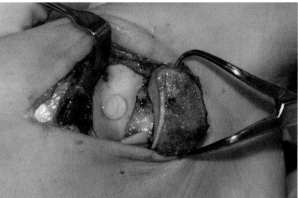

Figure 98-6

- Insert the cylindrical grafts carefully into the recipient hole using the designed extruder or collared pin through the donor harvester (Figure 98-6).
- Do not remove the OATS harvester before completion of full graft extrusion. Do not allow the harvester to deviate from the insertion angle. Either of these may cause fracture of the donor core.
- Use the sizer-tamp to tamp the core gently flush with the surrounding cartilage.
- Test range of motion of the ankle to ensure that the graft is well seated and secured.

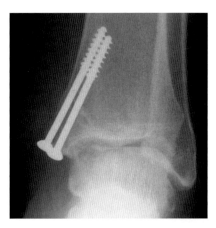

Figure 98-7

- Close the incision, and secure the osteotomy in the usual fashion. Place one drain in the knee, and apply a compressive dressing to the ankle. Apply a posterior splint with strips (Figure 98-7).

POSTOPERATIVE CARE

The patient is kept non–weight bearing for 10 weeks. At 2 weeks, the sutures are removed, and a short-leg non–weight-bearing cast is applied. At 4 weeks, a boot is fitted; the patient is kept non–weight bearing, and range-of-motion exercises are begun. At 6 to 8 weeks, pool therapy and stationary biking can be instituted.

ANTERIOR DÉBRIDEMENT

- With the patient under general anesthesia, apply and inflate a thigh tourniquet.
- Insert a needle just medial to the anterior tibial tendon, and distend the ankle joint with 15 to 20 mL of saline.

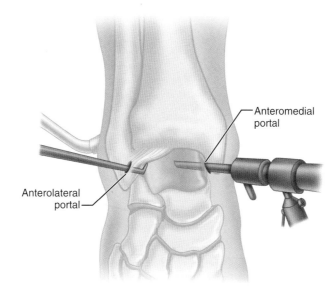

Anteromedial portal

Anterolateral portal

Figure 99-1

- Make a small longitudinal incision to allow insertion of a 2.7- or 4.0-mm, 30-degree angle arthroscope through an anteromedial portal just medial to the anterior tibial tendon. Take care to pass the arthroscope across the anterior aspect of the joint and not across the dome of the talus (Figure 99-1).
- Make a separate anterolateral portal just lateral to the peroneus tertius tendon to allow inflow and outflow of saline. Be aware of the superficial peroneal nerve in this area. Instruments and the arthroscope can be switched to either portal as necessary.

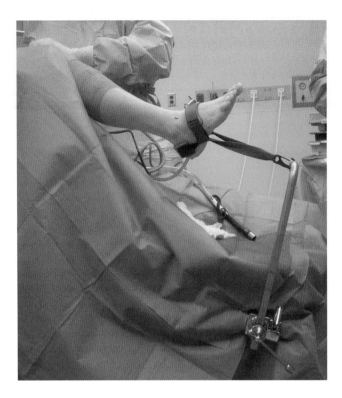

Figure 99-2

- Fully examine the ankle with the use of a noninvasive ankle distraction device as necessary. Distraction may need to be removed to identify and gain access to large anterior osteophytes, especially on the talus, because distraction may cause the anterior capsule to tighten (Figure 99-2).
- Use a pressure irrigation system with a 3.5-mm full-radius resector to clear the anterior synovium and define the anterior tibial and superior talar bony spurs.
- Use a 3-mm burr to remove the spurs, resecting them back to the level of normal cartilage.
- Smooth off the tibial surface with a 3.5-mm full-radius resector.
- Carry out a similar procedure on the superior neck of the talus.
- Examine the whole ankle by passing the arthroscope gently over the dome of the talus. This can be accomplished with the use of manual distraction in mid-plantar flexion or with a commercially available noninvasive ankle distraction device.
- After irrigation, place 20 mL of 0.25% bupivacaine into the joint, suture the incision, and apply a compression dressing.
- Davis described a modification of this technique in which a trough is made with a 3-mm arthroscopic burr approximately 1 mm proximal and parallel to the anterior edge of the tibia. This trough is taken down to subchondral bone to the level of surrounding normal cartilage. An arthroscopic bone-biter is used to remove the bony spur. This allows for more control of the burr with less potential for inadvertent damage to the articular surface than may occur with the use of an arthroscopic shaver, with which it often is difficult to gain purchase on the intact chondral surface of a spur.

POSTOPERATIVE CARE 〉

Ambulation is allowed immediately. A vigorous rehabilitation program is begun at 1 week, including ice packs and active and passive range-of-motion exercises. A tilt board is used for proprioceptive training and to strengthen the anterior and posterior muscles of the calf and foot. At 6 weeks, sports activities can be resumed in a gradual, protected fashion, taking care that the footwear is adequate for its purpose (e.g., properly fitted running shoes).

POSTERIOR DÉBRIDEMENT 〉

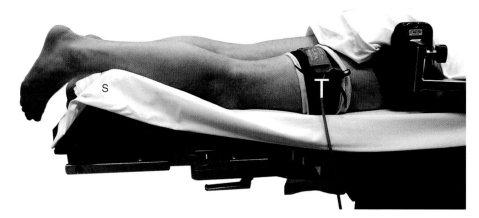

Figure 99-3

- Place the patient prone with the foot at the end of the bed and a support under the lower leg so that the foot hangs freely. Keeping the foot in neutral with respect to dorsiflexion/plantar flexion and varus/valgus is the safest position in which to avoid neurovascular damage (Figure 99-3).

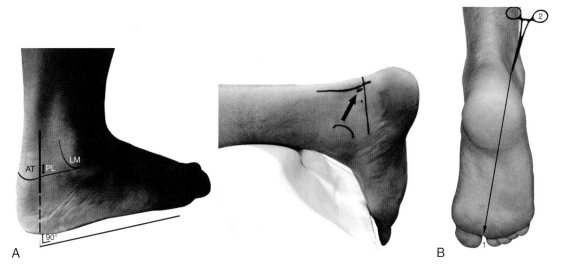

Figure 99-4

- Make the posterolateral portal just superior to a line from the tip of the lateral malleolus to the Achilles tendon, just lateral to the tendon (Figure 99-4, **A**). Insert a hemostat through a small skin incision, aiming along a line directed to the first web space of the forefoot, until it hits bone (**B**).

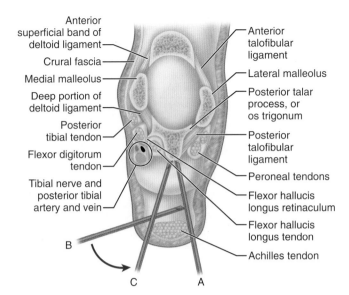

Figure 99-5

- Make the posteromedial portal at the same level, just medial to the Achilles tendon, and insert a hemostat through the skin incision, directing it to contact the arthroscope at a 90-degree angle. Once the hemostat contacts the arthroscope, move it down the shaft until it hits bone and can be seen through the scope. If desired, use fluoroscopy to confirm appropriate placement (Figure 99-5).

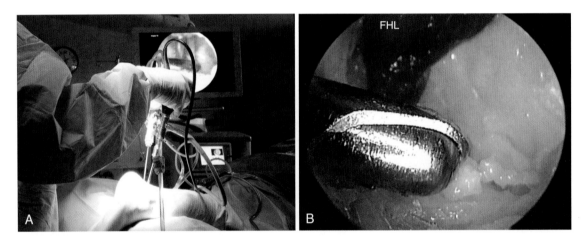

Figure 99-6

- Place a shaver in this portal and remove the posterior subtalar capsule (Figure 99-6, **A**). Take care to stay lateral to the flexor hallucis longus tendon to avoid damage to the neurovascular bundle (**B**).

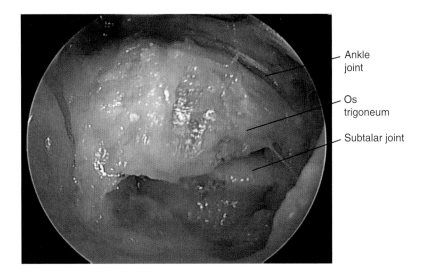

Ankle joint

Os trigoneum

Subtalar joint

Figure 99-7

- To remove the os trigonum, partially detach the posterior talofibular ligament and posterior talocalcaneal ligament and release the flexor retinaculum to expose the bone to be removed (Figure 99-7).
- If distraction is needed, a transcalcaneal traction pin can be hooked to a traction device.

Jeffrey R. Sawyer

Achilles tendon lengthening typically is indicated when the ankle cannot be brought into the neutral position in an ambulatory child and when it leads to difficulties with hygiene, foot wear, and standing programs in a nonambulatory child.

Z-PLASTY LENGTHENING OF THE ACHILLES TENDON ⟩

- Make a posteromedial incision midway between the Achilles tendon and the posterior aspect of the medial malleolus. The lower extent of the incision is at the superior border of the calcaneus and it continues cephalad for 4 to 5 cm.
- Expose the Achilles tendon with a sharp dissection directed posteriorly toward it.
- Incise the sheath of the Achilles tendon longitudinally from the superior to the inferior extent of the incision. Free the tendon from the surrounding tissues.

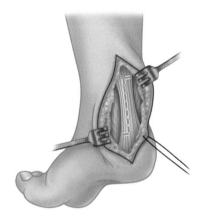

Figure 100-1

- Make a longitudinal incision in the center of the Achilles tendon from proximal to distal (Figure 100-1).
- Turn the scalpel either medially or laterally distally and divide that half of the tendon transversely. Make the distal cut toward the medial side for a varus deformity and toward the lateral for a valgus deformity.
- Hold this cut portion of the tendon with forceps and bring the scalpel to the proximal portion of the longitudinal incision in the tendon.
- Turn the scalpel opposite to the distal cut and divide that half of the tendon transversely to free the Achilles tendon completely.
- Divide the plantaris tendon on the medial aspect of the Achilles tendon transversely.
- Evaluate the passive excursion of the triceps surae muscle using a Kocher clamp to pull the proximal stump of the tendon to its maximally stretched length.

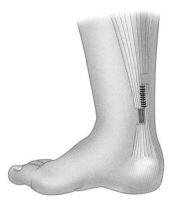

Figure 100-2

- Allow the tendon to retract halfway back to its resting length and suture it to the distal tendon end at that point (Figure 100-2).
- Control tension further by adjusting the foot position: neutral for mild spasticity; 10 degrees of dorsiflexion for moderate involvement; and 20 degrees of dorsiflexion for severe deformity.
- Perform the repair in a side-to-side manner with heavy absorbable sutures.
- Close the wound with absorbable sutures or subcuticular sutures and skin strips and apply a long-leg cast.

POSTOPERATIVE CARE 〉

Ambulation is allowed as soon as the patient is comfortable. When pain is gone (usually 5 to 10 days) the cast is changed to a short-leg cast and walking is continued. Cast immobilization is continued for a total of 6 weeks. Bracing is used if the anterior tibial muscle is not strong or is not under volitional control. If there is no function in the anterior tibial muscle, full-time bracing is required. If the anterior tibial muscle functions only with withdrawal, full-time bracing is required for several months and then only at night to prevent recurrence of the Achilles tendon contracture.

When performed as an outpatient procedure, percutaneous lengthening of the Achilles tendon is quick and inexpensive, with a low complication rate.

PERCUTANEOUS LENGTHENING OF THE ACHILLES TENDON 〉

- With the patient prone and the leg prepared to the midthigh to include the toes, extend the knee and dorsiflex the ankle to tense the Achilles tendon so that it is subcutaneous, easily outlined, and away from the neurovascular structures anteriorly.

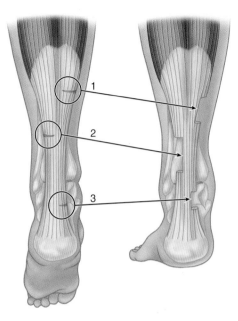

Figure 100-3

- Make three partial tenotomies in the Achilles tendon. Make the first medial cut just at the insertion of the tendon onto the calcaneus through one half of the width of the tendon. Make the second tenotomy proximally and medially just below the musculotendinous junction. Make the third laterally through half the width of the tendon midway between the two medial cuts (Figure 100-3).
- Place the two incisions on the medial side if the heel is in varus (as it usually is) and on the lateral side if the heel is in valgus.
- Dorsiflex the ankle to the desired angle.
- The incisions do not require closure only a sterile dressing and a long-leg cast with the knee in full extension.

POSTOPERATIVE CARE 〉

The patient is allowed to bear full weight on the leg postoperatively. The cast is left on for approximately 4 weeks. During this time knee extension is encouraged to maintain the lengthening of the gastrocnemius-soleus complex. The cast is removed and an ankle-foot orthosis is fitted with the ankle in maximal dorsiflexion. Alternatively a mold for a custom ankle-foot orthosis can be made at the time of the initial procedure so that it is ready at the time of cast removal. This is especially helpful if patient compliance and follow-up are questionable. The patient begins with a full-time brace and this is modified depending on the patient's growth remaining and progress in physical therapy.

INDEX

Page numbers followed by "f" indicate figures, "t" indicate tables, and "b" indicate boxes.